Neuromuscular Orthodontics

Fabio Savastano

Neuromuscular Orthodontics

A Clinical Guide

Springer

Fabio Savastano
Albenga, Italy

ISBN 978-3-031-41294-3 ISBN 978-3-031-41295-0 (eBook)
https://doi.org/10.1007/978-3-031-41295-0

Disclaimer: Several instrumentations and appliances are described in this book. I have no financial interest with any of the companies mentioned. Myotronics® U.S.A. is an official sponsor of the master's course on Neuromuscular Orthodontics at the University of Castellón, Spain. I have no financial interest from any sponsor participating at this program.

This Springer imprint is published by the registered company Springer Nature Switzerland AG
The registered company address is: Gewerbestrasse 11, 6330 Cham, Switzerland

Paper in this product is recyclable.

Thus, I became a madman.

And I have found both freedom and safety in my madness; the freedom of loneliness and the safety from being understood, for those who understand us enslave something in us.

Kahlil Gibran (جبران خليل جبران)

This book is dedicated to my wife Ilaria.
She has enlightened my life, supported my
passions, and encouraged me in this journey.

Preface

Neuromuscular Dentistry has been a topic of extensive debate spanning several years, captivating the attention of dental professionals and researchers alike. It was in 1967 that Dr. Bernard Jankelson, a pioneer in the field, laid the groundwork for this innovative approach. At that time, the technology required to implement this methodology was only accessible to a select few, but with advancements over the years, it has become readily available to dentists worldwide. Since its inception, Neuromuscular Dentistry has undergone remarkable transformations fueled by the evolving technology and the brilliant concepts introduced by Dr. Jankelson. This has given rise to a contemporary and physiological method of practicing dentistry that deviates from traditional approaches.

At the heart of this paradigm shift lies the crucial determination of the mandibular physiological rest position as the central focus in any diagnostic procedure. From this position, the ideal centric, referred to as MyoCentric, is achieved through the involuntary movement of the mandible, which is stimulated by electrical impulses using ULF-TENS. Placing emphasis on the muscles of the stomatognathic system as the foundation for constructing a new occlusion marks the genesis of this transformative approach. The significant impact of successful neuromuscular treatments over the past three decades has unquestionably validated and revolutionized this approach, forever transforming our understanding and knowledge in the field of dentistry. In fact, the surge in functional dentistry courses and the exponential increase in the usage of terms such as "muscular" and "muscles" within the dental community clearly attests to the profound influence of these achievements.

The idea of considering occlusion as a dynamic aspect of the stomatognathic system, rather than a static feature, fascinated me so much that in 1991, I started applying Neuromuscular principles to Orthodontics and studying my cases using the Myotronics® K5-AR. It was a more complicated process back then, without the convenience of personal computers and readily available technology. As a pioneer, I found myself somewhat isolated, facing the challenges that came with this groundbreaking approach. I vividly remember my reaction when I first saw the results of the initial diagnostics using the mandibular tracking system and TENS. It was astonishing to see how different they were from the traditional orthodontic teachings I had learned. I couldn't understand why the dental and orthodontic community was so reluctant and unwilling to recognize the transformative impact of the neuromuscular concept. It made me sad for patients in general and disappointed for my colleagues.

In the past couple of decades, the demand for high-quality treatments has significantly increased, largely influenced by the revolutionary changes brought about by social media. The influx of information, along with misinformation, has rapidly affected our practices and influenced our treatment decisions. The pursuit of aesthetic improvements at any cost has given rise to new philosophies in the dental and orthodontic field that often prioritize appearance over optimal functionality. While this demand has led to a focus on physiological treatment knowledge, it has also emphasized aesthetics as the sole objective for certain treatments. However, delivering a truly exceptional orthodontic treatment requires a fundamental principle: treatment goals should focus on preventing future dysfunctional problems rather than just achieving short-term aesthetic results. What matters most is not only the immediate outcome but also the state of patients' oral health years later.

Although there is a prevailing trend towards fast, inexpensive, and convenient solutions, true quality often follows a different path: it takes time, investment, and effort. Orthodontics deals with young children who represent our future, and the responsibility of providing high-quality therapies rests on the orthodontist's shoulders. There is no other dental specialty that demands such delicacy and difficulty. The Neuromuscular theory simplifies treatments by uncovering the underlying physiological requirements hidden by severe occlusions. It also emphasizes the importance of understanding the unique characteristics of each individual patient for optimal treatment calibration.

This book aims to guide orthodontists who are interested in exploring a fresh approach to treatment and, most importantly, a new method of diagnosis. While some explanations are provided throughout the text, it is recommended that readers have some familiarity with mandibular tracking. Unfortunately, mastering mandibular scanning techniques can only be achieved with specific equipment and guidance from experienced instructors.

I am grateful to my father Raul and my brother Alex, my family, my friends, and mentors that made me what I am today, passionate for what I do and curious about everything I encounter each day.

Albenga, Italy Fabio Savastano

Acknowledgments

Writing this book has been a challenging endeavor, far more difficult than I initially anticipated. It has been a long and arduous journey filled with debates and confrontations. I owe a debt of gratitude to my dear friend Piero Silvestrini Biavati, who has been my mentor, friend, and brother throughout this entire process. I am eternally grateful for the enthusiasm he has instilled in me and for teaching me to question what I see and to test my beliefs.

I would also like to express my appreciation to my colleagues Ira L. Shapira, Prabu Raman, Curtis Westersund, Stanislav Blum, Florin Constantinescu, and Konstantin Ronkin, whose constant inspiration has fueled my curiosity and motivated me to delve deeper into my research. I am indebted to Barry Cooper and Norman Randall Thomas for their pioneering studies, which have ignited my passion for this field. I would also like to remember Luigi Balercia, who, although no longer with us, guided me through my early steps in Kinesiography.

I extend my heartfelt thanks to Alison Wolf, who believed in my project and provided unwavering support for its publication. Without her, this book would not have come to fruition.

To my daughter Giulia and my son Filippo, I am profoundly grateful for their understanding and sacrifice of family time and space, allowing me to pursue this project. Their unwavering support has been invaluable.

To my remarkable wife Ilaria, you have been my role model in life. Your simplicity, pragmatism, and boundless love serve as a constant source of inspiration for me every day.

Lastly, I would like to express my gratitude to all my friends, doctors, and coworkers who have supported my ideas and provided me with opportunities to express them. Your encouragement and belief in my work have been instrumental in shaping this book.

Thank you all for being a part of this remarkable journey.

Fabio Savastano

Contents

Freeway Space (FWS) in Neuromuscular Dentistry

1

In the 1968 edition of the Nomenclature Committee of Prosthetic Terms, the Vertical Dimension (VD) is defined as “a vertical measurement of the face between any two arbitrarily selected points which are conveniently located, one above and one below the mouth, usually in the midline” (Fig. 1.1).

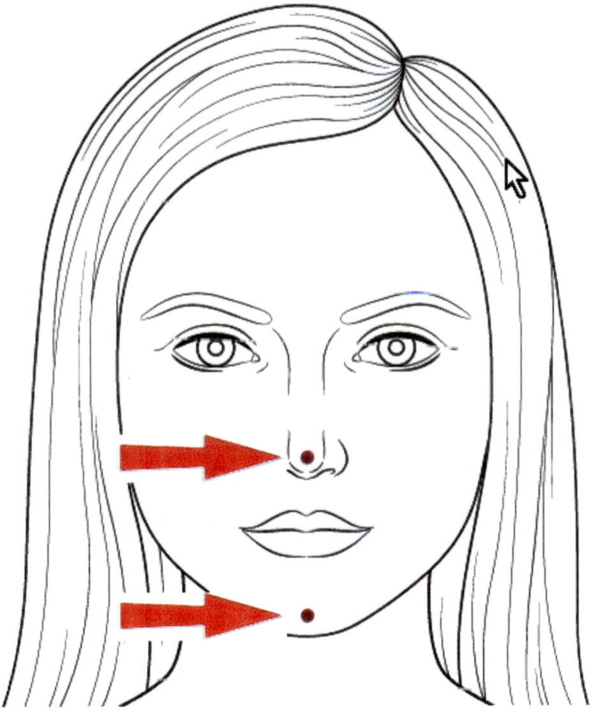

Fig. 1.1 Schematic representation of VD measurement

F. Savastano, *Neuromuscular Orthodontics*,
https://doi.org/10.1007/978-3-031-41295-0_1

VD measurement is obtained by calculating the distance of these two points on the soft tissues. VD is also referred to a more dental significance when applied to changes that occur with an increase or decrease of the vertical occlusal relationship for prosthetic or orthodontic therapies. Ideally, any increase of the VD measured between these two points from CO (Centric Occlusion, intended as ICP = Inter-Cuspal Position), would produce the same *proportional* amount of opening at the posterior teeth. For example, an increase of the VD of 3 mm measured as the vertical opening from CO between the maxillary and mandibular incisors, would produce a vertical opening in the molar region of about 1 mm.

Neuromuscular orthodontics is less focused on the changes in the vertical opening from CO. The major interest of NO is the resting position of the mandible once the postural muscles of the mandible have been relaxed and *deconditioned (from occlusal conditioning).* There are several procedures to relax the mandibular postural musculature, but the only accepted procedure in neuromuscular dentistry is by means of a TENS device (Transcutaneous Electrical Nerve Stimulator) with the application of an inter-occlusal media that avoids tooth contact during deglutition. In the coming chapters, the meaning of deconditioning will be clarified and explained thoroughly. When the mandible is at rest (and this happens 90% of the lifetime), there is an inter-occlusal space between the arches: freeway space. Freeway space is 3D for definition and varies according to muscle tone thus muscle accommodation. Muscles accommodate, adapt, to function according to the dental occlusion in ICP during a swallow. The spatial position of ICP is a fundamental factor that induces the CNS to position the mandible during habitual rest in the best starting position, HRP (Habitual Rest Position), from which the closing movement to ICP is most physiologically convenient.

VD has been long used as a one-dimensional measurement that is limited to the anterior portion of occlusal relationships of the dental arches. It can also be referred to as soft tissues for the definition of the lower facial height. It is an anterior vertical measurement of the individual occlusion in ICP with no other information. Considering freeway space widens the limited and useful concept of the vertical dimension because it includes a posterior VD (that can be different in the two molar regions on the left or right side of the dental arches), an anterior vertical dimension and a horizontal (transverse) as well as the anterior-posterior relationship between the dental arches. This means that as the mandible reaches a physiologic resting state due to muscle relaxation induced by TENS, the transverse and anterior-posterior relationships can change in respect of the habitual rest position. Freeway space is the result of muscle tone, and this is the result of the quantity of accommodation needed to adapt function to occlusion (malocclusion) during ICP and swallow. Since the ICP is present mainly during swallow, the stomatognathic system strives to create a RP, a ***starting point,*** to ICP where there is less energy consumption possible. This effort is not limited to deglutition needs but it involves complex closure pathways to ICP that avoid premature tooth contacts. The CNS may also modify cranio-cervical posture to facilitate mandibular posture (Rest Position). The *habitual rest position* is a ***physiological adaptive parameter*** and represents the resting vertical dimension [1–3].

While its quite clear what an increase or decrease of VD does on our patients (bite-opening or bite-closing), it is not always possible to foresee the changes in the maxillo-mandibular relationship after application of TENS according to the Neuromuscular methodology. The interruption of the occlusal contacts during the TENS application has an important effect, not only locally on the muscles of mastication but as well at the CNS. This effect on the CNS, is a depletion or strong reduction of the afferent signals that usually arise from the periodontal tissues, and that are responsible for mandibular spatiotemporal acquisition. It is like as if the CNS loses consciousness of the exact mandibular position. The constant development of engrams that arise from occlusal contact are interrupted [4]. The resulting muscle tone is usually lower than that before the 45′ application of TENS. There is an increase in the physical length of the muscle fibers. This rest position is called *Physiologic Rest Position* (PRP) and is *not conditioned by occlusion.* This is the ideal muscular rest position from which all functional tasks are energetically more effective. All biological systems tend to economize energy, all biological systems must be energy efficient [5]. Occlusion and cranio-cervical posture condition the mandibular rest position, and although the habitual rest position is the result of adaptation, it remains the most energy-efficient RP for that *specific occlusion.*

After muscle deconditioning with TENS, together with an inter-occlusal media, the PRP represents a cranio-mandibular *orthopedic relationship* and consequently a *condyle–fossa relationship* as well. Recording this rapport can be done with an occlusal silicone during a complete k7 assessment or it can be done with good approximation, during a bite registration with "TENS/Aqualizer®" only technique (see coming chapters). This occlusal recording embodies freeway space and can be used to setup dental casts on an articulator with facebow setup. The visualization of the PRP of the mandible in relation to the maxilla gives the practitioner important information on the adjustments needed for the occlusion to reduce muscle accommodation. Occlusal correction is guided toward muscle needs and not vice versa. Conceptually, any occlusion has a certain degree of malocclusion and so muscles adapt to functional demands in the short term but will try to overrun occlusal obstacles during functional and sometimes para-functional tasks (such as bruxism) in the long term. Orthodontic treatment without respecting muscle needs always relapses. Relapse is an "occlusal response" to adapt to muscle needs. When forceful retention is applied after orthodontic wrongdoing, relapse cannot be left to occlusion alone and continues through the TMJ anatomy that usually responds with arthrosis and related pathologies.

In most of the population, the HRP (Habitual Rest Position) is about 2–4 mm away from ICP [6, 7], and this has led the general dental knowledge to the idea that this range should be considered the norm. It should be taken into consideration the fact that there will be differences in muscle tone, however, thus erroneously regrouping different muscle lengths, facial morphologies, and cranio-cervical postures to one single norm. Freeway space is somewhat linked to facial morphology [8] and this makes this 2–4 mm norm questionable.

Long face skeletal open-bite individuals do not have freeway space and if any space is measured between the dental arches, it is probably a result of head extension to the point that the lower depressor muscles act on the mandible to separate the dental arches. Freeway space is necessary to avoid superfluous continuous tooth contact. There is no need for the CNS to constantly receive afferent signals from the most neuralgically represented peripheral system. Skeletal open bites are not necessarily to be considered long face syndromes without inter-occlusal space, and there is a variety of skeletal characteristics that occupy the different degrees that go to the extremes. It is in this purview, that the bioelectrical instrumentation is necessary to uncover skeletal open bite individuals with normal head posture and recordable freeway space. However, neuromuscular dentistry finds its limitation when there is no freeway space to record but at the same time remains very useful to monitor freeway space *creation*. In this perspective, VD and freeway space are linked by the fact that any decrease in VD in open-bite malocclusions, will create freeway space or at least reduce cranio-cervical compensation.

A complete deconditioning of the postural muscles of the mandible means that the postural muscles of mandible are fully relaxed. This can result in a different quantitative increase of the PVD (Posterior Vertical Dimension) and AVD (Anterior Vertical Dimension) than what could be expected or recorded without TENS relaxation. In Figs. 1.2, 1.3, 1.4, and 1.5 some example cases are schematically

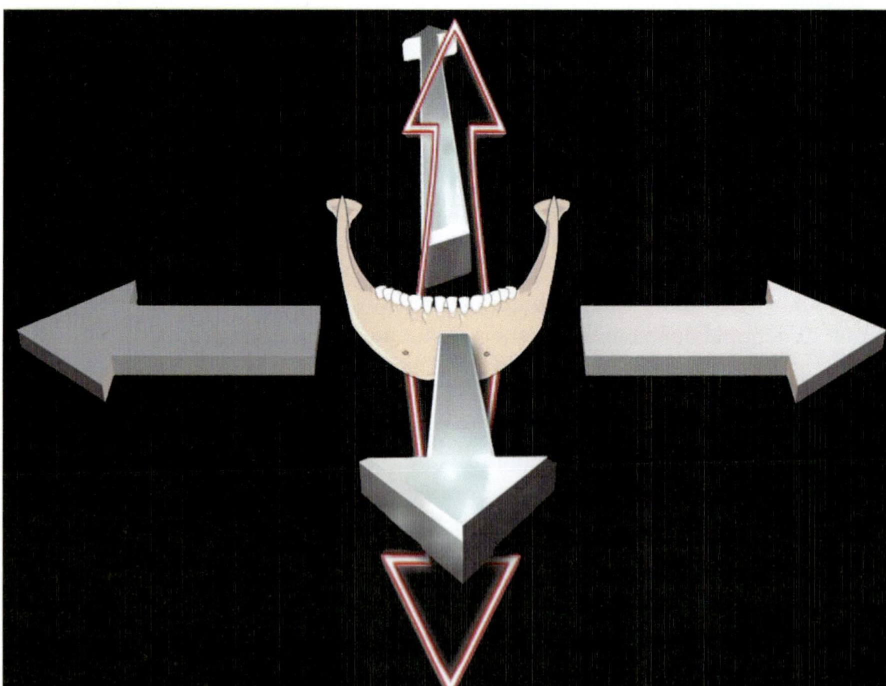

Fig. 1.2 Mandibular position after TENS application: it is important to consider a mandibular position after muscular deconditioning that can be directed in any of the 3 dimensions of space with different combinations and mixtures. Mandibular torquing and asymmetrical positioning in respect of the maxilla are frequent

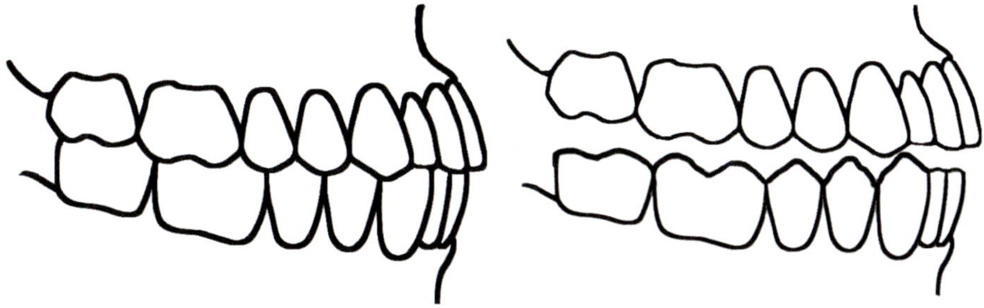

Fig. 1.3 Mandibular position in Class I occlusion and after TENS application, lateral view in ICP and after TENS application: the increase in posterior vertical freeway space can result as disproportional relatively to anterior vertical increase

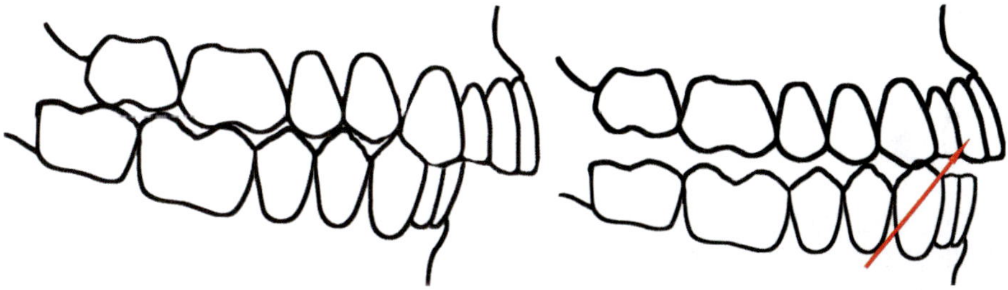

Fig. 1.4 Mandibular position after TENS application, Class II positional, lateral view before and after TENS application: mandible comes down and forward with a 2:1 ratio (Vertical = 2, AP = 1). This is the desired proportional ratio when freeway space is normal or slightly above normal. Red line indicates the approximate path of closure to Class I occlusion

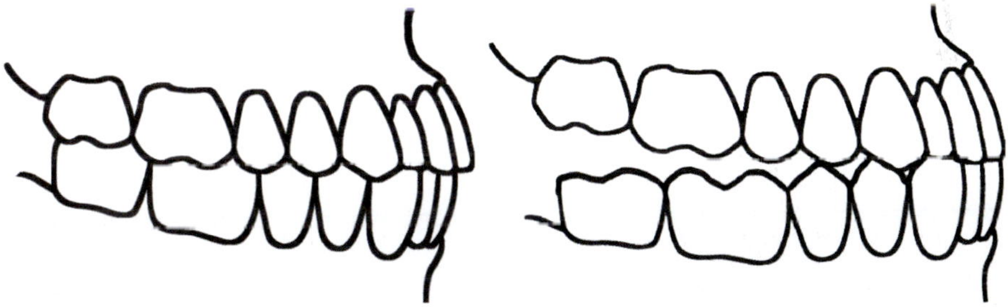

Fig. 1.5 Mandibular position after TENS application, Class I occlusion lateral view before and after TENS application: the anterior VD undergoes a slight change, while there is a substantive change in the posterior VD. This is a common finding in TMD patients

represented. When TENS is ***applied correctly*** to relax postural muscles, the mandibular rest position obtained is called *physiologic rest position* (PRP) or simply RP. This RP differs from a *habitual rest position* (HRP) which is seen regularly and habitually in each one of us without any TENS application. The RP (physiologic after TENS application) is always different from HRP.

The articulator mounting of mandibular rest position, as previously described, will be a way to visualize a malocclusion without looking at a misplaced mandible in CO. This concept is important. Orthodontic diagnosis, as it done today by most practitioners, is ***conceptually wrong*** because *its starting point is the* ***malocclusion***. The diagnostic procedure in neuromuscular orthodontics is different, the starting point is a ***correct mandibular position at rest. The Myocentric position determined by lower arch repositioning represents the ideal ICP at end of treatment.***

This new method of representing the relationship of the dental arches without occluding teeth, has the practitioner visualize the malocclusion in a new way. The practitioner understands that the muscular demands are different in respect of the current CO and *visualizes* the dental correction needed to support a new neuromuscular centric, the Myocentric. While there will be cases in which a considerable effort to correct freeway space with extrusion is fundamental, in others, freeway space is less important and leaves room for more fine adjustments such as dental torque and arch expansion. All of this can be visualized with a correct TENS bite occlusal registration and/or a complete k7 diagnostic procedure.

Dr. Piero Silvestrini and I have done extensive testing on TENS application with Aqualizer®. There is no neuromuscular procedure for administering TENS without inter-occlusal media. The main scope of Neuromuscular Dentistry diagnostics is the deconditioning of the muscles of mastication. The interruption of the afferent inputs to the CNS is an important step that can be done only with an occlusal media, that is, placing wax or other materials or appliances that interrupt occlusal contacts. Any accidental occlusal contact during TENS application immediately stimulates accommodation thus resulting in an erroneous RP at the end of the TENS application period. This compromises the final mandibular position. Special attention is necessary after the 40-minute period of application, as the occlusal media is taken out of the patient's mouth: if the patient distractively has an occlusal contact, the bite registration is then useless.

The bite registration obtained when recording the mandibular rest position (physiologic) ***is the freeway space.*** It is the inter-occlusal space between the dental arches with the mandible at physiologic rest. This recording is a *materialization* of the inter-occlusal space and represents a *cranio-mandibular relationship*.

Some dentists, in hoping to reduce time and expenses, avoid the use of inter-occlusal media and instruct the patient to avoid touching teeth together during the TENS session. This is absolutely wrongdoing for a very simple reason: it is important that the patient swallows during this relaxation period in the most natural position available and favoring all the necessary, physiologic reflexes that are fundamental for deglutition. If the patient is swallowing on an Aqualizer®, mandibular movement and swallow progress are quite "normal," meaning that the swallow automatism is not interrupted or compromised in any manner [9]. Instructing the patient to keep the dental arches apart forces an unnatural swallow procedure that is executed with the tongue between the teeth. Furthermore, after 40 min of tensing, there is no need to risk tooth contact because the patient could be tired, annoyed, or simply forget to keep teeth apart. Relying on patient truthfulness for not having tooth contact is simply an illusion. Controlling every second of patient compliance is simply impossible. There is no reason during this procedure to eliminate intra-occlusal media.

The Aqualizer® comes in three sizes. The size chosen should never exceed clinical freeway space. The decision on which size to choose should be done after a clinical evaluation of facial morphology/function and lateral cephalogram study. Any doubts on the quantity of freeway space in the low numbers should be a good indication to use the thinnest Aqualizer® available. Even if sEMG values drop within 5 min, it is always advisable to continue TENS application for at least 40 min. Other inter-occlusal media that have been used are either wax or cotton rolls. Wax such as Occlusal Indicator® from Kerr®, applied over the occlusal surface (double stratified) is a good method and has been used very much. The use of cotton rolls, cut and laid over the occlusal surfaces in the molar region is used by some doctors too. When TENS pulses in this case, there can be a lever effect with vertical condylar distraction. The author does not have experience with this methodology, but swallow again is completed with an unnatural occlusal balance.

Some freeway space concepts here are summarized in three main points:

Concept 1

There are two rest positions.

A. Habitual Rest Position (HRP). This is the mandibular rest position in a non-relaxed (TENS has not been applied) subject. This rest position varies with head posture, attitude, stress and so on. It is the CNS response to proprioception from the stomatognathic system.
B. Physiologic Rest Position (PRP or RP). This is obtained after relaxation of the mandibular postural muscles and can be checked via s-EMG. Procedures to obtain relaxed postural muscles of the mandible are discussed in the next chapters. This position is also influenced by postural strains, vision, stress, and attitude. This is important for a correct diagnostic, therapeutic, and follow-up point of view. Internal derangement (ID) of the TMJ can be an obstacle to finding this ideal rest position. PRP is the either the result of reduced proprioception to CNS or the result of a perfect occlusal treatment.

Concept 2

Freeway Space is three dimensional.

The only way to visualize this space is by recording the inter-occlusal relationship of the dental arches. This is usually done with a fast-setting silicone or a slower setting specific acrylic. This bite recording can be used to setup on an articulator the dental casts that will show the amount of neuromuscular discrepancy.

Concept 3

Like PRP and HRP, FWS can be either habitual or physiologic.

FWS in NO (Neuromuscular Orthodontics) is important for several reasons. In general, habitual FWS or inter-occlusal space is about 1.5–2 mm in its vertical dimension [10–14]. In most of the individuals, deconditioning the mandibular position, results in a different freeway space and rest position that is clinically significant. From a *kinesiographic point of view, the measurement of the vertical opening is referred to as vertical freeway space.* The vertical measurement is considered from the lower incisor edge as it comes to rest at ICP. The general population will have a larger FWS after TENS application, while in a small percentage (4.8) FWS is reduced [15]. The results vary from average increases of 0.8–0.9 mm in healthy subjects to greater increases up to 8 mm and more. FWS is not itself an indication of a neuromuscular disorder, but it can be used to understand the range of tolerance of the stomatognathic system.

The consequences of determining freeway space are important for therapeutic reasons. For example, if testing a patient with TENS determines a FWS of 1.5 mm., this can be a clear indication to avoid any procedure that may extrude teeth, such as some functional appliances do. If insufficient freeway space, as recorded in many open-bite individuals, is further reduced by erroneous orthodontic or prosthetic intervention, the result is generally a severe postural adaptation of the Cranio-Cervical district (hyperextension, neck pain, and so on). The consequences of this reduction/elimination of freeway will aggravate any pre-existing Temporo-Mandibular-Disorder (TMD) and put the patient at risk for new TMJ pathologies.

Recording P-FWS (Physiological FWS) with a resin or fast-setting silicone helps visualize where the rest position of the mandible should be at the *end* of treatment. The PRP has a deeper meaning. The condyles (being part of the mandible!) are repositioned in the glenoid fossa according to the muscular needs. In ***positional Class II*** cases (MCD: Morsus Coactus Distalis), and the majority of TMD cases as well, the condyle is repositioned in a lower and more advanced position in the fossa as a consequence of TENS deconditioning. Anterior disc displacement (ADD) is the most common internal derangement of the TMJ with pain and sounds and altered jaw movements [16–20]. ADD is the result of posterior condyle dislocation. This means that when TENS is applied correctly, the resulting condylar position must by logic, prevent ADD. Neuromuscular orthodontics is about the prevention of TMD and it makes sense that the determination of a new mandibular position generally affects the condyle setting it in a more forward and downward location.

There have been several studies on the condylar position in CO for Class I, II, and III occlusions [21–28]. Not without surprise, these studies from several authors state that Class II occlusions predominantly have an *anteriorly displaced condyle* [22, 27–32]. These studies do not use the same method for determining condylar positioning and so there is no way of comparison between them. This may seem difficult to understand when considering that most Class II occlusions are positional and not skeletal. In fact, the finding that Class II occlusions have a more forward position of the condyle, could be explained from a neuromuscular point of view, because cases with excess freeway space (generally more than 5 mm) in which the condyle does come down and forward with the use of TENS (the *mandible* does come forward) are characterized by a posterior vertical drop and rotation of the condyle of greater *proportional* entity in respect to the sagittal advancement. The general kinesiographic rule that vertical and anterior increase after TENS is at a 2:1 ratio relationship is outgone with a ratio close to 3:1 or even more. Consider a high increase in the posterior vertical dimension and a good increase in the sagittal relationship. Furthermore, not all studies indicate that the condyle is anteriorly displaced in Class II occlusion but posteriorly displaced [33–35]. There may be a direct link between Class II/TMD and posterior condylar displacement [16] and in general posterior condylar displacement and TMD [18, 19]. Posterior condylar displacement can be seen at the early stages of TMD when internal derangement is present with ADD without reduction (there is a reduction of the posterior condylar space) [36]. Therefore, freeway space and its recording after TENS/Aqualizer application represents essentially a cranio-*condylar*-mandibular relationship. Conceptually this is very important because it focuses on the condylar position that is now considered as an integrated part of malocclusion diagnosis and treatment.

Freeway Space a "Functional Space"

On a full or partial mouth rehabilitation that requires an increase in VD, there are usually fewer problems and difficulties if freeway space is, by the end of treatment, circa 1–2 mm (intended here in a neuromuscular fashion, after deconditioning muscles with TENS procedure). If, by any chance, the prosthetics use up all the freeway space available, the first reaction is head extension (needed to create missing freeway space) [37, 38]. If this extension is not sufficient to regain a functional freeway space, the consequences are an exaggerated head extension leading to continuous neck pain and TMJ stress.

Skeletal open-bite individuals in general, are linked to respiratory problems and have little or no freeway space with head extension as a functional reaction/adaptation [38–44]. Adult open-bite morphology varies in degrees of severity from a functional point of view. In less severe cases, a slight head extension is sufficient to guarantee a minimum of freeway space and avoid tooth contact at habitual mandibular rest. These subjects may not have a *dental* open-bite and may swallow correctly. As severity increases, head extension may not be sufficient to produce an adequate quantity of freeway space. As previously said, these patients are accompanied by TMJ pain, TMJ arthrosis, cervical arthrosis, and TMD [45–48]. Their dental open bite prevents them from swallowing correctly, aggravating and sustaining the malocclusion. Orthognathic surgery cases in which upper maxillary impaction is not done correctly and sufficiently, results in post-surgical trismus and worsening of open bite as a reaction to the loss of freeway space. Freeway space is necessary for a correct stomatognathic function.

Skeletal deep-bite morphology, on the other hand, is represented by an excess in freeway space. The more freeway space, the more tolerant the stomatognathic functions in relation to occlusal changes. The presence of the excess freeway space leaves a wide range of possibilities for occlusal correction of malocclusions. Functional appliances, build-ups, and so on, have all in common a mandibular positional correction dictated by muscular requests, in which the correction of the occlusal plane together with the selected extrusions/build-ups are carried out extensively [49]. Fortunately, most of the dental office population requesting a prosthetic correction/rehabilitation fall within the excess freeway space grouping.

The continuous reduction in VD (increase in freeway space) over time is due to several reasons, like tooth ware, clenching habits, and iatrogenic causes like lowering of prosthetic bridges and other erroneous maneuvers delivered by dentists. It is easier and faster for the practitioner to reduce posterior support when delivering bridges: it is easily accepted by the patient. Creating a sudden posterior support for patients that have been without prosthetic replacement for some time, requires muscular reactivation of the masseter and temporal muscles. Occlusal balancing is needed, and more precise prosthetic construction is required.

Skeletal deep-bite morphology cannot be changed. Skeletal changes can be achieved only via surgical procedures and a young adolescent with deep bite trait will continue to grow as a deep bite. It could be that very early interceptive treatment of skeletal deep bite can reduce skeletal severity. The everlasting question is, if early intervention with build-ups on deciduous teeth can in some way reduce skeletal deep-bite morphology. Interceptive orthodontics for severe deep bite children should focus not only by decreasing freeway space and increasing lower facial height but most importantly by assuring the mandible is not trapped by the upper dentition. Generally speaking, skeletal deep-bite individuals have and produce excess freeway space during their life span.

Freeway space obtained after deconditioning represents a quantitative measurement of space for functional tolerance. Deep bite individuals are characterized by a wide glenoid fossa, a large condyle, and a generous articular space, this represents the great anatomical tolerance linked to this morphological characteristic. On the contrary, in skeletal open bite morphology, the condyle is thin, joint space reduced and articular space scarce [50, 51]. The shape of the condyle is elongated and appears somewhat fragile. When taking CBCT scans of condyles in open bite adult individuals, shape alterations due to arthrosis are quite frequent [44, 52, 53]. So, defining freeway space as a "tolerance" index has some obvious advantages. One of which is to be very careful in not depleting freeway in patients that have little, and of course, trying to identify those patients that have a compensatory head extension to create a minimum functional space requirement. Skeletal deep bite morphology, on the other hand, is characterized by an anatomy that dictates tolerance. Replacing prosthetic bridges and placing implants is always easier in deep-bite individuals. Forward head posture with lordosis is somewhat present and participates as a compensation factor for excess freeway space [54, 55]. The reduction of excess freeway space reduces forward head posture [37, 56–60].

Between these extremes lie the skeletal individuals that we refer to as norm and that do not have an excess in freeway space and at worst, have a slight compensatory head posture. When clinically evaluated, habitual freeway space is quantitively slightly changed by TENS. Usually there is a vertical increase of a couple of millimeters. There is always a change in FWS and mandibular position after TENS application.

Freeway Space and Dental Occlusion

The comprehensive approach to understanding freeway space in its essential meaning must be ***unlinked*** to dental occlusion. Several studies on bite force and electromyographic output have dissimilar results because patient selection is based on groups allotted according to dental relationships (Angle classification). The Angle classifications are based on tooth relationship in ICP and lack of other important information like various morphological traits or stomatognathic muscular function. Studies that have tried to relate dental occlusion to head-neck and body posture are somewhat inconclusive. Literature is criticized by the scientific community and is not worthwhile to mention.

If any truth can be taken from studies that relate body posture to the stomatognathic system, then emphasis should be given to support those studies that relate body posture (mainly cranio-cervical posture) to craniofacial morphology and not to occlusion. This linkage between morphology and posture means that there is a direct link between posture and freeway space, and this means mandibular rest position. Immediate postural changes can be seen and can be verified during neuromuscular orthotic use in which swallow occurs on the Myocentric in ICP [61]. So cranio-facial morphology has an important link to freeway space. Severe skeletal open-bite will not have freeway space and severe skeletal deep-bite will have excess freeway space. Freeway space recording, bite recording, represents an orthopedic relationship of the mandible relative to the cranium and for this reason it cannot represent dental arch relationships. This is just one example of a potential bias that has led and will lead to erroneous conclusions of all those studies that have attempted to link occlusal relationships to posture without considering an attentive analysis of the vertical relationships. On the other hand, Neuromuscular Dentists measure freeway space on a daily basis during a full kinesiographic assessment and can confirm that an excess freeway space is a characteristic of skeletal deep bite individuals and that these individuals have a specific tendency to cervical lordosis. Freeway space change (correction) induced by dental/orthodontic treatment offers dramatic changes in head/body posture [55, 60, 61]. Too many variables compromise a direct relationship between dental occlusion and freeway space. The relationship is about mandibular posture (Physiologic Rest Position) and freeway space in relation to cranio-cervical posture and maybe to body posture.

References

1. Mohl ND. Neuromuscular mechanisms in mandibular function. Dent Clin N Am. 1978;22(1):63–71.
2. McNamara JA, Carlson DS. *Muskuloskeletal adaptation following orthognatic surgery.*, in *Craniofacial growth series*. 1978, Needham Press: University of Michigan, Ann Aror, 1978 U.S.A.
3. Niswonger ME. The rest position of the mandible and the centric relation. JADA. 1934;21:1572–82.

4. Lerman MD. A revised view of the dynamics, physiology, and treatment of occlusion: a new paradigm. Cranio. 2004;22(1):50–63.
5. Johnson AT. Teaching the principle of biological optimization. J Biol Eng. 2013;7(1):6–6.
6. Johnson A, Wildgoose DG, Wood DJ. The determination of freeway space using two different methods. J Oral Rehabil. 2002;29(10):1010–3.
7. Dosumu OO, Ikusika OF. An assessment of interocclusal space in a dentate Nigerian population. Niger Postgrad Med J. 2013;20(4):315–8.
8. Peterson TM, Rugh JD, McIver JE. Mandibular rest position in subjects with high and low mandibular plane angles. Am J Orthod. 1983;83(4):318–20.
9. Lerman MD. The hydrostatic appliance: a new approach to treatment of the TMJ pain-dysfunction syndrome. J Am Dent Assoc. 1974;89(6):1343–50.
10. *Neuromuscular dental diagnosis and treatment: Robert R. Jankelson Ishiyaku EuroAmerica, St. Louis: 1990. 687 pages, 1132 illustrations*. American journal of orthodontics and dentofacial orthopedics : official publication of the American Association of Orthodontists, its constituent societies, and the American Board of Orthodontics, 1991. **99**(3): p. 283–284.
11. Ferrario VF, et al. Statistical evaluation of some mandibular reference positions in normal young people. Int J Prosthodont. 1992;5(2):158–65.
12. Nielsen IL, et al. Patterns of mandibular movements in subjects with craniomandibular disorders. J Prosthet Dent. 1990;63(2):202–17.
13. Suarez D. Posiciòn de reposo mandibular. Revista Espanola de Ortodoncia. 1987;17:63–76.
14. Rugh JD, Drago CJ. Vertical dimension: a study of clinical rest position and jaw muscle activity. J Prosthet Dent. 1981;45(6):670–5.
15. Konchak PA, et al. Freeway space measurement using mandibular kinesiograph and EMG before and after TENS. Angle Orthod. 1988;58(4):343–50.
16. Owen AH 3rd. Orthodontic/orthopedic treatment of craniomandibular pain dysfunction. Part 2: posterior condylar displacement. J Craniomandibular Pract. 1984;2(4):333–49.
17. Weinberg LA. The role of stress, occlusion, and condyle position in TMJ dysfunction-pain. J Prosthet Dent. 1983;49(4):532–45.
18. Weinberg LA. Role of condylar position in TMJ dysfunction-pain syndrome. J Prosthet Dent. 1979;41(6):636–43.
19. Imanimoghaddam M, et al. Evaluation of condylar positions in patients with temporomandibular disorders: a cone-beam computed tomographic study. Imaging Sci Dent. 2016;46(2):127–31.
20. Shokri A, et al. Comparative assessment of condylar position in patients with temporomandibular disorder (TMD) and asymptomatic patients using cone-beam computed tomography. Dent Med Probl. 2019;56(1):81–7.
21. Alhammadi M, Fayed M, Labib A. Three-dimensional assessment of temporomandibular joints in skeletal class I, class II, and class III malocclusions: cone beam computed tomography analysis. J World Fed Orthod. 2016:5.
22. Katsavrias EG, Halazonetis DJ. Condyle and fossa shape in class II and class III skeletal patterns: a morphometric tomographic study. Am J Orthod Dentofac Orthop. 2005;128(3):337–46.
23. Kaur A, et al. Improved visualization and assessment of condylar position in the glenoid fossa for different occlusions: a CBCT study. J Contemp Dent Pract. 2016;17(8):679–86.
24. Merigue L, et al. Tomographic evaluation of the temporomandibular joint in malocclusion subjects: condylar morphology and position. Braz Oral Res. 2016;30
25. Gu YJ, et al. Comparison of condylar position between angle class I and class II malocclusion in teenagers. Shanghai Kou Qiang Yi Xue. 2016;25(6):694–6.
26. Gianelly AA, Petras JC, Boffa J. Condylar position and class II deep-bite, no-overjet malocclusions. Am J Orthod Dentofac Orthop. 1989;96(5):428–32.
27. Uzel A, Özyürek Y, Öztunç H. Condyle position in class II division 1 malocclusion patients: correlation between MPI records and CBCT images. J World Fed Orthod. 2013;2:e65–70.
28. Vitral RW, et al. Computed tomography evaluation of temporomandibular joint alterations in patients with class II division 1 subdivision malocclusions: condyle-fossa relationship. Am J Orthod Dentofac Orthop. 2004;126(1):48–52.

29. Pullinger AG, et al. Relationship of mandibular condylar position to dental occlusion factors in an asymptomatic population. Am J Orthod Dentofac Orthop. 1987;91(3):200–6.
30. Krisjane Z, et al. Three-dimensional evaluation of TMJ parameters in class II and class III patients. Stomatologija. 2009;11(1):32–6.
31. Rodrigues AF, Fraga MR, Vitral RW. Computed tomography evaluation of the temporomandibular joint in class I malocclusion patients: condylar symmetry and condyle-fossa relationship. Am J Orthod Dentofac Orthop. 2009;136(2):192–8.
32. Fraga MR, et al. Anteroposterior condylar position: a comparative study between subjects with normal occlusion and patients with class I, class II division 1, and class III malocclusions. Med Sci Monit. 2013;19:903–7.
33. Kinzinger G, Kober C, Diedrich P. Topography and morphology of the mandibular condyle during fixed functional orthopedic treatment—a magnetic resonance imaging study. J Orofac Orthop. 2007;68(2):124–47.
34. Fernández Sanromán J, Gómez González JM, Alonso del Hoyo J. Relationship between condylar position, dentofacial deformity and temporomandibular joint dysfunction: an MRI and CT prospective study. J Cranio-Maxillofac Surg. 1998;26(1):35–42.
35. Greven M, Cazacu I, Piehslinger E. Correlation of occlusal-plane-inclination with functional condylar displacement in different skeletal classes. Int J Dent Oral Health. 2020;6
36. Ozawa S, et al. Reconsideration of the TMJ condylar position during internal derangement: comparison between condylar position on tomogram and degree of disk displacement on MRI. Cranio. 1999;17(2):93–100.
37. Ohnmeiß M, et al. Therapeutic effects of functional orthodontic appliances on cervical spine posture: a retrospective cephalometric study. Head Face Med. 2014;10:7.
38. Daly P, Preston CB, Evans WG. Postural response of the head to bite opening in adult males. Am J Orthod. 1982;82(2):157–60.
39. Kim P, Sarauw M, Sonnesen L. Cervical vertebral column morphology and head posture in preorthodontic patients with anterior open bite. Am J Orthod Dentofacial Orthop. 2014;145:359–66.
40. Vig PS, Showfety KJ, Phillips C. Experimental manipulation of head posture. 1980;77(3):258–68.
41. Liu Y, et al. Relationships of vertical facial pattern, natural head position and craniocervical posture in young Chinese children. Cranio. 2018;36(5):311–7.
42. Kim P, Sarauw MT, Sonnesen L. Cervical vertebral column morphology and head posture in preorthodontic patients with anterior open bite. Am J Orthod Dentofac Orthop. 2014;145(3):359–66.
43. Leitao P, Nanda RS. Relationship of natural head position to craniofacial morphology. Am J Orthod Dentofacial Orthop. 2000;117(4):406–17.
44. Ioi H, et al. Relationship of TMJ osteoarthritis/osteoarthrosis to head posture and dentofacial morphology. Orthod Craniofac Res. 2008;11(1):8–16.
45. Byun ES, Ahn SJ, Kim TW. Relationship between internal derangement of the temporomandibular joint and dentofacial morphology in women with anterior open bite. Am J Orthod Dentofac Orthop. 2005;128(1):87–95.
46. Yan ZB, et al. Craniofacial morphology of orthodontic patients with and without temporomandibular disorders: a cross-sectional study. Pain Res Manag. 2022;2022:9344028.
47. Kuroda S, et al. Anterior open bite with temporomandibular disorder treated with titanium screw anchorage: evaluation of morphological and functional improvement. Am J Orthod Dentofac Orthop. 2007;131(4):550–60.
48. Williamson EH. Temporomandibular dysfunction in pretreatment adolescent patients. Am J Orthod. 1977;72(4):429–33.
49. Constantinescu FE, et al. Complete morphofunctional oral rehabilitation by physiological increase of occlusal vertical dimension according to computerized mandibular scanner. Romanian J Morphol Embryol. 2022;63(1):245–51.
50. Björk A, Skieller V. Normal and abnormal growth of the mandible. A synthesis of longitudinal cephalometric implant studies over a period of 25 years. Eur J Orthod. 1983;5(1):1–46.

51. Bjork A. Variations in the growth pattern of the human mandible: longitudinal radiographic study by the implant method. J Dent Res. 1963;42(1 Pt 2):400–11.
52. Tanimoto K, et al. Characteristics of the maxillofacial morphology in patients with idiopathic mandibular condylar resorption. J Clin Med. 2022;11:4.
53. Deng MZ, Leotta D, Huang GJ, Zhao ZH, Liu ZJ. Craniofacial, tongue, and speech characteristics in anterior open bite patients of east African ethnicity. Res Rep Oral Maxillofac Surg. 2019;3:021.
54. Solow B, Tallgren A. Head posture and craniofacial morphology. Am J Phys Anthropol. 1976;44(3):417–35.
55. Biavati, P.S., *Trattamento semplificato in gnatologia. Il metodo Global Occlusion*. 2019: Edra.
56. Urbanowicz M. Alteration of vertical dimension and its effect on head and neck posture. Cranio. 1991;9(2):174–9.
57. Moya H, et al. Influence of stabilization occlusal splint on craniocervical relationships. Part I: cephalometric analysis. Cranio. 1994;12(1):47–51.
58. Tecco S, et al. Evaluation of cervical spine posture after functional therapy with FR-2: a longitudinal study. Cranio. 2005;23(1):53–66.
59. Kamal AT, Fida M. Evaluation of cervical spine posture after functional therapy with twin-block appliances: a retrospective cohort study. Am J Orthod Dentofac Orthop. 2019;155(5):656–61.
60. Savastano F. Correction of a class II occlusion in an adult. J Dent Oral Disord Ther. 2014;4:1–10.
61. Silvestrini Biavati P. Trattamento semplificato in gnatologia: il metodo Global Occlusion. Edra: Milano; 2019.

Creating a Common Language

2

If you are an orthodontist and you are just starting to read on neuromuscular diagnosis and treatment, please understand that while I have a conventional orthodontic formation and vocabulary, I also use a neuromuscular terminology that is quite typical of Neuromuscular Dentistry. It is necessary to establish a common ground for communication purposes on some occlusal, morphological, and functional terminologies of our specialty.

Lateral Cephalograms

Lateral head X-rays are done in maximal intercuspation (Centric Occlusion). Besides cephalometrics, the clinician should be able to retrieve quite a bit of information from a visual examination of a lateral cephalogram. Lymphatic tissue as cause of suspected breathing problems and alterations of the sella turcica just to name a few, are left to the reader to consider for future studies. For orthodontic diagnosis, cephalometric results should be considered together with a skeletal interpretation of the morphological characteristics.

Cephalometrics

Conventional orthodontics relies greatly on cephalometrics for diagnostics and decision-making. It has even developed several analysis that try to predict growth and malocclusion development [1]. The lateral head X-ray is generally executed in an unnatural head posture and measurements are usually carried out with the help of cephalometric software [2]. Cephalometrics is operator dependent and potential bias is just around the corner [3–7]. If we consider that the validity and usefulness of the cephalometric evaluation is measured in millimeters, the reproducibility is compromised when results are more than 1 mm in difference between operators [8,

F. Savastano, *Neuromuscular Orthodontics*,
https://doi.org/10.1007/978-3-031-41295-0_2

9]. It is probably not important from a clinicaltherapeutic point of view as some authors have suggested [10, 11], but there continues to be endless discussions on this issue. Even different cephalometric analyses can result in different diagnostic interpretations [12]. Superimpositions are very arguable in assessing cephalometric results [13].

The question regarding Neuromuscular Orthodontics is not the preciseness of the cephalometric tracings (given that the execution is done correctly), but rather trying to gather from cephalometrics, information to integrate and help clinical decision-making. For this reason, it is preferable to assess patient lateral cephalometry with a more proportional rather than linear measurement type of cephalometric analysis. The Sassouni [14–16] Archial Analysis focuses on the identification of facial disharmony. It is a very simple method and widely used among functional orthodontists (Fig. 2.1).

Orthodontic schools teach to classify malocclusion once cephalometric analysis and casts have been assessed with the patient's occlusion in ICP. Cephalometric evaluation should guide the clinician to qualify results on skeletal class, vertical and horizontal relationships of the maxilla and the lower jaw. It represents a great method to calculate incisor inclination to skeletal references and calculate the amount of sagittal discrepancy as overjet. Overbite is also clearly visualized and calculated. All other recordings, angles between linear measurements, sum of angular measurements, distance between non-anatomical points just to name a few, are specific in most cases for each cephalometric methodology.

The definition of skeletal class, for example, is often misinterpreted because it is linked to dental relationships during centric occlusion. Centric Occlusion (CO) occurs only about 17 min in total during the 24-h day span and usually during swallow or voluntary clench. The lateral cephalogram cannot give us further information, like muscle function or TMJ integrity or swallow disorders. Conventional

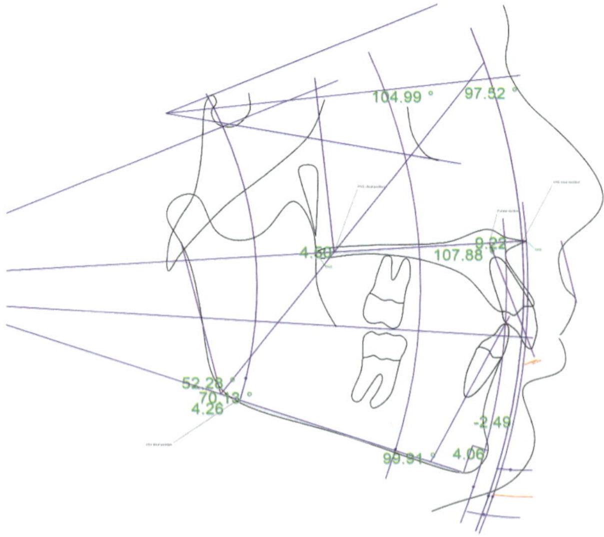

Fig. 2.1 Sassouni cephalometric analysis

orthodontics has relied way too much on cephalometrics and a lot less on clinical observation. The information obtained from lateral Cephalograms should be limited to *confirmation* of the clinical and bioelectric functional diagnosis and not considered a diagnostic method per se. The starting point is CO, this means that the ***starting point of this diagnostic procedure is the malocclusion***. Especially true for inexperienced orthodontists, cephalometric analysis can be misleading. The dental class, on the other hand, emphasizes occlusal relationship only. Our orthodontic training is still essentially anchored to the six keys of occlusion of Dr. Andrews [17]. We have been taught that our treatment objectives were essentially aesthetic, and that function was linked to occlusal interdigitation and alignment and that this could guarantee a very low probability of relapse. Since neuromuscular orthodontics has a different starting point, the mandibular posture, it is easily understood why the main objectives are shifted toward muscle and TMJ functional requests rather than achieving a Class I dental relationship.

Figures 2.2, 2.3, 2.4, and 2.5 represent some examples of lateral cephalograms and explain some differences in orthodontic interpretations. The Neuromuscular Orthodontist foresees vertical and sagittal repositioning of the mandible and uses a different diagnostic vocabulary. The reason is that neuromuscular diagnostics deals with a *dynamic occlusion* and reasonably limits static occlusion importance for swallow interpretation purposes.

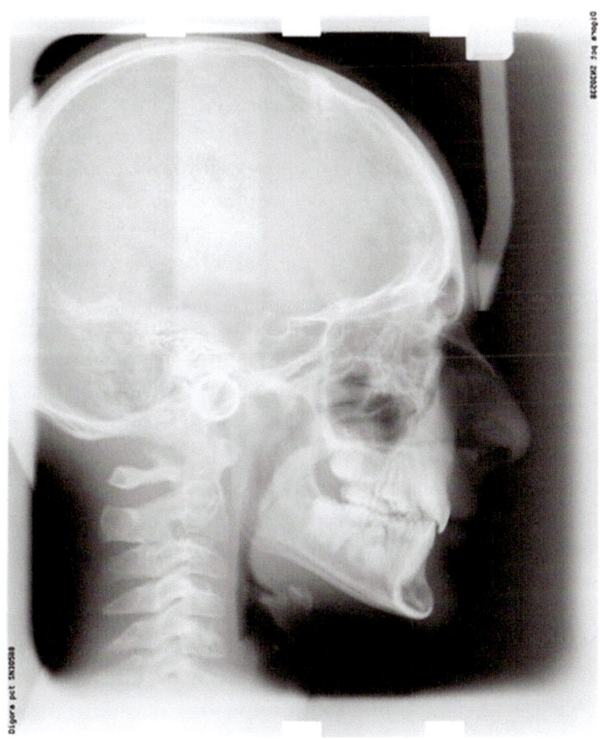

Fig. 2.2 Several experienced orthodontists who have analyzed this lateral cephalogram X-ray, agreed to diagnose it as a mild Class II, with slight dental deep bite. From a neuromuscular perspective, this is a Class III individual who has excess freeway space (or as you may prefer, deep bite). Note Witt's appraisal measurements within normal limits [18]. Unfortunately, the dental relationship is Class II, and this is one typical reason for which orthodontic errors occur. Any treatments that could have distalized the upper arch would have caused severe dental/orthodontic relapse and TMJ dysfunction. This clinical case will be discussed further on

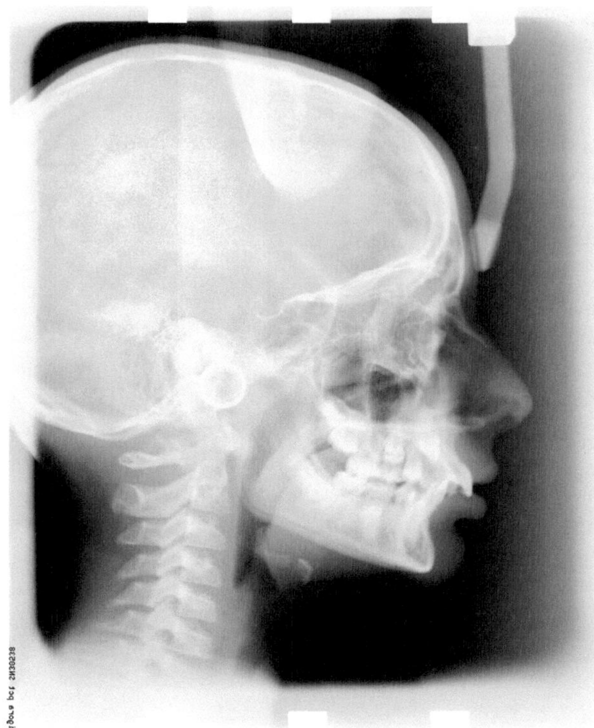

Fig. 2.3 Class II occlusion with increased overjet. Several treatments from experienced orthodontists suggested upper distalization, Extra-Oral Traction (EOT). In NO, this is a **Skeletal Class I**. Mandible is distally positioned, normal in size for age and sex, and cranial base and cannot be in a more forward position due to upper contraction and excess of posterior freeway space. This is a ***positional* Class II**

Table 2.1 recaps some differences in interpretation between the classical orthodontic diagnosis terminology and the neuromuscular one. This table describes briefly the skeletal/dental diagnosis from a Cephalometric analysis versus a correct interpretation in NO.

Neuromuscular Orthodontics is basically a functional approach in orthodontics, with the important aspect that in NO we *measure* function. The author avoids the use of static diagnostics, such as "deep bite," rather prefers to state diagnostically the missing or excess of function, say "excess of freeway space." This example statement contains already information for the correction in one direction, that is, "reduction of freeway space." There are anyways, certain terminologies that are typical of neuromuscular diagnosis. For example, referring to an occlusion as having a "front wall" is usually used to describe those occlusions characterized by mandibular entrapment determined from the upper arch contraction with reduced incisal toque or premaxilla contraction. Typically seen in Class II/2, front walls are very frequent in many malocclusions. Mandibular entrapment is one of the main issues of neuromuscular diagnostics.

Lateral cephalograms give other precious information to the orthodontist. Breathing problems may be suspected as well as neck issues especially when the lateral cephalograms are executed in natural head posture [22, 23]. Other problems too can be detected like tooth impaction and third molar positioning, cystis, and so

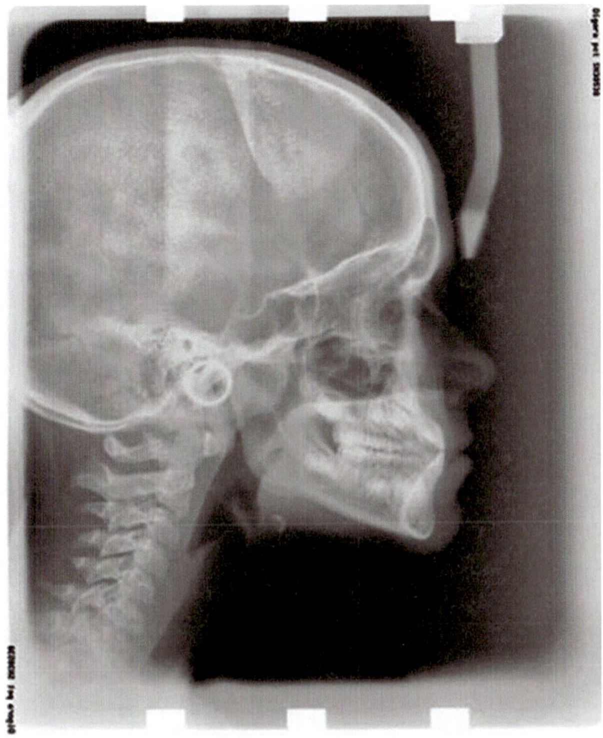

Fig. 2.4 Class III patient, dentally and skeletally. The mandible is longer than what you would expect for age, sex, cranial base, and race [19, 20]. Treatment cannot reduce the overall length of the mandible without risking articular damage, the only real treatment possibility in these Class III cases is to improve the length and the transverse deficiency of the maxilla. If there is an excess in freeway space, then there is an option to reduce it with extrusion, hence *reducing the sagittal discrepancy*

on. More severe problems like tumors and other rare potentially life-threatening pathologies may sometimes be seen [24].

Introducing a different terminology is not an easy task. This is because it takes a neuromuscular understanding of the diagnostics that is function oriented instead of occlusal oriented. Needless to say, clinical examination is key to any medical procedure although there is a certain percentage of orthodontists that mostly rely on cephalometric analysis for treatment planning [25, 26]. Even if it is understandable that orthodontic diagnosis and treatment teaching should have a starting point from cephalometric interpretation, it remains questionable as an orthodontic necessity for treatment decisions. Experience and other information derived from dental casts and panoramic X-rays may be sufficient for orthodontic diagnosis [27–29]. The validity of cephalometrics remains dubious [7, 30].

There is a rigid link existing between morphology of malocclusion and orthodontic necessity: the socially acceptable need for orthodontic treatment cannot be based solely on occlusal aspects of malocclusion. The IOTN (Index of Orthodontic Treatment Need) elaborated by the British Orthodontic Society together with their National Health System, focuses on solely dental/cephalometric aspects of occlusion up to grade 3 without any reference to any dysfunctional problem, as if functional problems can arise solely when severe visual malocclusion is present (grade

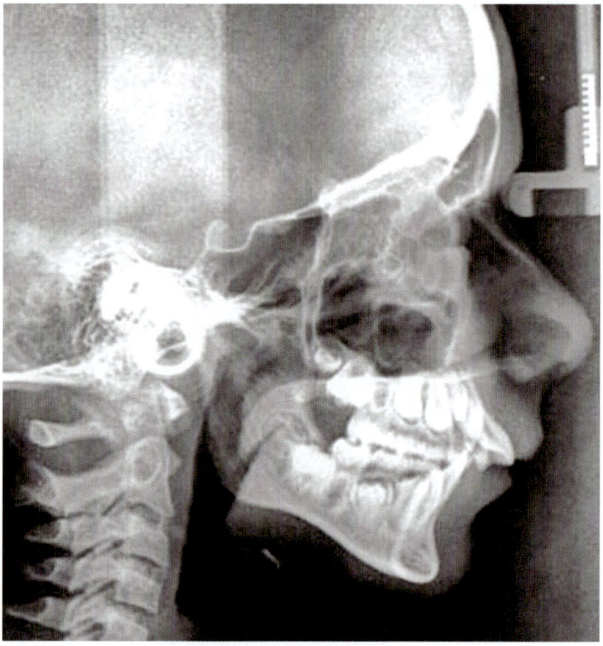

Fig. 2.5 This is a Class II skeletal malocclusion: mandible is very small. You can refer to the various tables in your orthodontic books for the normal mandibular length for age, sex, race, and cranial base, keeping in mind that below the sixth percentile you will be dealing with a very small mandible. Same is said for any measurement over the 94th percentile: mandible would be larger/longer for age, sex, and race [19–21]. This is a very different situation in respect of a *positional* Class II. Furthermore, note the curve of Spee, the compensation needed for the anterior open bite. This is not a patient with an excess in freeway space, but rather lacking in such. *Skeletal Class II are for definition surgical cases* and are usually severe. When mild cases are present, a "compensation" can be attempted by intrusion of the upper dentition together with a slight distalization. This improves the sagittal relationship but cannot improve the profile

Table 2.1 Summary of most common interpretation changes from a neuromuscular point of view

Cephalometric analyses	Neuromuscular orthodontics
Class I skeletal/dental	1. Can be an ideal Class I skeletal and occlusal 2. Could be a perfect occlusion but a dysfunctional patient. Could in fact be a *Class III functionally* and thus a distalized mandible/condyle, entrapped by upper arch. This is a Mandible Forced Distalized (MFD).
Class II skeletal/dental	Could be a skeletal Class II (mandible is shorter than normal for age and sex), or could be a ***positional*** Class II (normal skeleton, incorrect relation). 95% of Class II are positional.
Class III skeletal/dental	Could be a ***positional*** Class III, that is, a normal mandible that is positioned mesially. In NO, skeletal Class III is considered so only if mandible is longer than normal for age and sex, with upper maxilla normal or shorter than normal for age and sex.
Open bite	Reduced freeway space. No freeway space.
Deep bite	Excess freeway space

4). This discriminates dysfunctional patients that present a low grade of teeth irregularity and a high grade of TMJ dysfunction and associated symptoms. The IOTN index has been used as a reference by several countries within Europe [31, 32]. The objective of a national health system should be *in primis*, prevention.

Finally, the goal of this chapter is to introduce a common language between conventional orthodontics and its neuromuscular counterpart. Here are some diagnostic concepts and terminologies that summarize this chapter.

Diagnostic Concept 1

The Importance of the Cranio-Mandibular Relationship

Defining an occlusion by dental and skeletal class relationship is like taking a photo in CO, it is a static representation of the jaws during ICP. It does not provide any information on function and aesthetics. We need to unfold the hidden functional characteristics of our patients. CO forces the mandible to close and muscles to adapt according to occlusal needs. Muscles do adapt temorarily to preserve important functions of the stomatognathic system, like swallowing and chewing. The question is, what do we mean by temporarily? Whenever the mandibular position in CO is not ideal and requires accommodation, as time passes, muscular effort (elicited by the CNS) will show signs of adaptation to malocclusion *on the dentition*. The presence of wear facets is a tentative by the neuromuscular system to consume, overcome, occlusal interferences that limit mandibular repositioning according to muscle needs. As an example, excessive growth of the mandible may force the lower incisors to tip lingually. This represents the first line of defence against a skeletal discrepancy by teeth that are passive elements and adapt to a more lingual position to save TMJ function. A sudden occlusal interference may generate an avoidance pattern with a new adaptive engram, but prolonged malocclusions cannot force continuous muscular avoidance patterns permanently without signs opf muscular intolerance on the occlusal sufaces. For this reason, malocclusions are destinated to get worse because of unnatural tooth wear and dental compensation. Irregularities and misalignment are the result of malocclusion and muscle adaptation. Relapse happens when muscles do not accept the mandibular position during ICP, that is, *during swallow*. How many occlusions do we see with abnormal anterior lower tooth wear? If dental abrasions are part of our everyday experience while visiting young or adult patients, this means that the neuromuscular system is struggling to overcome occlusal interferences as a tentative procedure for a more physiological mandibular position during swallow. *We should be more interested in the Cranio-mandibular relationship, rather than defining the skeleton per se*. This relationship should be considered without any limitation of movement and in a *muscle-relaxed environment.*

Diagnostic Concept 2

Anterior-Posterior Relation

The three dimensions of space interact together. Every well-trained orthodontist understands these mechanisms. Any increment in the Anterior Vertical Dimension

(AVD) decreases the Anterior-Posterior (AP) relationship (sagittal) between mandible and maxilla and vice versa. This means that the more you extrude and open the bite, the more you will increase Overjet. The more you reduce facial height, the more you will reduce Overjet.

Diagnostic Concept 3

Vertical Relation

The use of "Skeletal Open bite," should be limited only to those cases in which it is identifiable the skeletal characteristics as referred to the *anatomy of the mandibular bone (and face)* (Bjork). For example, when studying a patient's cephalogram, we would like to consider it as an open-bite only when the mandible's anatomy is typical of this morphology. We are not considering a lack of freeway space *until we measure so*. Furthermore functional treatments should be reserved only for ideal-normal/deep-bite cases, for the fact that any extrusion in an open-bite case may very well aggravate the occlusion by opening the bite. Patients with all but unsevere typical skeletal characteristics you would expect in an open-bite case may have *some degree of freeway space* that allows the use of functional appliances and mandibular repositioning. Other judgments of open-bite anatomy patterns obviously complete this scenario, maxilla, cranial base, and anterior facial height and must be taken into account for diagnostic and treatment purposes.

Deep bite, on the other hand, is characterized by an excess of freeway space. Skeletal morphology is important too. The growth pattern cannot change dramatically with treatment, meaning that if this typology is linked to excess freeway space, it will remain so even with treatment. NO treatment objectives include extrusion when there is excess interocclusal space, but the treatment outcome remains limited by the skeletal discrepancy. Sometimes at best, extrusion limits the creation or worsening of freeway space.

Diagnostic Concept 4

Transverse Relation. Expansion

In the majority of malocclusions, there is a well-known discrepancy between the transverse relationship of the dental/skeletal arches. Maxillar insufficiency is not the only responsable for transverse discrepancies. When the mandible is larger than it should be, the result is similar. Since mandibular intervention is essentially surgical, it is nonsense to want to reduce the mandibular transverse dimension in this equation. So maxillary *expansion* is really needed in most malocclusions. This abused orthodontic terminology has only one meaning in Neuromuscular Orthodontics: the expansion of the upper arch should be achieved limiting the loss of torque/tipping of teeth and with ***opening of the mid-palatal suture*** [33–37]. If we accept the modern idea that malocclusions are the result of maxillary deficiency, then more bone is needed for the maxilla. When expansion is needed it is needed because there is a *skeletal discrepancy*. This is the main reason why expansion should be obtained *only* by means of a fixed palatal expander and RPE. A removable appliance may easily obtain reversible expansion through loss of upper torque/tip in the premolar/molar region. This does not create a larger maxilla but an overexpanded dental malocclusion with loss of upper lateral/posterior sector torque. This simply means that you should use an upper removable appliance for expansion only in cases where you can justify the loss of torque/tip in the upper arch. The author is extremely critical toward removable expansion appliances and prefers referring to well-established literature.

References

1. Abdullah R, et al. Steiner cephalometric analysis: predicted and actual treatment outcome compared. Orthod Craniofac Res. 2006;9(2):77–83.
2. Polat-Ozsoy O, Gokcelik A, Toygar Memikoglu TU. Differences in cephalometric measurements: a comparison of digital versus hand-tracing methods. Eur J Orthod. 2009;31(3):254–9.
3. Durão APR, et al. Cephalometric landmark variability among orthodontists and dentomaxillofacial radiologists: a comparative study. Imaging Sci Dent. 2015;45(4):213–20.
4. Baumrind S, Frantz RC. The reliability of head film measurements. 1. Landmark identification. Am J Orthod. 1971;60(2):111–27.
5. Chen YJ, et al. Reliability of landmark identification in cephalometric radiography acquired by a storage phosphor imaging system. Dentomaxillofac Radiol. 2004;33(5):301–6.
6. Kamoen A, Dermaut L, Verbeeck R. The clinical significance of error measurement in the interpretation of treatment results. Eur J Orthod. 2001;23(5):569–78.
7. Durão AR, et al. Validity of 2D lateral cephalometry in orthodontics: a systematic review. Prog Orthod. 2013;14(1):31.
8. McClure SR, et al. Reliability of digital versus conventional cephalometric radiology: a comparative evaluation of landmark identification error. Semin Orthod. 2005;11(2):98–110.
9. Gonçalves FA, et al. Comparison of cephalometric measurements from three radiological clinics. Braz Oral Res. 2006;20(2):162–6.
10. Proffit WR. Contemporary orthodontics. 5th ed. Elsevier/Mosby: St. Louis, MO; 2013.
11. Santoro M, Jarjoura K, Cangialosi TJ. Accuracy of digital and analogue cephalometric measurements assessed with the sandwich technique. Am J Orthod Dentofac Orthop. 2006;129(3):345–51.
12. Hurmerinta K, Rahkamo A, Haavikko K. Comparison between cephalometric classification methods for sagittal jaw relationships. Eur J Oral Sci. 1997;105(3):221–7.
13. Coben SE. The spheno-occipital synchondrosis: the missing link between the profession's concept of craniofacial growth and orthodontic treatment. Am J Orthod Dentofac Orthop. 1998;114(6):709–12. discussion 713-4
14. Sassouni V. A roentgenographic cephalometric analysis of cephalo-facio-dental relationships. Am J Orthod. 1955;41(10):735–64.
15. Gerber JW, Magill T. NFO diagnostics: a modified Sassouni Cephalometric Analysis. Funct Orthod. 2006;23(2):32–4. 36-7
16. Phillips JG. Photo-cephalometric analysis in treatment planning for surgical correction of facial disharmonies. J Maxillofac Surg. 1978;6:174–9.
17. Andrews LF. The six keys to normal occlusion. Am J Orthod. 1972;62(3):296–309.
18. Jacobson A. The "Wits" appraisal of jaw disharmony. Am J Orthod. 1975;67(2):125–38.
19. Bailey KL, Taylor RW. Mesh diagram cephalometric norms for Americans of African descent. Am J Orthod Dentofac Orthop. 1998;114(2):218–23.

20. Singh IJ, Savara BS. Norms of size and annual increments of seven anatomical measures of maxillae in girls from three to sixteen years of age. Angle Orthod. 1966;36(4):312–24.
21. Woodside DG, Linder-Aronson S. The channelization of upper and lower anterior face heights compared to population standard in males between ages 6 to 20 years. Eur J Orthod. 1979;1(1):25–40.
22. Cooke MS, Orth D, Wei SHY. The reproducibility of natural head posture: a methodological study. Am J Orthod Dentofac Orthop. 93(4):280–8.
23. Solow B, Tallgren A. Head posture and craniofacial morphology. Am J Phys Anthropol. 1976;44(3):417–35.
24. Moffitt AH. Discovery of pathologies by orthodontists on lateral cephalograms. Angle Orthod. 2011;81(1):58–63.
25. Bruks A, et al. Radiographic examinations as an aid to orthodontic diagnosis and treatment planning. Swed Dent J. 1999;23(2–3):77–85.
26. Atchison KA, Luke LS, White SC. Contribution of pretreatment radiographs to orthodontists' decision making. Oral Surg Oral Med Oral Pathol. 1991;71(2):238–45.
27. Ritschel R, Bechtold TE, Berneburg M. Effect of cephalograms on decisions for early orthodontic treatment. Angle Orthod. 2013;83(6):1059–65.
28. Nijkamp PG, et al. The influence of cephalometrics on orthodontic treatment planning. Eur J Orthod. 2008;30(6):630–5.
29. Durão AR, et al. Influence of lateral cephalometric radiography in orthodontic diagnosis and treatment planning. Angle Orthod. 2014;85(2):206–10.
30. Helal NM, Basri OA, Baeshen HA. Significance of cephalometric radiograph in orthodontic treatment plan decision. J Contemp Dent Pract. 2019;20(7):789–93.
31. Borzabadi-Farahani A. An insight into four orthodontic treatment need indices. Prog Orthod. 2011;12:132–42.
32. Shaw WC, Richmond S, O'Brien KD. The use of occlusal indices: a European perspective. Am J Orthod Dentofac Orthop. 1995;107(1):1–10.
33. Davidovitch M, et al. Skeletal and dental response to rapid maxillary expansion with 2- versus 4-band appliances1. Am J Orthod Dentofac Orthop. 2005;127(4):483–92.
34. Van de Velde A-S, et al. Short term effects of interceptive expansion treatment: a prospective study. Eur J Orthod. 2021;43(3):324–31.
35. Tanaka OM, et al. Complete maxillary crossbite correction with a rapid palatal expansion in mixed dentition followed by a corrective orthodontic treatment. Case Rep Dent. 2016;2016:8306397.
36. Lima AC, et al. Spontaneous mandibular arch response after rapid palatal expansion: a long-term study on Class I malocclusion. Am J Orthod Dentofac Orthop. 2004;126(5):576–82.
37. Geramy A, Shahroudi AS. Fixed versus removable appliance for palatal expansion; a 3D analysis using the finite element method. J Dent (Tehran, Iran). 2014;11(1):75–84.

3 Neuromuscular Theory and the Stomatognathic Triad: Treatment Objectives in Neuromuscular Orthodontics

Research has produced many publications on malocclusion. Orthodontic schools teach at their specialty classes that a good occlusion must respect the six keys of a normal occlusion as described by Dr. Andrews [1]. Any missing key of this equation equals a *malocclusion*. This description of dental occlusion in ICP (Inter-Cuspal Position), that is, a Centric Occlusion (CO), is achieved almost exclusively during deglutition and is present only for about 17.5 min in the 24 h [2].

The final goal of our orthodontic training was achieving the six keys of occlusion at the end of treatment, and we are still being taught to judge results on the analysis of occlusal intercuspation in ICP. Most publications focus on tooth contacts and premature contacts, tip, torque, anchorage, and alignment. Today's orthodontics' main goal remains a Class I dental relationship or a Class II relationship in case of upper premolar extractions. The analysis of dental occlusal relationships in ICP is still thought to be the best way to identify the major causes of relapse. Post-treatment growth and parafunctional habits may be responsible for relapse, but frequently the focus remains on unstable cuspal interdigitation [3–9]. Other authors have identified and classified several important reasons why relapse occurs, like arch dimension and tooth extraction. This has in some way divided the orthodontic community into expansionists and non-expansionists, against and for extractions. If it is true that NO focuses on correct deglutition in ICP, then we should always be sure that the treatment procedures preserve tongue space. The etiology of malocclusion should be updated as generations pass. It seems that environmental factors change continuously over time and have a greater importance than what previously thought (diet, allergies, pharmacology, etc.) [10–12]. Therefore, maxillary insufficiency has increased, and this questions extraction therapy orthodontics while supporting expansion orthodontics. Correct breathing and head posture contribute to malocclusion and morphological changes in the individual to the point where interceptive treatments become mandatory.

The neuromuscular paradigm includes muscles that have been somewhat disregarded from the occlusal equation. Muscles have been seen mainly as the engine of the system and as *adaptive to occlusal needs*. Interestingly, it can be noted that the

F. Savastano, *Neuromuscular Orthodontics*,
https://doi.org/10.1007/978-3-031-41295-0_3

literature terminology, when referring to occlusion, has changed in the past 20 years or so. Journal articles now specify "static occlusion" to wisely avoid any link with a "balanced function". In some way, there is scientific recognition that a good static occlusion might not guarantee a good function of the stomatognathic system. Furthermore, the importance of muscle function has gained momentum, and this is proved by several surface EMG systems that have hit the market.

As straight wire technique and NiTi wires came to the profession, bracket prescription seemed to focus on "locking up" the lower arch, with reduced torque for the upper anterior incisors and canines. The idea was rather oriented that relapse could also be caused by the lack of upper arch "occlusal control" over the lower arch. The author also observed that some cases that were well finished respecting cephalometric and occlusal key requests were presenting TMJ clicking during or at the end of treatment; mainly Class II cases in which the choice to distalize the upper arch was imperative according to orthodontic school teachings and conventional orthodontic logic. The "diagnostic criteria" was put to doubt by observing treated patients with perfect Class I dental Occlusion accompanied by TMJ clicking or TMD. Just recall that at the beginning of the 1990s there was no access to the Internet as we know it today and essentially the practitioner had to rely on publications and phone calls to seek confrontation on clinical cases. Several subscriptions to scientific orthodontic journals were necessary to keep the practitioner updated. There were many scientific journal articles stating that occlusion had little or nothing to do with TMD [13–19]. The orthodontic community was on the defense for malpractice issues. That was great news for us orthodontists but bad news for our patients. Several orthodontists, including me, were feeling in a way responsible for some TMJ pain or signs/symptoms of TMD after orthodontic therapy for our patients even if canonic treatment procedures were conducted without hesitation. Besides all, it was an uncommon procedure to listen to children or adults TMJ during orthodontic diagnosis and follow-up. Anyways, there were also some timid approaches trying to link occlusal problems and TMD by some brave professionals [20–26]. It was only in 1997 that Dr. Barry Cooper started a less timid approach to occlusal problems and dysfunction of the TMJ [27].

So, what is relapse in orthodontics? Relapse is a major muscle issue. Muscles do not accept the position teeth are trying to keep the mandible at during swallow and attempting ICP. Simple as that. When there is relapse after treatment has terminated, it is because respect for muscle needs is missing. Transforming a Class II occlusion to a Class I that after 6 months of retention just swings back to a Class II, is obviously a treatment that missed something in diagnostics. Muscular functional requests have been disregarded. This has been questioned quite some time ago [28], incorrect muscle function is the main reason for relapse [29].

To better understand the Neuromuscular Theory, we should consider the Stomatognathic Triad: Muscles-TMJ-Teeth (Fig. 3.1).

This concept based on the representation of the stomatognathic triad is not new in Neuromuscular Dentistry (ND). Teeth have always been considered as dominant while TMJ and Muscles adapt to occlusion. This was and will remain true because this theory was developed for and from prosthetics. Full mouth rehabilitation or

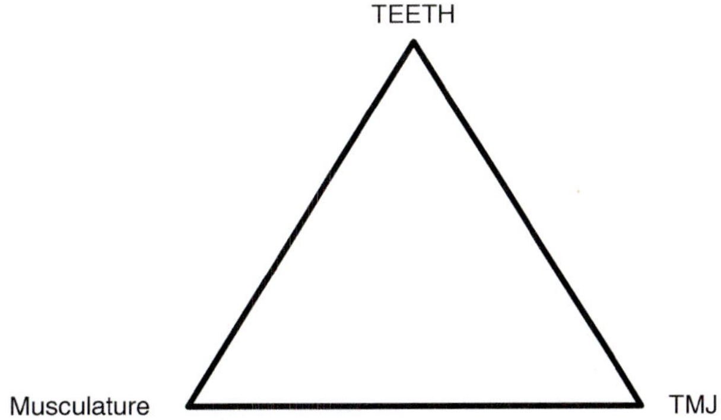

Fig. 3.1 The stomatognathic triangle in Neuromuscular theory

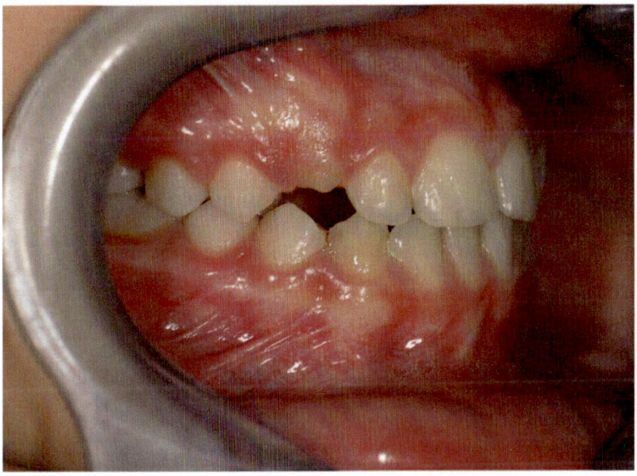

Fig. 3.2 Class III occlusion in skeletal Class III. Mandibular growth and posture requests from musculature must be compensated by lower incisors that are tipped lingually

multiple implants effectively create a very "unmovable" or "unadaptable" dental occlusion. *There is no choice for muscles and TMJ but to adapt as passive elements*. Even though some doubts can arise about this concept (bridge cracking, implant failure…etc... etc.), accepting the idea of accommodation to malocclusion within the structural tolerance of the individual sounds quite acceptable (muscles that adapt to occlusal needs). With Neuromuscular Orthodontics, the idea that muscles are passive adaptive elements simply does not stand. The practitioner can move teeth thus *changing the anatomical relationships within the* TMJ but will *never be able to modify muscle insertion and function* (except for surgery). Intervention can be directed *only* to teeth with mandibular (and TMJ) re-positioning as a starting point. The only possibility to create harmony in the Stomatognathic Triad is therefore obeying to muscle needs. Teeth are passive elements that will articulate and thus compensate muscular needs, and this is seen on an everyday basis (for example, Figs. 3.2 and 3.3). Agreeing that the position of the teeth changes due to functional requests, equals admitting that reverting the process (alignment) without repositioning the mandible and improving freeway space leads to a reaction, (muscular) relapse. When teeth are not properly aligned for a muscular functional occlusion,

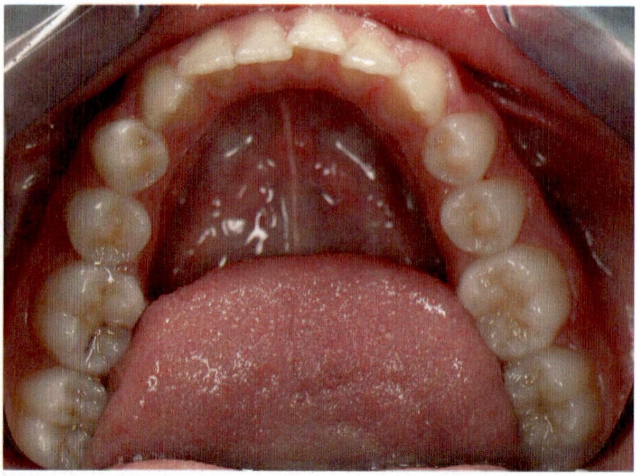

Fig. 3.3 Detail of lower incisor compensation. Click upon aperture is a clear sign of TMJ compensation (not shown)

musculature, and consequently TMJ are ready to accommodate this deficiency in their range of tolerance. Posterior Condylar displacement is one of the many compensations within the TMJ when the sagittal relationships between the upper maxilla and the mandible are unsustainable by the lower arch dental compensation. In this case, the practitioner can usually detect a TMJ click upon the aperture.

TMJ-Masticatory Musculature-Teeth: This triad represents a unique functional entity that is not independent from the anatomical surroundings but rather blends with other body functions to become in some way inseparable. Afferent inputs from stimuli of the periodontium ligaments arrive to the Central Nervous System (CNS), and after being processed from the cortex determine the fine coordination and activity of the masticatory musculature.

The pterygoideus, the masseter, the zygomaticomandibularis, and the temporalis all connect directly to the articular disk (Figs. 3.4 and 3.5) [30–33]. These anatomical features may not necessarily play an active role in disk alignment but could participate as control systems for condylar/disk coordination. These muscles are also postural muscles of the mandible, and their modulation is sustained via a signals that originate as afferential inputs from the TMJ, muscles, tendons, and fascia to the CNS [34]. The CNS balances, via efferential signals, specific muscles to perform intra-oral physiological tasks. Some, as swallowing, will include conscious and predetermined automatic actions from the CNS. Other tasks such as chewing, speaking, and biting, are well-controlled conscious actions that do not require automatisms but rely on muscle memory [35, 36]. This system is a complicated symphony in which every musical instrument plays a specific and very delicate role.

Centric Occlusion (dental) represents an exact and repeatable mandibular (bone) position. This position reflects a specific condyle/fossa relationship as well. Centric Occlusion represents the maximum intercuspation of the teeth at the lowest VD. This ICP is necessary and usually present during a good deglutition. All the muscles that are involved in the swallowing process will adapt in any possible way if

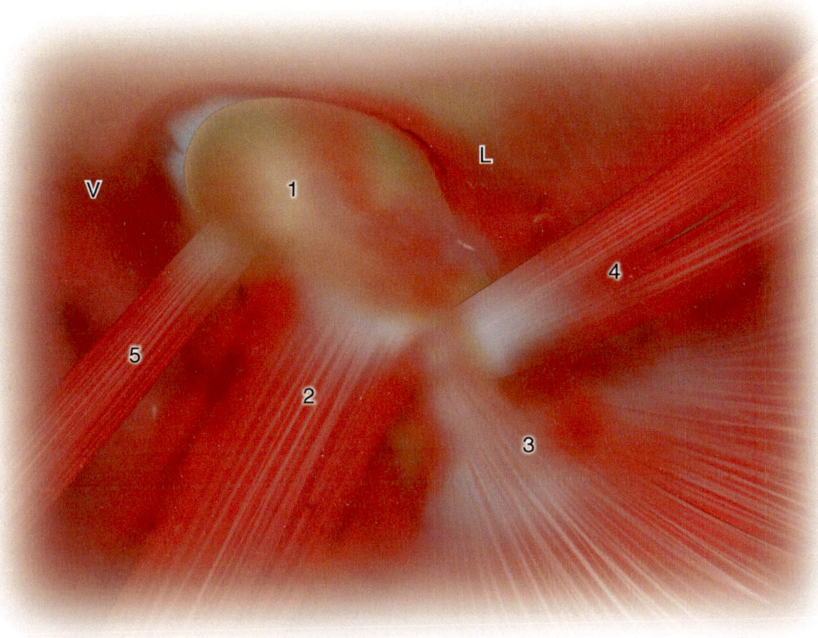

Fig. 3.4 Upper superior access of temporomandibular joint: 1: articular disk, 2: masseter muscle, 3: temporalis muscle, 4: lateral pterygoid muscle, 5: zygomaticomandibularis, V: ventral, L: lingual

Fig. 3.5 Prediscal lamina, 1 on which muscles are inserted, 2: masseter muscle, 3: temporalis muscle, 4:lateral pterygoid, 5: articular disk

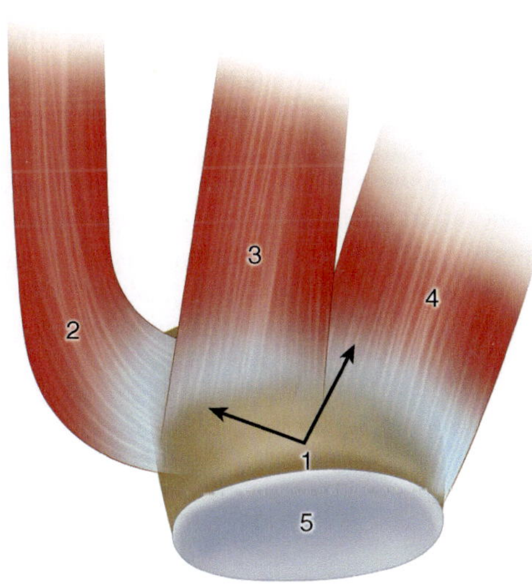

malocclusion is present, since this function is necessary for survival. A major role is played by the tongue, which will modify posture and swallow behavior according to any malocclusion present. Tongue function plays a major role in adapting to occlusal deficiencies. Secondary tongue thrust is easily seen in Class II occlusions with large overjets or open bites. These are adaptive neuromuscular patterns that usually disappear when occlusal corrections are made.

Orthodontics has focused too much on one vertex of the Triangle: Teeth. There are very few lectures at dental school on muscles of mastication and their role in occlusion/relapse. Its time orthodontics includes muscle physiology and TMJ function in its diagnostic procedures.

The Neuromuscular Paradigm represents revenge for the functional orthodontist. This holistic view centers the dental practitioner, with the Stomatognathic Triad, within in the human body and not away from it. The multidisciplinary dental/orthodontic treatment that derives from this concept includes other medical specialists to rebalance compensation of postural strains and to rehabilitate muscle functions that have derived as a reaction to malocclusion (so-called descending pathologies). In other cases, other medical specialties identify primary dysfunctions that act and create/sustain malocclusion and TMJ pathology (so-called ascending pathologies). In real life, most identifiable etiologic factors usually will classify complex malocclusion/posture pathologies as mixed between ascending and descending causes. The diagnostics are therefore related to the sensibility and ability of the practitioner and to computerized postural analysis. Luckily, children and adolescents do not usually have important postural problems and misdiagnose is frequent.

The information obtained from the musculature is extensive. Surface EMG can interpret quantitively and qualitatively muscle adaptation to occlusion; this is called in ND, *accommodation* [36]. With functional appliances (i.e., Frankel appliance) the idea is to act directly on the musculature (changing the mandibular position) to reduce accommodation: the disocclusion is the first step for a new muscular function. The goal is, therefore, establishing with treatment, a Neuromuscular Mandibular Position (NMP), a position in which muscle accommodation is *minimum*. Functional appliances such as the Frankel 2, will guide the growing patient to an optimal relationship of the dental arches. The orthodontist therefore will guide occlusion to obtain minimal accommodation from the neuromuscular system. The construction of the Frankel appliance is based on a bite recording of the PRP and not as described in orthodontic literature with a mandibular advancement bite recording with wax. When properly constructed and applied on a full-day basis, the occlusal and profile changes are impressive.

From a Neuromuscular point of view, whenever there is no muscle balance, no correct tongue posture or tongue function, there is a malocclusion regardless of the position and alignment of teeth [37]. Each of us has some level of accommodation, and each of us is somewhat maloccluded. The ideal neuromuscular occlusion is that of an occlusion without any level of muscular accommodation and an ideal swallow sequence. Therefore, this concept does include the idea of a “static occlusion” but defines occlusion as a result of balanced physiological dynamics: the neuromuscular occlusion. By understanding the importance of muscle and TMJ function, posture and related factors, and by including these analyses in our orthodontic diagnostics, we elevate the orthodontic specialty to a much higher level within the medical profession. Treatments that include the preservation of TMJ function, the correction of swallow disorders, the correction of cranio-cervical posture, the correction of breathing issues, and so on, should therefore be integrated into orthodontic treatment planning.

As said, we are all maloccluded to some extent, we all have some degree of accommodation.

Neuromuscular orthodontics has several therapy objectives.

Treatment objectives for Neuromuscular Orthodontics regarding the stomatognathic system:

1. Reduce muscle accommodation
2. Re-establish a correct swallow pattern
3. Preserve TMJ function
4. Class I dental occlusion (when and if possible)

The reduction of accommodation is obtained by targeting treatment toward the Myotrajectory and the Myocentric. Once this is obtained at best, there will be an improvement of the tongue environment thus re-establishing a correct swallow pattern if previously compromised. Trying to establish a correct swallow pattern when the environment is not ideal for the tongue, is a waste of time (Form-Function). Most tongue dysfunctions are secondary to alterations of the maxilla and loss of their functional space. Since maxillary deficiency is the main cause of orthodontic malocclusions, improving tongue space and correcting overjet are two main goals for treatment. The everlasting dilemma Form-Function is an Ouroborus under many aspects. A skeletal and dental open bite will always have a tongue dysfunction with anterior thrust. Can this skeletal alteration after a certain period of time preclude any possibility of swallow correction? Can a primary tongue dysfunction (uncorrectable) be a consequence of a chronic secondary cause? Can a severe malocclusion compromise, for some sort of peripheral adaptation, central activation circuits of a normal swallow? Probably we will never know the answers to these questions. There are though some considerations to do: **first**, the recovery of function, if ever possible, lies in the early stages of life, and is reduced as time passes. The later we correct severe malocclusions, the less opportunity we have for a permanent correction in all its functional and morphological aspects. The correction of malocclusion is essentially a correction of form. After this first correction, functional improvements occur spontaneously. The holistic and more modern idea that there is always autonomous and spontaneous healing occurring is true if the body is given an opportunity. Sometimes it is necessary to work on some sort of re-education to cancel parafunctional habits, but overall function follows form correction and correct function supports form [38]. **Second**, if we recognize swallow behavior as probably the most important of oral functions, we are confirming that the neuromuscular theory should be the pillar of orthodontic diagnosis and treatment. This is explained by clinical and bioelectric findings, in which TMD patients undergoing orthotic treatment improve deglutition dramatically. Swallow remains the key factor in the determination of occlusal harmony. There is a higher incidence of Dysphagia and tongue habits in TMD patients with respect to the general population [39, 40]. If TMD can be considered a clear indicator of stomatognathic dysfunction, swallow alterations and disorders, in general, must be key to stomatognathic function homeostasis. So, reducing muscle accommodation (point 1) and re-establishing a correct swallow pattern (point 2) preserves TMJ function (point 3). The anatomy of the TMJ, as previously discussed, is coupled to muscles of mastication and mandibular posture that are also attached to the articular disk. The coordination of the disk and the condyle must in some way be linked to the muscles attached to it. Finally, point 4 includes Class I dental occlusion only when permitted by muscle requirements. If there is a skeletal discrepancy that does not allow the combination of muscle needs together with a Class I dental occlusion, any other dental occlusion can fulfill the first three therapy objectives.

The reduction of accommodation should result in a new mandibular Rest Position. From this physiologic rest position, the TENS spike permits the computer (in anyways the practitioner) to prolong/draw the neuromuscular trajectory. It is on this muscular pathway that the Myocentric is determined by the practitioner (Fig. 3.6).

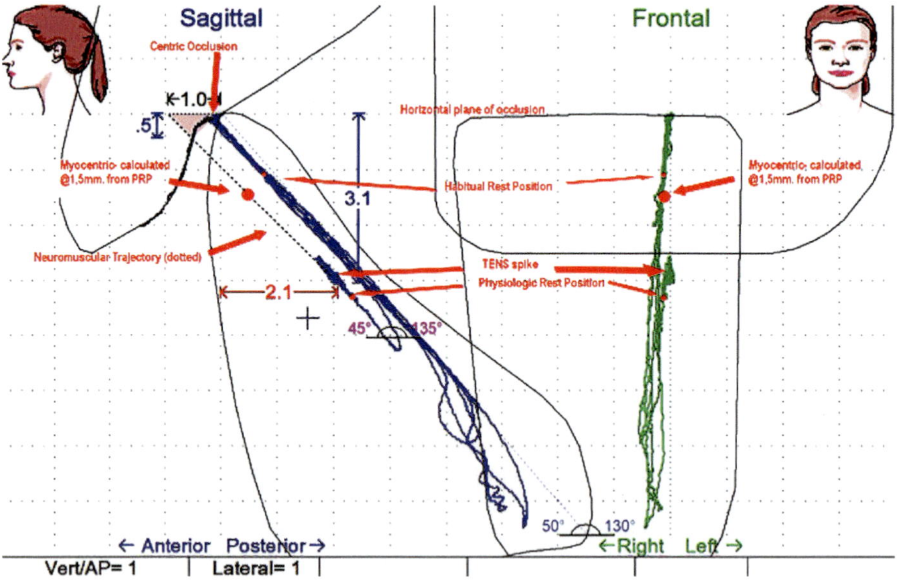

Fig. 3.6 Scan 5 tracing. From the Physiologic Rest Position (PRP) note the TENS spike (length about 1 mm). From the spike is drawn by computer the dotted line that represents the Neuromuscular Trajectory. The Myocentric is calculated on the neuromuscular trajectory at circa 1.5–2.0 mm vertically from PRP. The habitual path of closure passes over the Habitual Rest Position (HRP)

The Myocentric (the ideal Neuromuscular Centric) is always calculated on the Myotrajectory. While this is easier to accomplish when fabricating an orthotic or full mouth rehabilitation on adults, with orthodontic treatment it is much more difficult to achieve. Orthodontic treatment is usually carried out on growing patients, and in general tooth movement is quite slow when compared to prosthetic treatment. Treatment may even include orthopedic appliances. The Myocentric is not a stable and constant point during growth and during life. During growth, the changes due to craniofacial development, that include not only bone but soft tissues and fascia, result in a continuous changes in the position of the calculated and ideal Myocentric. Body growth too with the inuous adjustments in cranio-cervical posture influences changes of the Myocentric position. Probably, it could be that the path drawn by multiple point recordings of the Myocentric over time resemble the direction of mandibular growth in young individuals. In the adult, tooth wear, parafunctions, and loss of teeth can obviously modify this *ideal centric with respect to CO*. The malocclusions that arise after tooth loss, for example, are not predictable. Each one of us reacts differently to specific stimuli. For these reasons, the Myocentric cannot always be considered as a mandatory treatment objective in Neuromuscular Orthodontics. The Myocentric in the growing patient is a good indication of where the muscles are developing the occlusion and clearly indicates the ***direction*** of where treatment should be oriented.

Orthodontic treatment should be considered terminated when growth is finished. One cause of orthodontic relapse is unexpected and expected mandibular growth after treatment. The advantage of NO, is the possibility, with the *specific bioelectrical investigation*, to actually *visualize quantitively mandibular positional discrepancy relative to ICP*. This advantage is used by the practitioner to foresee *at least* the risk of mandibular entrapment, thus condylar distalization. From this point of view, *TMD preservation*, during adult treatment is easier to accomplish because growth is terminated. Follow-up is needed for orthodontic patients up to age 21 years if male and 15 years if female. There are no shortcuts for orthodontic treatments in growing patients. The final occlusion is final only when all growth of the supporting structures has terminated.

There are some practical limitations to succeeding in creating a perfect occlusion on the Myocentric. This happens when craniofacial morphology, i.e., skeletal discrepancy poses a limit to the neuromuscular intervention and guides the operator to the closest tolerable occlusion. In other circumstances, skeletal discrepancy is too severe for a neuromuscular (acceptable) mandibular position, so neuromuscular dentistry and thus the Myocentric with bite registration are utilized for surgical setup procedures. The ideal path of closure is the Myotrajectory. In many cases of orthodontic therapy, it is difficult to reduce freeway space adequately and for this reason the Myotrajectory remains the most important orthodontic objective for mandibular repositioning because the *Myocentric is always calculated on the Myotrajectory*. As an example in severe skeletal deepbite, an habitual path of closure that is close or overlaps the Myotrajectory at the end of treatment with an excess in freeway space, remains the most functional option available for treatment. Simply said, there is no orthodontic way to treat skeletal deep-bite or open-bite by transforming them into average skeletal morphology with an ideal freeway space.

Treatment objectives regarding the other systems:

1. Improve cranio-cervical posture.
2. Improve breathing/reduce sleep-disordered breathing (SDB).
3. Improve vision.

Improving cranio-cervical posture can be achieved by two actions:

1. Correction of mandibular rest position by improving, positioning on/close to the Myocentric. Cranio-cervical posture is linked to facial morphology [41–47], and in general facial morphology is linked to freeway space (decrease/increase in freeway space is generally associated with severeness of skeletal open-bite and deep bite). Orthodontic objectives of Neuromuscular treatment include normalization of freeway space and mandibular repositioning on the Myotrajectory, for this reason, improvement of the cranio-cervical posture is a consequence of the correct application of neuromuscular orthodontic treatment procedures. When there is no freeway space and head extension is present such as in chronic mouth breathers who have developed a skeletal/dental open bite, recreating freeway space (and of course treating the respiratory problems) immediately improves cranio-cervical postural compensation [41, 48]. In the coming chapters, Class II occlusion with overjet will be discussed. Most of these malocclusions are represented by a normal mandibular size and a posterior mandibular displacement. Functional orthodontic therapy, which includes mandibular advancement for these malocclusions, generally improves all aspects of cervical spine posture by reducing forward head posture and improving cervical straightening [49]. Several other studies do give mixed results when seeking cervical spine curvature changes in relation to different treatment modalities, but these studies do not include patient selection in relation to morphology or vertical development but focus on the angle class relationship of the first molars. As previously said, selection criteria of these studies remain unacceptable.
2. Physical therapy [50–52]. Osteopathic treatments are important in any rehabilitation regarding the spine and are equally important in patients with TMD [53–55]. Although not all authors agree that there is an association between TMD and cervical spine postural alterations [56–58], general agreement subsists for physical therapy as a positive aid to treatment. From a morphological point of view, skeletal open-bite patients benefit the most from these treatments, since pain is more frequently associated with this facial typology [59].

Improvement of breathing in general and the reduction of any sleep disorder breathing is a major issue in neuromuscular orthodontic diagnosis and treatment. Orthodontic treatment should not be initiated without a complete ENT assessment. Furthermore, the author has implemented a home sleep analysis with PAT (Peripheral Arterial Tone-Tonometry) technology for ***the majority*** of orthodontic patient diagnosis. This is a noninvasive methodology and very simple home testing for sleep-related breathing problems [60]. Although validated for ages 12 years and up, it can be used to *screen* patients younger than 12 years. This is a great opportunity for intercepting serious disordered breathing in children. When PAT technology devices report high AHI values in children, it is necessary to refer these young patients to pulmonary or sleep specialists for hospital polysomnography, which remains the gold standard for impaired breathing pathologies. This technology is also useful to monitor follow-up after adenoidectomy and tonsillectomy surgery. PAT technology is an excellent screening method in young children to monitor breathing improvement after RPE or other orthodontic treatments.

Functional appliances that advance the mandible always improve breathing. If this is or not a permanent result depends on several factors. First, functional appliances that advance the mandible are used to treat positional Class II [1] [61–66]. The increase seen, in practically all treated patients, regarding air lumen on the lateral cephalograms and other evaluation methods must mean an improvement of some sort [67–70]. RPE should be done prior to functional mandibular advancement, and this procedure is known to improve breathing in OSAS too [71–75]. The sure advantage of functional non-extraction therapy on improving breathing alone seems to be proof that this treatment modality is respecting physiologic needs while others who reduce overjet with extraction or distalization of the upper sectors are not. Secondly, functional appliances are generally constructed to increase posterior vertical dimension, that is, reduce posterior inter-occlusal space. The increase in vertical opening *during* mandibular advancement is gaining momentum as the most effective way to reduce OSAS with removable appliances [76, 77]. A reduction of sagittal advancement for the non-orthodontic MAD (Maxillary Advancement Device) treatment of OSAS is a positive move since this therapy is probably not free of collateral TMJ damage.

Improvement of vision is another result of neuromuscular balance of the stomatognathic system. The practitioner should identify or suspect any vision alteration that could affect cranio-cervical posture [78, 79]. Adding multiple factors that participate in the overall postural complexity of the individual, complicates the identification of the primary triggering causal pathology. It is a complex procedure to identify a *primum movens* for severe alterations of body posture accompanied by symptomology. This is because all physiological systems tend to compensate for any fault, in the sense that the compensation is a response of the biological system (the body) to heal spontaneously. For this reason, it is advisable to cooperate with other specialists to complete a thorough diagnosis with a neuromuscular taste.

[1] Skeletal Class II definition, in general, orthodontics refers to a discrepancy in the relationship of the skeletal bases and does little to consider the total development of the maxilla and mandible. For this reason, in N.O. positional Class II represents the majority of Class II with OJ and Class II/2, while a very small amount of Class II skeletal are considered so because of a small mandible in relation to age, sex, and cranial base. The sagittal position of the maxilla in positional Class II is usually normal.

References

1. Andrews LF. The six keys to normal occlusion. Am J Orthod. 1972;62(3):296–309.
2. Graf H. Bruxism. Dent Clin N Am. 1969;13(3):659–65.
3. Pancherz H. The nature of class II relapse after herbst appliance treatment: a cephalometric long-term investigation. Am J Orthod Dentofac Orthop. 1991;100(3):220–33.
4. Lewis B. Orthodontic retention. Dent Nurs. 2008;4(9):496–503.
5. Thilander B. Biological basis for orthodontic relapse. Semin Orthod. 2000;6(3):195–205.
6. Moro A, et al. Stability of class II corrections with removable and fixed functional appliances: a literature review. J World Fed Orthod. 2020;9(2):56–67.
7. Strang RHW. The fallacy of denture expansion as a treatment procedure*. Angle Orthod. 1949;19(1):12–22.
8. Lundström AF. Malocclusion of the teeth regarded as a problem in connection with the apical base. Int J Orthod Oral Surg Radiogr. 1925;11(10):933–41.
9. Breckon J. The 20 principles of the Alexander discipline (2008). Eur J Orthod. 2009;31(2):213.
10. Moimaz SAS, et al. Longitudinal study of habits leading to malocclusion development in childhood. BMC Oral Health. 2014;14(1):96.
11. Mew JRC. The postural basis of malocclusion: a philosophical overview. Am J Orthod Dentofac Orthop. 2004;126(6):729–38.
12. Meyers A, Hertzberg J. Bottle-feeding and malocclusion: is there an association? Am J Orthod Dentofac Orthop. 1988;93(2):149–52.
13. Lipp MJ. Temporomandibular symptoms and occlusion: a review of the literature & the concept. N Y State Dent J. 1990;56(9):58–66.
14. Bales JM, Epstein JB. The role of malocclusion and orthodontics in temporomandibular disorders. J Can Dent Assoc. 1994;60(10):899–905.
15. Seligman DA, Pullinger AG. The role of functional occlusal relationships in temporomandibular disorders: a review. J Craniomandib Disord. 1991;5(4):265–79.
16. Greene CS. Etiology of temporomandibular disorders. Semin Orthod. 1995;1(4):222–8.
17. McNamara JA Jr, Seligman DA, Okeson JP. Occlusion, Orthodontic treatment, and temporomandibular disorders: a review. J Orofac Pain. 1995;9(1):73–90.
18. Conti PC, et al. A cross-sectional study of prevalence and etiology of signs and symptoms of temporomandibular disorders in high school and university students. J Orofac Pain. 1996;10(3):254–62.
19. Rodrigues-Garcia RC, et al. Effects of major Class II occlusal corrections on temporomandibular signs and symptoms. J Orofac Pain. 1998;12(3):185–92.
20. Kerstein RB. Treatment of myofascial pain dysfunction syndrome with occlusal therapy to reduce lengthy disclusion time—a recall evaluation. Cranio. 1995;13(2):105–15.
21. Raustia AM, Pirttiniemi PM, Pyhtinen J. Correlation of occlusal factors and condyle position asymmetry with signs and symptoms of temporomandibular disorders in young adults. Cranio. 1995;13(3):152–6.
22. Willis WA. The effectiveness of an extreme canine-protected splint with limited lateral movement in treatment of temporomandibular dysfunction. Am J Orthod Dentofac Orthop. 1995;107(3):229–34.
23. Hobo S. Occlusion in temporomandibular disorders: treatment after occlusal splint therapy. Int Dent J. 1996;46(3):146–55.
24. Sonnesen L, Bakke M, Solow B. Malocclusion traits and symptoms and signs of temporomandibular disorders in children with severe malocclusion. Eur J Orthod. 1998;20(5):543–59.
25. Fushima K, Inui M, Sato S. Dental asymmetry in temporomandibular disorders. J Oral Rehabil. 1999;26(9):752–6.
26. Liu ZJ, et al. Electromyographic examination of jaw muscles in relation to symptoms and occlusion of patients with temporomandibular joint disorders. J Oral Rehabil. 1999;26(1):33–47.

27. Cooper BC. The role of bioelectronic instrumentation in the documentation and management of temporomandibular disorders. Oral Surg Oral Med Oral Pathol Oral Radiol Endod. 1997;83(1):91–100.
28. King EW. Relapse of orthodontic treatment. Angle Orthod. 1974;44(4):300–15.
29. Picchioni P, Soli P, Pirini D. Treatment of orofacial musculature imbalance. Mondo Ortod. 1990;15(1):71–90.
30. Gaudy JF, et al. Functional anatomy of the human temporal muscle. Surg Radiol Anat. 2001;23(6):389–98.
31. Kageyama M, Itoh I. Orientation of the deep part of the human temporal muscle and morphological study of the infratemporal crest. Jpn J Oral Biol. 2003;45(6):397–406.
32. Bravetti P, et al. Histological study of the human temporo-mandibular joint and its surrounding muscles. Surg Radiol Anat. 2004;26(5):371–8.
33. Matsunaga K, et al. An anatomical study of the muscles that attach to the articular disc of the temporomandibular joint. Clin Anat. 2009;22(8):932–40.
34. Schmolke C. The relationship between the temporomandibular joint capsule, articular disc and jaw muscles. J Anat. 1994;184(Pt 2):335–45.
35. Lerman MD. The muscle engram: the reflex that limits conventional occlusal treatment. Cranio. 2011;29(4):297–303.
36. Lerman MD. A revised view of the dynamics, physiology, and treatment of occlusion: a new paradigm. Cranio. 2004;22(1):50–63.
37. Foletti J-M, et al. Is atypical swallowing associated with relapse in orthognathic patients? A retrospective study of 256 patients. J Oral Maxillofac Surg. 2018;76(5):1084–90.
38. Brand RA. Biographical sketch: Julius Wolff, 1836-1902. Clin Orthop Relat Res. 2010;468(4):1047–9.
39. Gilheaney O, Stassen LF, Walshe M. Prevalence, nature, and management of oral stage dysphagia in adults with temporomandibular joint disorders: findings from an Irish cohort. J Oral Maxillofac Surg. 2018;76(8):1665–76.
40. Maffei C, et al. Videofluoroscopic evaluation of mastication and swallowing in individuals with TMD. Braz J Otorhinolaryngol. 2012;78(4):24–8.
41. Solow B, Siersbæk-Nielsen S, Greve E. Airway adequacy, head posture, and craniofacial morphology. Am J Orthod. 1984;86(3):214–23.
42. Solow B, Tallgren A. Head position and craniofacial morphology. Mondo Ortod. 1977;19(6).75–99.
43. Solow B, Tallgren A. Head posture and craniofacial morphology. Am J Phys Anthropol. 1976;44(3):417–35.
44. Sandikçioğlu M, Skov S, Solow B. Atlas morphology in relation to craniofacial morphology and head posture. Eur J Orthod. 1994;16(2):96–103.
45. Leitao P, Nanda RS. Relationship of natural head position to craniofacial morphology. Am J Orthod Dentofac Orthop. 2000;117(4):406–17.
46. Kim P, Sarauw M, Sonnesen L. Cervical vertebral column morphology and head posture in preorthodontic patients with anterior open bite. Am J Orthod Dentofac Orthop. 2014;145:359–66.
47. Hellsing E, et al. The relationship between craniofacial morphology, head posture and spinal curvature in 8, 11 and 15-year-old children. Eur J Orthod. 1987;9(1):254–64.
48. Vig PS, Showfety KJ, Phillips C. Experimental manipulation of head posture. Am J Orthod. 1980;77(3):258–68.
49. Ohnmeiß M, et al. Therapeutic effects of functional orthodontic appliances on cervical spine posture: a retrospective cephalometric study. Head Face Med. 2014;10:7.
50. Falla D, et al. Effect of neck exercise on sitting posture in patients with chronic neck pain. Phys Ther. 2007;87(4):408–17.
51. Kielnar R, et al. The influence of cervical spine rehabilitation on bioelectrical activity (sEMG) of cervical and masticatory system muscles. PLoS One. 2021;16(4):e0250746.
52. Dennis AK, et al. Alleviation of neck pain by the non-surgical rehabilitation of a pathologic cervical kyphosis to a normal lordosis: a CBP(®) case report. J Phys Ther Sci. 2018;30(4):654–7.

53. Flores HF, Ottone NE, Fuentes R. Analysis of the morphometric characteristics of the cervical spine and its association with the development of temporomandibular disorders. Cranio. 2017;35(2):79–85.
54. Silva RMVD, et al. The influence of temporomandibular disorders in neck pain and posture. Man Ther Posturology Rehabil J. 2016;14
55. Wolford LM, Cardenas L. Idiopathic condylar resorption: diagnosis, treatment protocol, and outcomes. Am J Orthod Dentofac Orthop. 1999;116(6):667–77.
56. Iunes D, et al. Craniocervical posture analysis in patients with temporomandibular disorder. Braz J Phys Ther. 2009;13:89–95.
57. Matheus RA, et al. The relationship between temporomandibular dysfunction and head and cervical posture. J Appl Oral Sci. 2009;17(3):204–8.
58. Olivo SA, et al. The association between head and cervical posture and temporomandibular disorders: a systematic review. J Orofac Pain. 2006;20:1.
59. Tanimoto K, et al. Characteristics of the maxillofacial morphology in patients with idiopathic mandibular condylar resorption. J Clin Med. 2022;11:4.
60. Schnall RP, Sheffy JK, Penzel T. Peripheral arterial tonometry–PAT technology. Sleep Med Rev. 2022;61:101566.
61. Xiang M, et al. Changes in airway dimensions following functional appliances in growing patients with skeletal class II malocclusion: a systematic review and meta-analysis. Int J Pediatr Otorhinolaryngol. 2017;97:170–80.
62. Ali B, Shaikh A, Fida M. Changes in oro-pharyngeal airway dimensions after treatment with functional appliance in class ii skeletal pattern. J Ayub Med Coll Abbottabad. 2015;27(4):759–63.
63. Hourfar J, et al. Effects of two different removable functional appliances on depth of the posterior airway space. J Orofac Orthop. 2017;78(2):166–75.
64. Han S, et al. Long-term pharyngeal airway changes after bionator treatment in adolescents with skeletal Class II malocclusions. Korean J Orthod. 2014;44(1):13–9.
65. Ganesh G, Tripathi T. Effect of fixed functional appliances on pharyngeal airway dimensions in skeletal class II individuals—a scoping review. J Oral Biol Craniofac Res. 2021;11(4):511–23.
66. Pavoni C, et al. Orthopaedic treatment effects of functional therapy on the sagittal pharyngeal dimensions in subjects with sleep-disordered breathing and Class II malocclusion. Acta Otorhinolaryngol Ital. 2017;37(6):479–85.
67. Mirhashemi A, Bahrami R. Long-term stability of growth modification treatment in children with obstructive sleep Apnea; a systematic review. Iran J Orthod. 2021;16(1):1–7.
68. Giuca MR, et al. Pediatric obstructive sleep Apnea syndrome: emerging evidence and treatment approach. ScientificWorldJournal. 2021;2021:5591251.
69. Kannan A, Sathyanarayana HP, Padmanabhan S. Effect of functional appliances on the airway dimensions in patients with skeletal class II malocclusion: a systematic review. J Orthod Sci. 2017;6(2):54–64.
70. Bariani RCB, et al. Effectiveness of functional orthodontic appliances in obstructive sleep apnea treatment in children: literature review. Braz J Otorhinolaryngol. 2022;88:263–78.
71. Castillo JL. Maxillary expansion may increase airway dimensions and improve breathing. J Evid Based Dent Pract. 2012;12(1):14–7.
72. Taki AA and Thabit A. *Changes in pharyngeal airway dimensions, hyoid position, and head posture after rapid palatal expansion and face mask therapy*. 2014. Journal of American Science 2014;10(10). http://www.jofamericanscience.org.
73. Ahn H-W, Kim S-J. Surgical maxillary expansion for OSA adults with nasal obstruction. In: Kim S-J, Kim KB, editors. Orthodontics in obstructive sleep Apnea patients: a guide to diagnosis, treatment planning, and interventions. Cham: Springer International Publishing; 2020. p. 65–79.
74. Quinzi V, et al. Efficacy of rapid maxillary expansion with or without previous adenotonsillectomy for Pediatric obstructive sleep Apnea syndrome based on polysomnographic data: a systematic review and meta-analysis. Appl Sci. 2020;10(18):6485.

75. Remy F, et al. Management of the pediatric OSAS: what about simultaneously expand the maxilla and advance the mandible? A retrospective non-randomized controlled cohort study. Sleep Med. 2022;90:135–41.
76. DDS, D.E.R. *A more effective Bite Registration technique for Dental Sleep Appliances; the inclusion of increased vertical dimension (3D) over the traditional 2D techniques.* Pantera Dental Clinical Study Series, 2016.
77. Hu JC, Comisi JC. Vertical dimension in dental sleep medicine oral appliance therapy. Gen Dent. 2020;68(4):69–76.
78. Boricean ID, Bărar A. Understanding ocular torticollis in children. Oftalmologia. 2011;55(1):10–26.
79. Silvestrini-Biavati A, et al. Clinical association between teeth malocclusions, wrong posture and ocular convergence disorders: an epidemiological investigation on primary school children. BMC Pediatr. 2013;13(1):1–8.

Updates on Functional Anatomy

4

The inexhaustible nature of anatomical revelations pertaining to the cranium and cervical region continues to astound us. Recently, novel muscular structures have been discerned within the temporomandibular joint and its encompassing surroundings. In light of this, a contemporary elucidation of the intricacies of our bodily mechanics during movement is imperative. To fully apprehend the nuances of these anatomical and functional characteristics, a succinct explication is indispensable.

Temporo-Mandibular Joint

The Tempo-Mandibular Joint (TMJ) is a very peculiar joint (Fig. 4.1). Its two bony components, the mandibular fossa-articular tubercle and the mandibular head are separated by the articular disk. The articular disk is connected posteriorly via the posterior ligament to the bilaminar zone and the posterior part of the glenoid fossa. This disk splits the joint in two, creating two distinct sliding surfaces in the joint, the first (upper) with the glenoid fossa (translation) and the second with the mandibular condyle (lower, rotation). The articular surfaces of the bone are covered by fibrocartilage and not hyaline cartilage as in other joints of the body. Anteriorly the disk is connected to the superior part of the external pterygoid, while the inferior component of this muscle connects directly to the condylar head. The articular disk is thin in the center and thicker along the external border. This anatomy favors the sliding and rotational movements that occur when the condyle changes position during mouth opening. During these movements, the condylar head remains in contact with the center of the disk (intermediate zone). The disk is composed of a compact and fibrous connective tissue and is attached laterally and medially to the TMJ.

Several tissues compose the complex joint capsule conferring stoutness to the anatomical structure of the TMJ. The retro-discal tissue and the insertion of the superior belly of the lateral pterygoid muscle are enveloped by the articular capsule that extends superiorly from the mandibular fossa to just under the condyle. The synovial fluid provided by specific cells lubricates the inside of the joint.

F. Savastano, *Neuromuscular Orthodontics*,
https://doi.org/10.1007/978-3-031-41295-0_4

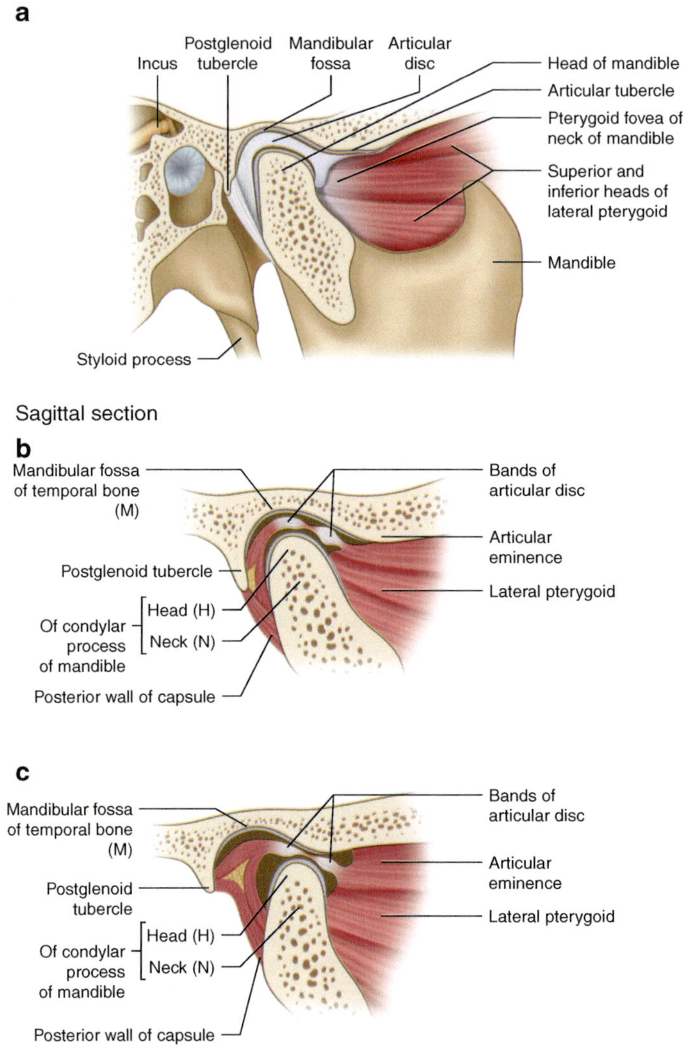

Fig. 4.1 Anatomy of TMJ. From top to bottom, (**a**) Sagittal section during ICP, (**b**) shows muscles, and (**c**) during aperture of the mouth

This aspect is very important for TMJ function and it has been hypothesized that a reduction of lubrication can be an important factor in TMD [1].

Remodeling capabilities of the articular surfaces are limited to the anterior portion of the glenoid fossa and the condylar head. Here, the bone ***is morphologically ready for remodeling*** due to its spongy nature. The posterior part of the glenoid fossa is not covered by fibrocartilage while the bilaminar zone is rich in nerve and blood vessel tissues. This indicates that this part of the articular surface ***is not dedicated to functional activity and so not anatomically predisposed to functional loading.*** A synovial membrane covers the internal surface of the TMJ capsule and is composed of endothelial cells that permit lubrication and nutrition of the articular components. Some fibers of the articular capsule are inserted into the articular disk to stabilize the condylar head.

Recent studies have proved that the pterygoid muscle is not the only muscle connected to the articular disk, but via the pre-discal lamina, the masseter, and temporalis muscles have a direct connection with the articular disk. Also, the zygomaticomandibularis muscle seems to be quite frequently connected to the disc as well [2–5] (Fig. 4.2).

Upon examining the pre-discal lamina of the articular disc, one would observe the lateral pterygoid muscle connecting medially, the temporalis muscle anteriorly, the masseter muscle connecting in a lateral-medial orientation, and the zygomatico-temporalis muscle laterally. Such intricate anatomical linkages have ignited a contentious discourse among physiologists with regard to the contribution of these muscles to the coordination of the articular disc during temporomandibular joint (TMJ) function (Table 4.1).

The glenomandibular muscle originates from the condylar head and its insertion lies medially and distally in the glenoid fossa. The function and meaning of this

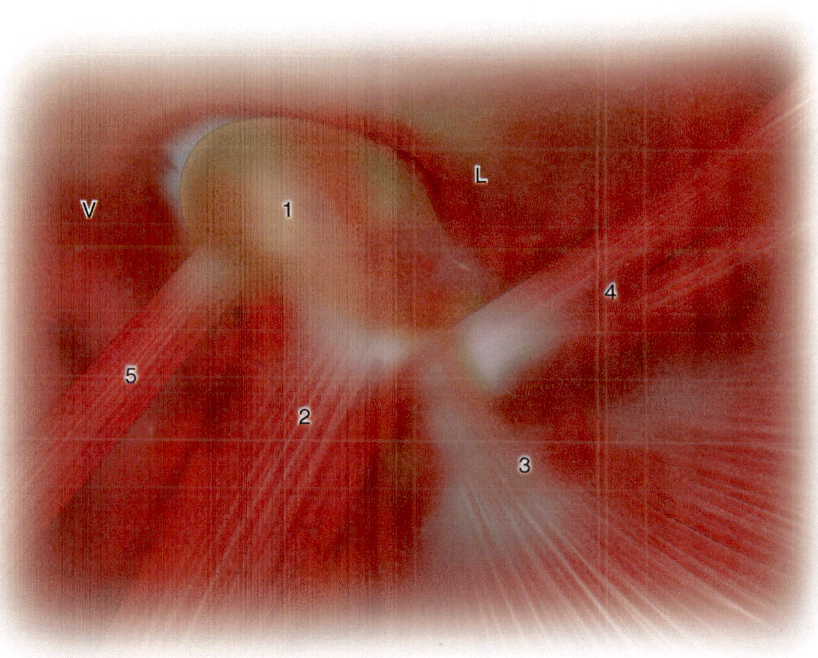

Fig. 4.2 Muscular insertions on the articular disk. The pre-discal lamina is connected to: 1 = external pterygoid muscle, 2 = temporal muscle, 3 = masseter muscle, 4 = zygomaticotemporalis muscle. L = lingual, V = ventral. Articular disk in light blue. Reproduced with permission from *Simplified treatment in Gnathology, the Global Occlusion Method*, author Dr. Piero Silvestrini, ©Edra 2019

Table 4.1 Summary of muscles linked to TMJ and their functions

Temporalis	Closure and mandibular retrusion
Masseter	Vertical closure
External Pterygoid	Condylar protrusion and/or lateral counter side
Glenomandibular	Condylar repositioning
Sphenomandibular	Vertical serration
Temporalis pre-belly	Not defined
Zygomaticomandibularis	Lateral movement of mandible

muscle are not clear yet, but it could be that its role could lie in the control of the condylar position, especially after rotation-translational movements of the condylar head. In fact, no other muscle has this function, and it would be an exceptional effort if only the posterior lamina is responsible for this seating process [6].

Considering the muscular system overlying the mandible, the sphenomandibular muscle (or a deep bundle of the temporalis muscle) originates from the anterior face of the pyramidal process and inserts on the medial face of the temporal crest of the mandible [7]. According to recent studies, this muscle is part of the temporalis muscle, its fibers run in a more vertical fashion and seem to work together with the masseter muscle [8]; its function could be to mitigate the retrusive effect of the overall temporalis muscle, which determines some mandibular retrusion during activation.

Muscles and Function

The muscular system under the mandible is mainly responsible for lowering and retruding the mandible through insertions with the hyoid bone.

Suprahyoid Muscles

They are the digastric, stylohyoid, geniohyoid, and mylohyoid muscles. The digastric connects the mandible to the hyoid bone to the cranium via the mastoid process of the temporal bone (Table 4.2).

The stylohyoid muscle also connects to the cranium via the stylohyoid process, that is, important for its stylomandibular and stylohyoid ligaments that can cause pathologies related to calcifications. Insertions on hyoid bone include muscles of the tongue, the hyoglossus-genioglossus-chondroglossus muscles. This complex muscular system of the tongue includes the palatoglossus and styloglossus. The first inserts from the palatine aponeurosis and is a depressor of the soft palate and elevates the back of the tongue during swallowing, while the second inserts on the styloid process of the temporal bone and is also involved in the act of swallowing. The genioglossus remains the only muscle to protrude the tongue, while the

Table 4.2 Suprahyoid muscles, origin, insertion, and innervation

Muscle	Origin	Insertion	Innervation
Digastric (anterior belly)	Digastric fossa of Mandible	Intermediate Tendon	Mylohyoid nerve—branch of CN V3 (Mandibular division of Trigeminal nerve)
Digastric (posterior belly)	Mastoid notch	Intermediate Tendon	Facial nerve (CN VII)
Geniohyoid	Inferior mental spine of Symphysis menti	Hyoid	Cervical Spinal Nerve 1 via the hypoglossal nerve (CN XII)
Stylohyoid	Temporal styloid process	Hyoid	Facial nerve (CN VII)
Mylohyoid	Mylohyoid line of mandible	Hyoid	Mylohyoid nerve—branch of CN V3 (Mandibular division of Trigeminal nerve—CN V)

Table 4.3 Summary of infrahyoid musculature

Muscle	Origin	Insertion	Innervation
Sternohyoid	Manubrium sterni, clavicle and the posterior sternoclavicular ligament	Medial of lower border of hyoid bone	Ansa cervicalis (C1-C3)
Sternothyroid	Posterior surface of manubrium sterni and first costal cartilage	Oblique line of thyroid cartilage	Ansa cervicalis (C1-C3)
Thyrohyoid	Thyroid cartilage	Lower border body and greater cornu of the hyoid bone	Cervical spinal nerve (hypoglossal nerve)
Omohyoid (superior belly)	Intermediate tendon	Hyoid bone	Superior root of ansa cervicalis (C1)
Omohyoid (inferior belly)	Superior border of scapula	Intermediate tendon	Ansa cervicalis (C1-C3)

hyoglossus is a tongue depressor. The innervation of the tongue consists of three types of fibers: motor, special sensory for taste, and general sensory for sensation. The hypoglossal nerve (CNXII) supplies all motor innervation to all muscles of the tongue with exception of the palatoglossus muscle which is innervated by the vagus nerve (CNX). The anterior two-thirds of tongue: taste via chorda tympani of facial nerve (CNVII) and taste via the trigeminal nerve (CNV). The posterior third of the tongue: taste/sensation via glossopharyngeal nerve (CN IX). Base of the tongue: taste/sensation via superior laryngeal nerve (vagus nerve CN X).

Infrahyoid Muscles

The thyrohyoid, omohyoid, and sternocleidohyiod (sternohyoid) muscles all lower the hyoid bone. From the clavicula origins the sternocleidomastoid muscle inserts to the cranium via the mastoid process. All the muscles described interact in a complex weaving that modulates movements of the cranio-mandibular-hyoid-sternum-scapular chain (Table 4.3).

Tongue

The anatomy of the tongue is complex because it absolves the most important function of the stomatognathic system: swallow. Tables 4.4 and 4.5 briefly describe muscles and innervation of the tongue.

Extrinsic musculature extends outside the organ and is important because it anchors to the bony structure surrounding the tongue. The intrinsic muscles alter tongue shape and are responsible for tongue orientation.

Table 4.4 Intrinsic muscles summary

Muscles	Origin	Insertion	Blood supply	Innervation
Sup. Longitudinal	Lingual septum, post part tongue	Apex/antero-lat margins	Lingual branch of ext. carotid artery	Hypoglossus (CNXII)
Inf. Longitudinal	Root of tongue	Apex	Lingual branch of ext. carotid artery	Hypoglossus (CNXII)
Transverse	Lingual septum	Lat margins	Lingual branch of ext. carotid artery	Hypoglossus (CNXII)
Vertical	Root of tongue, genioglossus	Lingual aponeurosis	Lingual branch of ext. carotid artery	Hypoglossus (CNXII)

Table 4.5 Extrinsic muscles summary

Muscles	Origin	Insertion	Blood supply	Innervation
Genioglossus	Mental spine mandible	Dorsum,lingual aponeurosis, hyoid bone	Lingual artery, submental b. facial artery	Hypoglossus (CNXII)
Hypoglossus	Body, greater horn of hyoid bone	Inferior/ventral parts lateral tongue	Lingual artery, submental b. facial artery	Hypoglossus (CNXII)
Styloglossus	Styloid process of temp. Bone	Inf long m./ hypoglossus	Lingual artery, submental b. facial artery	Hypoglossus (CNXII)
Palatoglossus	Palatine aponeurosis	Lateral margins, blends with intrinsic m.	Palatine branch of facial artery, the pharyngeal artery	Vagus nerve (CNX)

The extrinsic muscles have more complex functions. The genioglossus depresses and protrudes the tongue, while the hypoglossus depresses and retracts the tongue. The other two, the styloglossus and the palatoglossus, act more as elevators. The palatoglossus has also a constriction effect on the isthmus. This muscle is very important for the swallow process as it is responsible for occluding the oral cavity after food propulsion toward the esophagus. This muscle is the only of the extrinsic group that is innervated by the Vagus nerve. It has been proved that electrical stimulation of the hypoglossus nerve may have an indirect effect on this muscle and that there is an increase in the retropalatal space, therefore, potentially being an important muscle in the treatment of OSAS [9].

The Fascial System

A fascia is a sheath, a sheet, or any other dissectible aggregation of connective tissue that attaches, encloses and delineates muscles, bones, organs, blood vessels, and nerves [10]. The fascial system represents the hidden part of the body architecture. Too often our attempts to understand and interpret function from anatomical features have failed because we tend to break down the human body into parts. It is the sectorization of the muscle-skeletal system and it is breakdown to single movements that distract us from a wider perspective of movement fulfilled with harmonic features and complex interactions [11]. The musculoskeletal system is so complex that it is not possible to act or change any part of the human body without affecting the complex as a whole [12]. A more *holistic* approach is necessary to understand the human body's function and movement.

In general, three main types offasciae should be described (Table 4.6 and Fig. 4.3):

- Deep: Like tendons and ligaments, aponeurosis. This is dense and strong.
- Medium: Like visceral fascia.
- Superficial: Just under the skin, density is low, so this is considered loose fascia.

Table 4.6 Boston nomenclature for fascial tissues. Terminology proposed by Huijing and Langevin 2009

Superficial fascia	The back of the skin
Deep fascia	Surrounding the inner body
Intramuscular septa	Tissue between muscles
Interosseal membrane	Tissue between bones
Dense Connective tissue	Densely packed, irregular
Areolar Connective tissue	Non-dense, between skin and deep fascia
Epimysium	Around muscle fibers
Intra-extra-muscular aponeurosis	Multilayered tissue
Endomysium	Microscopic Fibrils, honeycomb structure
Neurovascular tract	Blood, lymph, and nerve vessels
Periost	Tissue around bone

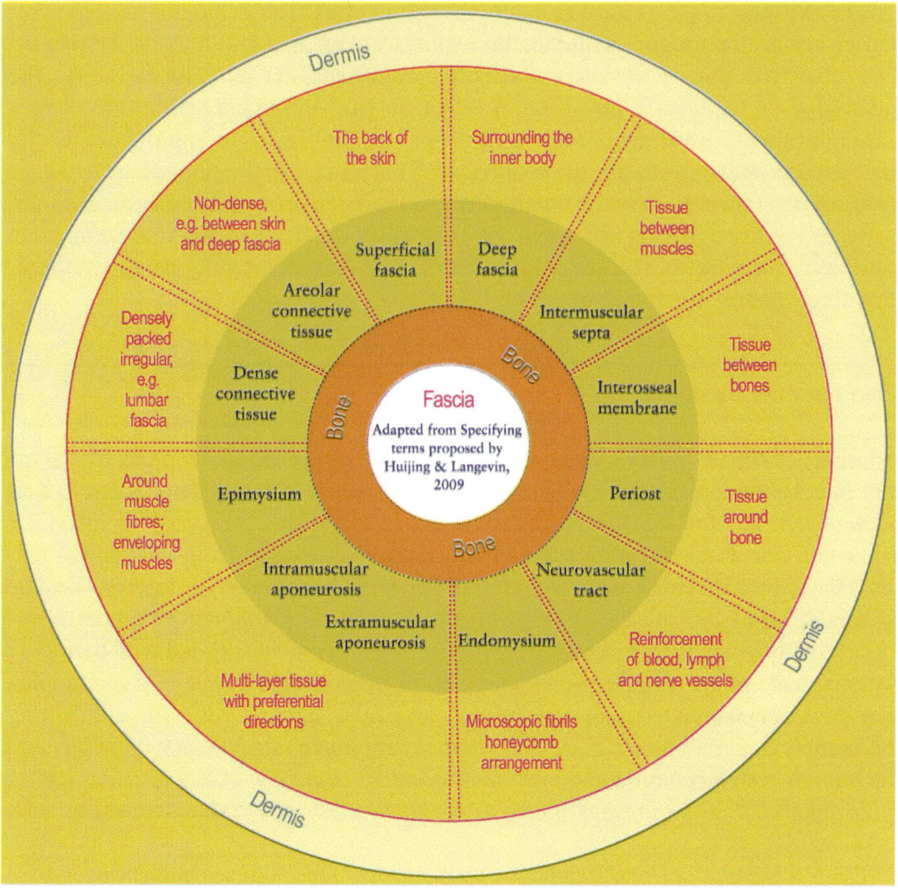

Fig. 4.3 Fascia Mandala by Joanne Avison, Yoga Fascia Anatomy & Movement, 2nd edition, 2021, Handspring Publishing, Edinburgh. Updated to include adaptation from Huijing & Langevin, with reference to Interstitium and Dermis (added by Dr. Neil Theise) and Bone (John Sharkey, Clinical Anatomist, and Emeritus Assoc. Professor of Anatomy & Embryology Dr. Jaap van der Wal) for Myofascial Magic in Action, due 2024, Handspring / Singing Dragon, Edinburgh. Reproduced with kind permission from Art of Contemporary Yoga Ltd.)

The deep cervical fascia is usually divided into a superficial, middle, and deep portion. While the superficial layer is attached to the inferior margin of the mandibular body and posteriorly to the mastoid process and to occipital bone and its lower portion is connected to the sternum, claviculae, scapula, and hyoid bone, the middle layer is stretched between the two omohyoid muscles and up between the hyoid bone and sternum and down to the thoracic girdle. The deep layer is superiorly attached to the occipital bone, laterally to the cervical vertebrae. The posterior fascia is distributed to the pharynx, larynx, and esophagus.

What is interesting about the anatomy of this region (head and neck) is important to understand some implications that dental and oral surgery treatments can have on farther anatomical districts. The anterior deep fascia insertion just under the tongue extends to the lungs and down to the pelvic bones. From here down posteriorly through the legs ends to the foot soles, in the arches. Connective tissue from here is distributed to the flexor hallucis longus. While this confirms our suspicion that the body should be considered as a whole, it also poses interesting debates on the efficacy of tongue-tie release procedures in adults. It is not infrequent to solve tongue ties in adults and immediately notice a long-lasting relief of patient head/neck painful symptomatology.

The fascial system is a complex tension network that wraps organs, blood vessels, nerves, and quite all content of the human body. It is the *tensional* component that together with the *compressional* component, the bone, defines the biotensegrity model of the human body [13]. Biotensegrity represents a modern model of interpretation of anatomical structures of living beings that can blend function and structure to a higher level of comprehension of bodywork. The centuries-old concept of the human body formed by a skeleton on which "soft tissue is draped" should leave space for new visions on biological structures.

The fascial system, an oft-overlooked yet crucial anatomical component, has long been undervalued within the medical field. Serving as a sheath that envelops muscles and other anatomical structures, it facilitates smooth and effortless sliding of muscular tissues against each other, thereby augmenting their capacity to adapt to various movement demands. Moreover, this wrapping of muscles and muscle groups prevents the dissipation of muscle force by confining excessive changes in muscle shape. This results in a mechanical enhancement or envelopment, which favors the redirection of force to anatomical segments that are specifically designed to perform a particular task.

The idea that the TMJ works as a lever system should be considered a surpassed idea too. Biotensegrity and an updated view of the TMJ functional anatomy should resolve unexplained clinical observations on TMJ loading [14]. In fact, the glenoid fossa is mainly composed of thin bone that does not represent an anatomical structure designed to withstand heavy compressional forces. This brings us to another chronic debate in dentistry, that is, defining normal TMJ loading. The stimulation of growth and development is essentially supported by functional loading, but unlike forces that overload anatomical structures and can create joint degeneration, functional loading is a result of a normal anatomical structure in conjunction with a balanced muscular function [15]. Like an athlete is used to lift hundreds of kilos on back-lift without any damage to knees and other joints of the body, the same can be said about TMJ loading. The human body is designed to resist loads and compression beyond the logical sum of the capacity of the single elements that compose the anatomical structures involved in an effort. The Biotensegrity model delivers a logical explanation of functional load by demonstrating that these forces are distributed among the structure as a whole and not to single anatomical parts. The lever system interpretation would of course result in excessive loading of the TMJ, but this view must now be abandoned. The understanding of what *excessive loading is* remains a speculative issue, but it can be seen occasionally with consequent joint degeneration that seemingly is not linked to any apparent pathological muscle or occlusal pathology [14]. From an occlusal point of view, excessive loading and consequent damage to TMJ structures are caused by changes that arrive from a malocclusion that modifies the spatial relationship of the mandible relative to the maxilla, therefore distributing load to specific parts rather than to the functional entity. This overcomes structural tolerance resulting in degenerative reactions.

Fascia mechanoreceptors are important for change in tonus of the muscular system. Other receptors that participate, like the Pacini, are important for proprioceptive feedback and kinesthesia [16]. The Golgi tendon receptors within the fascia are activated only when there is muscle contraction [17], and this could explain how and why ULF-TENS application is effective in lowering muscle tone. The Golgi receptors are found as less than 10% within the tendon, the remaining 90% are located in aponeurosis, capsules, ligaments, and myotendinous junctions. The Pacini/Paciniform and Ruffini bodies are located in greater numbers in the myotendinous junctions rather than in the muscles, like the Golgi. These mechanoreceptors are more sensible to pressure changes and are also found in the masseter muscle. Surprisingly, the most abundant intrafascial mechanoreceptors are the interstitial types III and IV. *They make up for the largest sensory organ of the human body and send to the CNS the greatest amount of afferential sensory inputs*. This means that the myofascial tissues are the most responsible for all afferential inputs. "..research conducted as early as 1974 revealed that the type III and type IV receptors in the fasciae of the temporalis, masseter, and infrahyoid muscles show "responses to the mandibular movement and the stretching of the fascia and the skin"; furthermore "with the sensation of position and movement of the mandible" [18]. This adds up

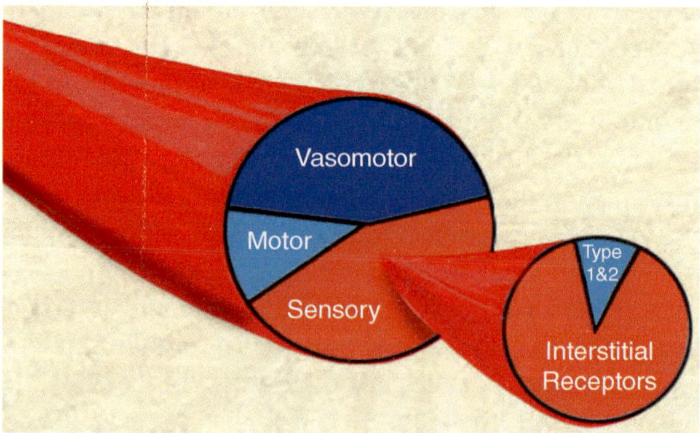

Fig. 4.4 From "Fascia as a Sensory Organ" *A Target of Myofascial Manipulation* Robert Schleip, Ph.D. Within a typical muscle nerve there are almost three times as many sensory neurons than motor neurons. Note that only a small portion of the sensory information comes from the type I and II receptors originating in muscle spindles—Golgi receptors, Pacinian corpuscles, and Ruffini endings. The majority of the sensory input comes from the group of type III and IV receptors, or interstitial receptors, which are intimately linked with the autonomic nervous system. With friendly permission of www.somatics.de

Receptor type	*Preferred location*	*Responsive to*	*Known results of stimulation*
Golgi 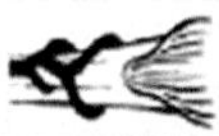 Type I b	• Myotendinous junctions • attachement areas of aponeuroses • ligaments of peripheral joints • joint capsules.	Golgi tendon organ: to muscular contraction. Other Golgi receptors probably to strong stretch only	Tomus decrease in related striated motor fibers.
Pacini & Pac inform 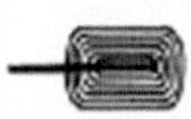 Type II	• Myotendinous junctions • deep capsular layers • spinal ligaments • investing muscular tissues.	Rapid pressure changes and vibrations	Used as proprioceptive feedback for movement control. (Sense of kinesthesia).
Ruffini 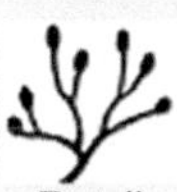 Type II	• Ligaments of peripheral joints, • Dura mater • outer capsular layers • and other tissues associated with regular stretching.	Like Pacini, yet also to sustained pressure. Especially responsive to tangential forces (lateral stretch)	Inhibition of sympathetic activity.
Interstitial 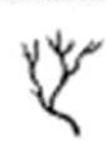 Type III & IV	• Most abundant receptor type. Found almost everywhere, even inside bones. • Highest density in periosteum.	Rapid as well as sustained pressure changes. 50% are high threshold units and 50% are low threshold units	Changes in vasodilation plus apparendy in plasma extravasation

Fig. 4.5 Mechanoreceptors in Fascia: from: Schleip R 2003: Fascial plasticity – a new neurobiological explanation. Journal of Bodywork and Movement Therapies 7(1):11–19 and 7(2):104–116. With friendly permission of www.somatics.de

to an intricate sensory network, and the complexity of the motor response from the CNS is far from being a single muscle activation. Rather the functional units of the motor system are the *motor units*. These can be activated and fine tuned for very precise movements. The activation can even be of a single motor unit [19]. The fascial system is quite alive, and while it is clear how manual therapy can reduce stiffness and relax muscles by stimulating these receptors, it could be hypothesized that the activation of the Golgi receptors by ULF-TENS reduces muscle tone. At the same time, the activation of the interstitial Types III and IV terminations could be responsible for a local increase in blood flow. The Autonomous Nervous System (ANS) is probably linked to fascial stiffness via the TGF-beta1, a transforming growth factor that controls numerous cellular responses, that could act directly on fascial myofibroblasts [20, 21] (Figs. 4.4 and 4.5).

A more modern view of the anatomical structures is necessary. The classical concept of the body as a mechanical object must be substituted with a neurobiological model, in which the body is considered a *self-regulating biological system*, involving nonlinear system dynamics, complexity, and autopoiesis [20, 21]. The consequences for diagnostics and therapy in this aspect, change the attitude of the neuromuscular dentist that acts and solves problems related to occlusion in a different manner in respect of what has been traditional, classical. There is a less clear distinction between structure and function and the nervous system is now included in treatment modalities. There is reduction of problem-solving attitude in favor of "enhancing" the self-regulation processes that are naturally present in every human being. What more is needed to withstand functional approaches to orthodontic treatment? The concept of the stomatognathic system as an integrated part of a self-regulating biological system, means that we should not only apply lesser forces for orthodontic tooth movement but most importantly guide occlusion and function to a point in which these forces of self-regulation are *sufficient to act in stabilizing occlusion and functions related to.*

The importance of the fascial system cannot be disregarded and must be considered as an active entity of the regulatory effects of muscular movement. If so, the mandibular rest position obtained after muscular deconditioning with ULF-TENS is the *result of muscular tone reduction and associated fascial response*. ULF-TENS, therefore, remains irreplaceable in this aspect and must be applied in an environment with *the lowest possible tooth/periodontium proprioception*. Reducing or eliminating all possible afferential signals to the CNS reduces mandibular kinesthesia and increases loss of functional engrams.

The afferent pulses arising from the tongue are complex too. The mandibular division of the trigeminal nerve (CN V, third branch) carries impulses from the dorsal part and lateral parts of the tongue. Branches from the facial nerve (CNVII) carry special signals for taste. The vagus nerve carries sensory stimuli from the base of the tongue, while glossopharyngeal nerve carries sensory signals from the vallate papillae. Sensory input to the CNS is responsible for the activation and modulation of the cascade of events that characterize deglutition. These stimuli modify swallow intensity, trigger peristalsis, and subconscious pharyngeal swallow [22]. Some sensory inputs can induce cortical reflexes, and this is important because it could prove that *peripheral therapeutic stimuli* could enhance, modulate or change swallow disorders [23]. The intraoral stimuli are sensory inputs that can have specific features when a treatment tentative is carried on. As an example, the FroggyMouth® appliance is used to normalize late transition of infant swallow to adult swallow. This appliance provokes an oral stimuli that could increase synapsis production and stimulate cortical and subcortical pathways to favor this transition [24]. Other sensory inputs can stimulate nociceptive receptors like lingual spikes bonded to the lingual surface of the lower and upper incisors for the treatment of anterior tongue thrust. These treatments are directly related to the duration/interruption of the stimuli to be more or less effective. There is always an individual response that may vary and there is no guarantee that these treatments are successful. It is important to underline that there is a proprioceptive response to any stimuli in the oral setting anyway, and this can give a positive outcome to swallow behavioral disorders. Swallow itself is a complicated cascade of events, and it could be that altering peripheral stimuli for the correction of tongue thrust or postural related anomalies be an effective measure in tongue reeducation for the cortical, voluntary swallow. Further investigation is needed to sustain such treatments as efficient in the correction of swallow defects during spontaneous swallow of saliva and related disorders.

Spontaneous swallow of saliva is a more sub-cortical response to peripheral stimuli, like saliva accumulation.

So, to draw a conclusion about the importance of the neural pathways that afferent oral stimuli take to the CNS and that are of interest to the neuromuscular clinician, it must be outlined that any intraoral stimuli that will improve swallow are a positive step toward treatment objectives and that since the duration of such stimuli to be effective is unknown, it must be prolonged as much as possible. Furthermore, such stimuli can come from nociceptors or simply stimulate proprioception to increase stereognosis for tongue position/posture. Tongue posture is a fundamental factor in malocclusion, and therefore should be addressed aggressively [25–27]. There has been some debate on the definition of bad tongue posture, but in general, when at rest, the tongue should not have any contact with lower or upper front incisors. Tongue rest position should be with the cranium, the *fixed* component of the maxilla-mandibular complex. The anatomy of the upper maxilla is clearly designed to receive this organ.

References

1. Nitzan DW. The process of lubrication impairment and its involvement in temporomandibular joint disc displacement: a theoretical concept. J Oral Maxillofac Surg. 2001;59(1):36–45.
2. Matsunaga K, Usui A, Yamaguchi K, Akita K. An anatomical study of the muscles that attach to the articular disc of the temporomandibular joint. Clin Anat. 2009;22(8):932–40.
3. Gaudy JF, Zouaoui A, Bravetti P, Charrier JL, Laison F. Functional anatomy of the human temporal muscle. Surg Radiol Anat. 2001;23(6):389–98.
4. El Haddioui A, Laison F, Zouaoui A, Bravetti P, Gaudy JF. Functional anatomy of the human lateral pterygoid muscle. Surg Radiol Anat. 2005;27(4):271–86.
5. Bittar GT, Bibb CA, Pullinger AG. Histologic characteristics of the lateral pterygoid muscle insertion to the temporomandibular joint. J Orofac Pain. 1994;8(3):243–9.
6. Dias GJ, Kieser J, Oliver J. Glenomandibular muscle band in the human TMJ: a muscular antagonist to Bennett movement? Cranio. 1999;17(1):38–43.
7. Palomari ETP, Ronaldo L, Tobo MP, Isayama NR, da Cunha MR. Sphenomandibular muscle or deep bundle of temporal muscle? Int J Morphol. 2013;31(4):1158–61.
8. Kageyama M, Itoh I. Orientation of the deep part of the human temporal muscle and morphological study of the infratemporal crest. Jpn J Oral Biol. 2003;45(6):397–406.
9. Safiruddin F, Vanderveken OM, de Vries N, Maurer JT, Lee K, Ni Q, et al. Effect of upper-airway stimulation for obstructive sleep apnoea on airway dimensions. Eur Respir J. 2015;45(1):129–38.
10. Scarr G. Defining the fascial system. J Bodyw Mov Ther. 2016;
11. Levin S, de Solorzano SL, Scarr G. The significance of closed kinematic chains to biological movement and dynamic stability. J Bodyw Mov Ther. 2017;21(3):664–72.
12. Scarr G. Biotensegrity. United Kingdom: Handspring Publishing; 2014.
13. Levin SM, Martin D-C. 3.5-Biotensegrity: the mechanics of fascia A2—Schleip, Robert. In: Findley TW, Chaitow L, Huijing PA, editors. Fascia: the tensional network of the human body. Oxford: Churchill Livingstone; 2012. p. 137–42.
14. Scarr G, Harrison H. Resolving the problems and controversies surrounding temporo-mandibular mechanics. J Appl Biomed. 2016;14(3):177–85.
15. Scarr G, Harrison H. Examining the temporo-mandibular joint from a biotensegrity perspective: a change in thinking. J Appl Biomed. 2017;15(1):55–62.

16. Sampallo-Pedroza RM, Cardona-López LF, Ramírez-Gómez KE. Description of oral-motor development from birth to six years of age. Revista de la Facultad de Medicina. 2015;62:593–604.
17. Jami L. Golgi tendon organs in mammalian skeletal muscle: functional properties and central actions. Physiol Rev. 1992;72(3):623–66.
18. Sakada S. Mechanoreceptors in fascia, periosteum and periodontal ligament. Bull Tokyo Med Dent Univ. 1974;21(Suppl):11–3.
19. Muscles alive—their functions revealed by electromyography. Postgrad Med J. 1963;39(449):162.
20. Schleip R. Fascial plasticity–a new neurobiological explanation part 2. J Bodyw Mov Ther. 2003;7(2):104–16.
21. Schleip R. Fascial plasticity–a new neurobiological explanation: part 1. J Bodyw Mov Ther. 2003;7(1):11–9.
22. Steele CM, Miller AJ. Sensory input pathways and mechanisms in swallowing: a review. Dysphagia. 2010;25(4):323–33.
23. Hamdy S, Rothwell JC, Aziz Q, Singh KD, Thompson DG. Long-term reorganization of human motor cortex driven by short-term sensory stimulation. Nat Neurosci. 1998;1(1):64–8.
24. Patrick F, editor The role of biochemistry and neurophysiology in the re-education of deglutition 2017.
25. Primozic J, Farcnik F, Perinetti G, Richmond S, Ovsenik M. The association of tongue posture with the dentoalveolar maxillary and mandibular morphology in class III malocclusion: a controlled study. Eur J Orthod. 2013;35(3):388–93.
26. Yamaguchi H, Sueishi K. Malocclusion associated with abnormal posture. Bull Tokyo Dent Coll. 2003;44(2):43–54.
27. Guay AH, Maxwell DL, Beecher R. A radiographic study of tongue posture at rest and during the phonation of/s/in class III malocclusion. Angle Orthod. 1978;48(1):10–22.

5 Transcutaneous Electrical Nerve Stimulator (TENS) and Surface Electromyography: Important Diagnostic Aids for Bite Registration and Skeletal Discrepancies

Transcutaneous Electrical Nerve Stimulator

TENS application is a widely recognized methodology in dentistry for treating general musculoskeletal pain [1–6]. Our particular interest lies in exploring the diagnostic applications of Ultra-Low Frequency TENS (ULF-TENS). While other types of TENS have been used to address conditions such as TMJ pain and myofascial pain syndrome, ULF-TENS is unique in that it employs a high-intensity and very low-frequency current, similar to that of acupuncture. This makes it an effective tool for treating craniofacial pain [5, 6]. Notably, conventional TENS employs a low-intensity and high-frequency current, while intense TENS utilizes high intensity and high-frequency current. The clinical efficacy and utility of ULF-TENS have been accepted by the scientific community and its use can be summarized in these five points:

1. TMJ pain treatment.
2. Reduces symptoms associated with muscle spasm.
3. Relaxes muscles and increases blood circulation.
4. Used for occlusal registrations.
5. Used for denture impressions.

Without doubt, the efficacy of ULF-TENS in the treatment of TMJ-related pain is probably the most popular characteristic of this device and its use can be monitored with surface EMG [5–19]. ULF-TENS is very useful for the management of TMD disorders and muscle spasms related to the stomatognathic system. The **J5® Dental TENS** (Myotronics, USA) is particularly useful in relieving pain related to TMD when muscle spasm is not present. Pain originating from the muscles is called *myalgia* and the causes may be related to vasoconstriction of the arteries with consequent reduction of blood flow and accumulation of metabolic waist products, so pain *usually* accompanies chronic muscle hyperactivity and consequent muscle fatigue. Jaw movements induced by hyper function and parafunctional tasks

F. Savastano, *Neuromuscular Orthodontics*,
https://doi.org/10.1007/978-3-031-41295-0_5

produce pain. Muscle dysfunction may originate in the muscles of mastication with consequent reduction of the range of motion of the mandible. The CNS may be responsible for changes in muscle function. Hypertonicity can be described as an increase in muscle tonus. Muscle *splinting* is a physiologic reaction to acute changes in occlusion or muscle traumas that increase nociception. It is a reaction of the *antagonist musculature* to protect injured muscles and neighboring anatomical structures. Muscle splinting decreases pain by reducing muscle function and shortening of the muscle, thus reducing movement that could induce pain. It is a protective effect of the CNS to create an ***avoidance pattern*** of a functional task, thus increasing the level of the usual stomatognathic muscle accommodation to its limit. Muscle splinting is a muscle contraction of the antagonist muscles elicited for *protection*. ULF-TENS is especially useful in these cases in which there is no evident reduction of muscle length but there is a need to relax muscle tonus. The efficacy of ULF-TENS on chronic pain has also been demonstrated [1, 20].

Myospasms are characterized by a continuous increased central activation of some motor units (with reduction of muscle length) and may be a consequence of prolonged muscle splinting. Myospasms are sudden, brief, and often painful contractions of a muscle or group of muscles. They may be caused by overuse, fatigue, dehydration, or electrolyte imbalances, among other factors. Myospasms can occur spontaneously or in response to physical activity or movement. They can be quite painful and may cause the affected muscle to twitch or spasm involuntarily. Sometimes an acute malocclusion will result from myospasms. When myospasms affect the temporalis or the masseter muscles, there is limited, consequent, mouth opening, and acute continuous pain. For this reason, ULF-TENS therapy, generally associated with the treatment of emotional stress, are important remedies ***for the prevention of muscle spasms***. Increased sEMG output is rarely associated with Myospasms [21, 22] and s-EMG is a questionable diagnostic aid in myospasms. ATP reserves are depleted and there is no energy available to separate actin and myosin filaments. The reduction of oxygen then stimulates the anaerobic production of ATP that produces lactic acid as a byproduct of the anaerobic oxidation. The build-up of noxious products causes pain and reduces muscle function, and until the underlining causes are addressed, a self-sustaining pathological pain cycle remains to deteriorate muscle function.

Other treatments may include local anesthetic injections to reduce pain. Prolonged muscle spasms can cause *myositis*, an inflammation of the muscle tissues. With myositis, pain is not only functional but is present on a 24-h basis, accompanied with general symptoms and signs related to inflammation (calor, rubor, tumor, dolor, functio laesa). Myositis is a centrally mediated myalgia with a chronic characteristic. The author does not have sufficient evidence that ULF-TENS therapy is useful during myospasms and myositis since any activation of the muscle can cause pain. Muscle tissue, besides being inflamed, may be depleted from most of the energy reserves (ATP) and any forced activation of the fibers is therefore not a reasonable action. Rest and anti-inflammatory drugs could be good treatment modalities. Control of emotional stress is very important. When myositis is caused by a viral or bacterial infection, treatment is limited to antiviral and antibiotic drugs. So, it is important to correctly diagnose the muscle state and understand the limitations of ULF-TENS application on pain reduction. The author suggests avoiding the use of ULF-TENS when TMJ pain and myospasms are a consequence of a closed lock (with limited opening) or *locking* (reduction of overall opening). This is because there is a disk interference to condylar movement and the activation of the masseter and temporalis during ULF-TENS provokes pain by stretching the posterior tissues attached to the disk. This can bring pain from the retro discal tissues and the surrounding muscles and has a negative effect on muscle relaxation.

Myofascial pain is usually referred to as a painful area involving structures other than muscles, like tendons and ligaments, that have a direct relationship with myofascial trigger points [23]. Splinting and central hyperalgesia can be associated with Myofascial pain. The treatment and existence of trigger points are still under debate, but several authors have illustrated some possible explanations of ULF-TENS efficacy [24], while others sustain the use of high-frequency TENS on trigger points for pain treatment [25].

The efficacy of ULF-TENS in pain treatment is not necessarily associated with hypertonic muscles. As previously said, pain is *usually* associated with muscle hyperactivity. The rhythmic activation of the elevator muscles during ULF-TENS application acts like a "pump" that *increases blood flow and reduces waste products* [26, 27]. Most if not all publications on the use of TENS for craniofacial pain treatment lack a specific diagnosis on the muscle *starting physiological or pathological state*. This is the reason why there is not enough evidence of the efficacy of ULF-TENS on non-infectious myositis and myospasms. *Chronic myositis* is the result of an untreated noxious cause centrally mediated that causes hyperalgesia during palpation and function. It is more likely that these publications gather patients based on symptoms rather than signs or objective data.

The J5® Dental TENS (Myotronics, USA) is an Ultra-Low Frequency TENS and its use has gathered popularity in the dental field. TENS application during Neuromuscular diagnostic procedures represents the key step for reducing or cancelling mandibular accommodation induced by the Central Nervous System (CNS). This is obtained via the application of ULF-TENS to Vth and VIIth cranial nerves through the coronoid notch where specific electrodes are placed. This electrical stimulation is neurally mediated and stimulates all the muscles innervated by the Vth and VIIth cranial nerves, including the lateral pterygoid muscles. Table 5.1 shows the effects of ULF-TENS application when electrodes are placed on the coronoid notch *and* on the "Prabu" point [28].

An inter-occlusal media like the Aqualizer® appliance is necessary to interrupt afferential inputs from the periodontal ligaments to the CNS that may arise if teeth come together during the procedure (during swallow or other mandibular movements). ULF-TENS reduces muscle activity of hyperactive and *relaxed muscles* [13, 29]. This is one of the important additional reasons for the application of ULF-TENS even if muscles are relatively relaxed with low EMG output. The role of ULF-TENS on muscle deconditioning is essential for neuromuscular bite registration procedures [30] as well as for the determination of the Myo-trajectory and the

Table 5.1 Muscle innervation for nerves V, VII, and XI affected by ULF-TENS application

Mandibular nerve V	Facial nerve VII	Accessory nerve XI
Masseter	Muscles of nose	Sternocleidomastoid (motor neurons situated c1-c2)
Temporalis	Buccinator	Trapezius muscles (motor neurons situated c3-c4
Medial Pterygoid	Risorius	Motor control of soft palate, larynx, and pharynx
Lateral Pterygoid	Orbicularis oris	
Tensor Veli Palatini	Lower lip/chin muscles	
Mylohyoid	Platysma	
Anterior belly Digastric	Posterior belly Digastric	

Myocentric [6–9, 31–33]. Furthermore, there is increasing evidence that TENS is useful for TMD treatment by effectively aligning the cervical spine [28, 34, 35]. This finding is of great importance because it expands the use of ULF-TENS stimulation to other cranial districts thus enhancing postural rehabilitation in TMD and non-TMD patients [36]. Some authors have not concluded that there is an effective alteration of cervical spine posture in TMD patients [37, 38], while others have found that TMD patients correlate positively with cervical posture alterations [39]. This is a very delicate matter that needs further investigation. Since neuromuscular orthotic treatment is highly effective in alleviating joint pain, clicking, and neck pain in patients with temporomandibular disorders (TMD), and since this procedure brings about changes in cranio-cervical posture, there must be a significant connection between the correction of cervical posture and signs and symptoms of TMD [40, 41].

The main objective in Neuromuscular Dentistry is determining the Physiologic Rest Position (PRP), a rest position that is not conditioned by occlusion. There are several ways to do this and several ways to relax the muscles of mastication. When teeth come to contact during swallow or voluntary C.O., the periodontal ligaments and other organules in muscles, tendons, and fascia, send afferent inputs to the CNS that will consequently fine-tune mandibular postural muscle activity to adjust mandibular position to a ***habitual rest position*** (HRP). This HRP is the expression of a compensation, an accommodation, to occlusal needs and the result of highly detailed *processing* by the CNS that establishes the most ergonomic "starting position" for the mandible to explicate functional tasks (the most important being deglutition). Mandibular postural elevator muscles are continuously activated selectively in order to maintain an adequate freeway space of circa 2 mm. Muscle memory (engram) is key in creating a functional adaptation to occlusal needs that determines reduction of energy consumption.

Dr. Piero Silvestrini and I have tested several inter-occlusal media including the Aqualizer® [42, 43] during the deconditioning procedure with ULF-TENS. The Aqualizer has changed dramatically the quality and speed to relaxation and has simplified the overall procedure of deconditioning. Over 90% of randomly selected patients have normal s-EMG outputs after 20 min of TENS/Aqualizer application. The protocol is to apply ULF-TENS for 40 min even if muscles are well relaxed because the effect of TENS on the tissues that surround and support the mandible cannot be monitored by s-EMG (fascia, ligaments, and tendons). The application of ULF-TENS, according to the described procedure, will *always* modify the maxilla/mandibular relationship. This is in contrast with some previous studies, but the described protocol, TENS/Aqualizer®, has not been thoroughly investigated yet. Bite registration with the use of ULF-TENS and wax as inter-occlusal media on teeth has been well described in literature [7, 8, 17, 33, 44].

The J5® Dental TENS from Myotronics, provides four patient stimulation channels, each left and right pair with independent controls. This provides a unique capability of stimulating the V and VII cranial nerves together with cervical/upper shoulder muscles. The efficacy of this TENS unit with the addition of two extra channels represents the state-of-the-art of ULF-TENS (Figs. 5.1, 5.2, and 5.3).

Procedures for obtaining dental impressions with the use of ULF-TENS for full mouth removable prosthetics, as well as their significance, are beyond the scope of this book. However, it is worth noting that these impressions are not limited to teeth and passive structures; rather, they are characterized by a muscle "imprint" that enhances the quality of the final casts.

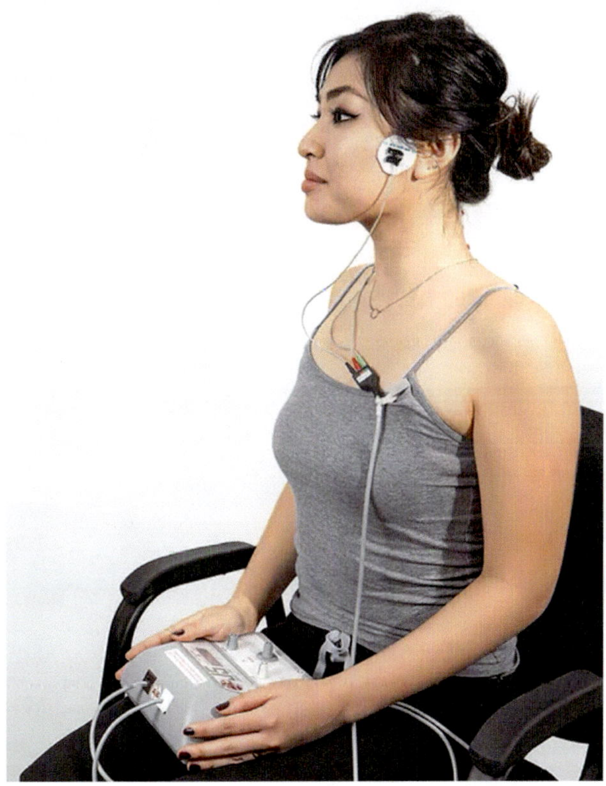

Fig. 5.1 Lateral electrode placement and connection to J5 Myomonitor®, Myotronics, Seattle, USA

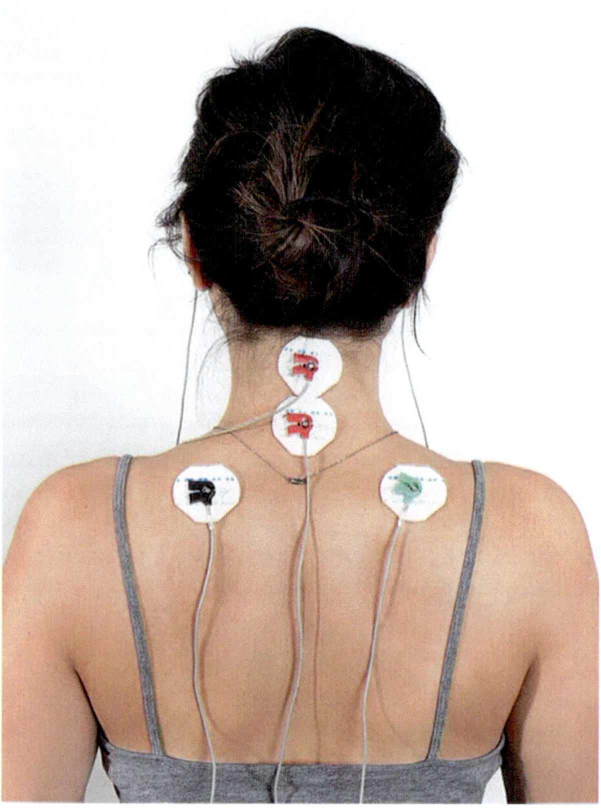

Fig. 5.2 Cont. showing posterior electrode placement

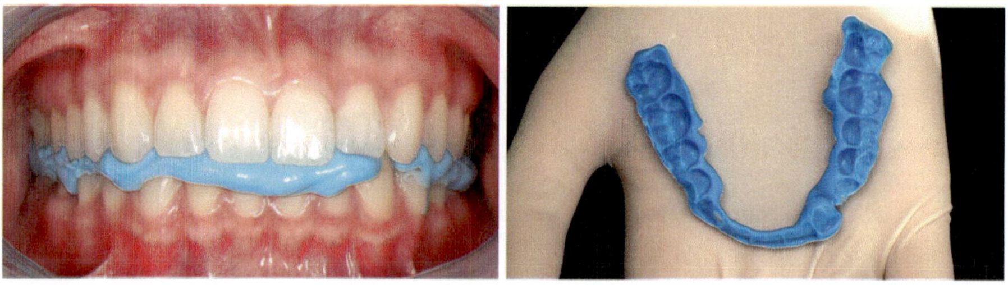

Fig. 5.3 On the left showing silicone setting bite registration and on the right hardened bite registration

Procedure for Bite Registration Technique

The following procedure applies to both the full **K7 diagnostic protocol** and the **"Tens only"** bite registration technique. Although the second requires some specific skill and experience since there is no kinesiographic control, both techniques are considered valid. The author supports the use of Myoprint® and similar techniques for bite registration even if these methods have been slowly replaced by other materials/techniques (and similar). The importance of head posture has been previously discussed, the patient should sit comfortably upright and natural head posture checked by a mirror.

1. **Clean skin** with 90% alcohol and apply electrodes according to manufacturer's specifications.
2. **Insert in the oral cavity an Aqualizer®.** The size and height of the Aqualizer *must* be determined clinically by the practitioner. If you are not sure which volume to use, always choose the lowest. The volume of the pads should never be so that they occupy all the vertical freeway space available. This is easy to determine, for example, in very deep bite individuals, in which the skeletal discrepancy is evident. It becomes trickier on those patients who tend to be slightly open bite. This is the reason why including a lateral cephalometric X-ray in all diagnostic procedures facilitates clinical diagnosis of freeway space. In general, skeletal morphology can reasonably give a good indication of freeway space.
3. If doing the "TENS only" technique, instruct the patient to **relax having their mandible fall due to the force of gravity**. Now turn on the J5® after being sure that the intensity is set to zero, and slowly increase the intensity on the channel you have chosen for the Vth and VIIth (coronoid notch) stimulation. To be sure you are tensing at the correct amplitude, place your finger on the lower incisors of your patient and feel the pulse just as you reach an intensity that is sufficient to feel the upward movement of the mandible. There is no way to check and measure the mandibular movement but clinically with your finger. On the other hand, if you are doing a complete diagnostic series with a K7® diagnostic system, you are proceeding with the ULF-TENS application ***only*** if the scan 9 (s-EMG at rest) has been documented and stored. You can use any scan you prefer to measure the ULF-TENS activity on mandibular movement. The spike seen during the sweep scan should always be sufficient for the computer to calculate the myo-trajectory (0.5–0.7 mm). Once the intensity has been set, it is important to check the patient; as the patient relaxes, you will have to lower the threshold accordingly. Frequent adjustments may be necessary. After 45′ of tens application, you should be ready to complete your bite registration.
4. **Bite registration**

   For the "Tens only" procedure, *simply pinch the Aqualizer with a long tweezer and pull and have it slide away*. Be sure to have instructed your patient to pretend you were not there and to avoid any movements of the mandible, like opening their mouth to facilitate Aqualizer® removal. Remember to lower the TENS intensity before removing the Aqualizer and *having instructed the patient not to swallow after removal; teeth must not come in contact in any way.* If you are not sure of the PRP because maybe the patient indivertibly has opened the mouth a bit, turn on the TENS progressively until you can **see** a slight mandibular movement. Wait until you feel the patient has regained the PRP from excessive opening. At this point of the procedure, if the patient for any reason has upper and lower tooth/teeth touch, you *must* relax with the Aqualizer® *again*. Unfortunately, reaccommodation takes only one quick tooth contact while mandibular distraction procedure takes much more time.

Now that you feel that the patient is or has regained the PRP, inject enough registration material (silicone) only on the front teeth to record and fix the aperture. You are turning off the Tens and manually accompanying and sustaining the mandible at about 1–2 mm closure **from** PRP. It only takes enough time for whatever silicone you have chosen to harden. Faster silicones work at about 30 s setting time and should be preferred. As soon as the silicone is set, have the patient open wide and complete the bite registration by adding silicone laterally and having the patient occlude on the front hardened occlusal silicone guide. This procedure can also be done with a full occlusal injection/preparation of a slow-working acrylic like Myoprint® or Blue Sapphire™ from Bosworth. Since the working time of these resins is longer and passes through an elastic phase, after relaxation with ULF-TENS, remove the Aqualizer and instruct the patient to open it wide enough to apply the prepared resin in a soft elastic state on the lower occlusal surface. The ULF-TENS spike is then increased to a visually detectible mandibular movement to about 2 mm. This creates an imprint recording on the resin of the relationship of the dental arches. This recording method remains the most precise for the "TENS only" procedure. As soon as the patient does not tolerate the increasing acrylic temperature, set it on fresh casts after trimming.

The K7 diagnostic steps of the mandibular recording of the Myocentric are different. You can proceed to scan 4/5 (bite registration) ***only*** if scan 10 demonstrates that the Aqualizer®/ULF-TENS procedure has been a success in relaxing muscles. This said, the Myocentric is calculated on the Myotrajectory, and this position will be the new centric for bite registration. Silicone is used and patient instructed to close on Myocentric, either by visual feedback on the computer screen or by guiding the patient to the Myocentric manually. Using the K7 and recording the Myocentric has obviously many advantages. You can check that the bite registration is correct. You can check that an orthotic resembles the bite registration (and not only on the articulator), and you can keep a record of the bite registration scan and procedure. This is not possible with the "TENS only" technique (Fig. 5.3).

There are some aspects that should be discussed on the most and accepted bite registration technique used during K7 use. During scan 4/5, at one point and before bite registration, the patient is instructed to close to CO and tap-tap to secure ICP position and then design the protrusive border: the patient **de facto** reaccommodates muscle function. While this is a standard procedure because it gives the possibility of an immediate visual analysis of the CO location relative to PRP, there is no way of controlling the change in posterior vertical dimension/position before and after closing in CO. This means that even though the sagittal mandibular position may be respected for the Myocentric registration, the posterior vertical freeway space may be compromised. In other words, recording is limited to the vertical opening on the Myotrajectory and does not guarantee proper 3D alignment of the mandible. The solution is to reapply the Aqualizer and Tensing for a few minutes to *reduce* the possibility of compromising posterior vertical dimension and mandibular torque registration. This method of bite registration is widely accepted by the neuromuscular community, and while it is sufficient for orthodontic diagnosis, it can still be debated if a few minutes of reapplication of TENS and occlusal media are sufficient to regain an ideal posterior vertical freeway space equal to that obtained after 45 min. of ULF-TENS application. The best way to perform an ideal Myocentric bite recording with the K7® system (always after minimum 45' TENS and Aqualizer application and scan 10 check) is to:

(a) Scan 4/5. After taking away the Aqualizer® from the patient's mouth, have the patient relax to levels seen before Aqualizer removal on scan 4 sweep.
(b) On scan 5 identify PRP. Be sure to see at least 1–1.5 mm. TENS spike and then turn off the TENS. Press space bar to stop sweep and recording of scan 5.
(c) Instruct patient to move slowly to a mandibular position on Myotrajectory (not yet calculated by the computer), *that you have set at the tip of the spike*, or, if you need more freeway space, at the calculated Myocentric on the Myotrajectory with visual positioning. The same is said for the frontal view.
(d) Inject silicone on front teeth only. When hardened, complete the dental arch relationship by applying silicone on the remaining teeth *without asking the patient to open their mouth widely*. Do not remove the front silicone guide before this procedure. When all silicone is hardened, remove silicone, and *immediately re-insert the Aqualizer®*. Reapply Tens to be sure the patient is relaxing and then complete scan 4/5 as by book. This is needed to design protrusive borders and canine disocclusion.
(e) With a complete 4/5 scan, check to see where your bite registration positions the mandible. This should be on the Myotrajectory and at chosen Myocentric.

The method of occlusal recording just described should be considered the best approach for achieving a precise registration on the MyoCentric, without posing the risk of compromising the posterior vertical dimension. It is essential to emphasize the significance of rechecking the recently completed cranio-mandibular recording, as this meticulous verification ensures the highest level of precision. Using the K7 is the only possible way to measure and visualize the Myocentric relative to ICP.

The "TENS only" technique, when done by expert hands, is a very good, fast, and inexpensive method for bite registration, but some limitations must be understood.

1. The Myocentric can be obtained on the neuromuscular trajectory only if the TENS pulsing is present. The spike cannot be measured, and silicone should not be used. For this reason, Sapphire™ Acrylic Peripheral Impression Material from Bosworth®is needed, which when mixed properly, has a good time lasting elastic phase that accommodates mandibular movement with tooth impressions. The result is a very good approximation on the neuromuscular trajectory. The approximation is generally within 1 mm tolerance in expert hands. The use of

silicone is not recommended because the practitioner should guide the patient to the MyoCentric at vertical opening given by spike, which is not an easy procedure.

2. There is no way to check if the recording is correct. Some practitioners choose to check the recording with muscle testing [45–48]. These techniques, although fascinating, are not proven by any scientific study. Since Neuromuscular dentistry relies on the neuromuscular trajectory and an established Myocentric, how can muscle testing be a precise method to check a *very* precise mandibular position? Rather, although unexplained, it could be a quick method to check if the recorded bite is beyond or within structural and physiological individual tolerance [49–51].
3. The insertion of Sapphire resin in the oral cavity is not always fully accepted from the patient. Bad taste can accompany bite recording procedures, and when in the advanced elastic phase, the patient can feel the increase in temperature of the acrylic: it is time to transfer the registration on complete dental casts. Final trimming is needed and done by simply cutting off excess material.

The TENS only technique is very useful in children when either a diagnostic bite is taken or a PRP recording is needed. In this last case, it will be useful for the construction of functional neuromuscular repositioning appliances or for the fabrication of the SAVA1 appliance.

Surface Electromyography

In these recent years, stand-alone surface electromyography instruments have started to penetrate at high numbers in the dental office. Affordable units are part of the reason for this gained popularity, while other factors like aggressive marketing, make the other. These EMG instruments do not incorporate any real scientific progress in detecting and representing the electrical activity of the muscle. *No important publications support sufficiently the stand-a-lone* use of surface electromyography (s-EMG) for the analysis of dynamic occlusion. Surface electromyography has proven to be useful in orthodontics and TMD-related issues [48, 49, 52] especially when used *in conjunction with jaw tracking instruments*.

The K7® Evaluation System, used by clinicians and researchers, incorporates eight-channel s-EMG and a jaw tracking module. Surface electromyography should not be a stand-a-lone procedure for occlusal analysis, but wisely coupled with mandibular movement analysis (CMS). Electromyography is a procedure to detect, record, and graphically represent a muscle's electrical activity. When a muscle works, it is mechanical function uses ATP as a source of energy. ATP is also used for other cell functions, like synthesis of chemical components and transfer of cell constituents across the cell membrane. So, contraction, a mechanical work, is the result of the sliding of two main proteins over each other of the muscle, actin, and myosin, with the reduction of ATP to ADP to ensure energy. The main event is triggered by the *action potential*, a depolarization of the cell membrane due to electrical stimuli.

These stimuli can arise as a voluntary activation of the muscle fibers (volitional movement), by a reflex, or even from trauma or involuntary muscle activation (heart contraction). This action potential releases calcium that again activates the ATP activity of myosin which starts contraction.

The cell membrane is semipermeable allowing a continuous exchange between the constituents of the cell and the environment. Some ions are restricted across the cell membrane while others are allowed to pass with ease. This creates a *potential difference* which is called *resting membrane potential*. Sodium, potassium, and chloride ions are in different concentrations across the cellular membrane, and this is achieved through the sodium-potassium pump that keeps sodium mainly outside the cell membrane while keeping potassium inside. The pump works five times more in concentrating the sodium outside the cell than the potassium inside, thus creating a polarization in which the inside of the cell is negative and the outside positive. This resting potential is about −85 mV and at these levels most sodium channels are closed. When depolarization reaches a predetermined threshold, an action potential is triggered that activates the sodium channel. A ~ 20 mV difference is needed as stimuli to depolarize the membrane, assuring that the fibers remain silent and react only if they are triggered to fire by an action potential [53]. Resting potentials do differ according to cell types, for example, skeletal muscle cells have a resting potential of -95 mV while neurons between −60 and −70 mV. Smooth muscle cells have a lower resting potential at −60 mV. If stimulus continues to depolarize the cell membrane without a proper resting phase, there is a consequent reduction of excitability due to several factors. The increase in external potassium concentrations causes a membrane depolarization to be characterized by a reduced threshold and reduced peak for action potential with an increase in overall duration. If stimulus is continued, the action potential is no longer *all or none* but there is a grading of the amplitude and output depending on the stimulus. Eventually, muscle fibers become no longer excitable.

Without speculating further on muscle physiology, it is important to understand that the action potential can be interpreted as an electrical current that, like a wave, is transported on the muscle fiber or the nerve to different parts of the body. The action potential propagates along the muscle fiber from the point of origin. The depolarization starts the action potential and this current travels along the fiber rather than in any other direction meaning that the bipolar surface electrode placement used in s-EMG should be placed carefully ***along/parallel*** to the muscle fibers. Figure 5.4 is a schematic summary of the cascade of these events.

There is always electrical activity in the muscle at rest. This is in contrast with *all or none* reactions to stimuli of the muscle fiber. In fact, muscle tone is represented by the continuous activation of several muscle fibers in the whole muscle that are fully contracted until fatigued. Muscle fibers alternate in activation to maintain muscle tone and consequently a fixed muscle length. Muscle tone is dependent on many factors, from psychological/emotional to conscious regulation. These are important factors because there are several studies on muscle tone of the stomatognathic system in relation to TMD [54–58]. When testing *resting muscle tone*, there is an EMG normative data we refer to, with widely accepted parameters [58, 59]:

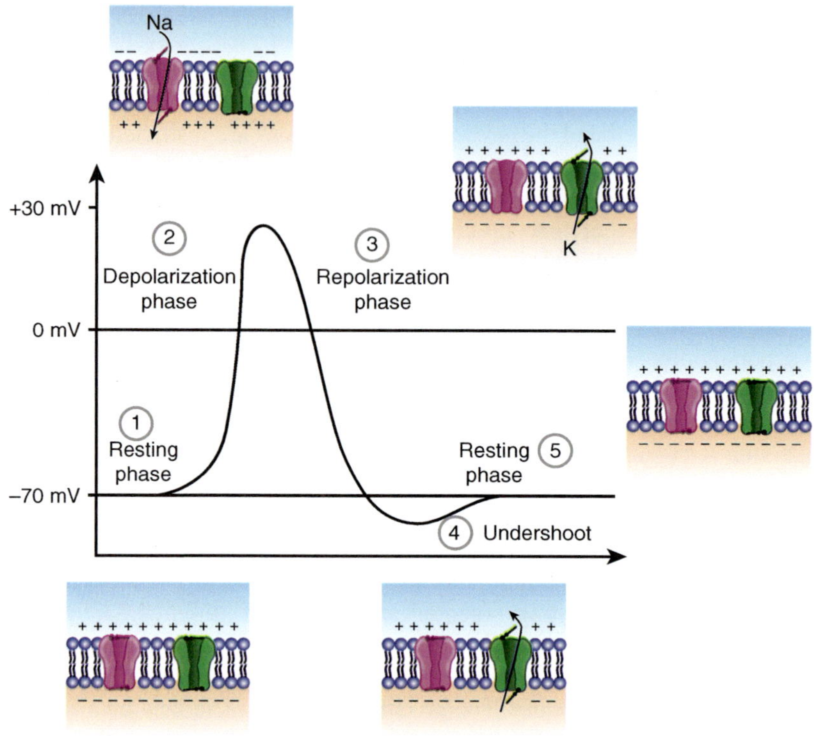

Fig. 5.4 From: Energy Production Bahar Hazal Yalçınkaya, ... Mustafa Özilgen Bayram Yılmaz, in Comprehensive Energy Systems, 2018 A 3.15.4.1.2. Action potential: Schematic description of action potential and voltage-gated ion channels. (1) Resting state: the $Na^{þ}$ and $K^{þ}$ channels closed. (2) Depolarization (rising phase): this upcoming stimulus opens $Na^{þ}$ channels. $Na^{þ}$ influx through the channels depolarize the potential when the depolarization reaches to threshold value it initiates an action potential. (3) Repolarization: $Na^{þ}$ channels are no longer voltage sensitive and close at maximum voltage and $K^{þ}$ channels fully open, out flux of $K^{þ}$ ions makes voltage become negative. (4) Undershoot: fully open $K^{þ}$ channels make voltage further negative, and channels eventually turn its mostly closed but leaky state with establishing resting potential. (5) Resting state: the $Na^{þ}$ and $K^{þ}$ channels are closed

Temporalis	1.5–2.5 μV
Masseter	1.0–2.0 μV
Temporalis Posterior	1.5–2.5 μV
Sub-Mandibular	1.5–2.5 μV
Sternocleidomastoid	1.5–2.5 μV

The sEMG is part of the K7® diagnostic system. It consists of a pre-amplifier that is connected to the K7 central unit on one side and to the patient on the other through the eight-channel wiring connected to the surface electrodes (Fig. 5.5).

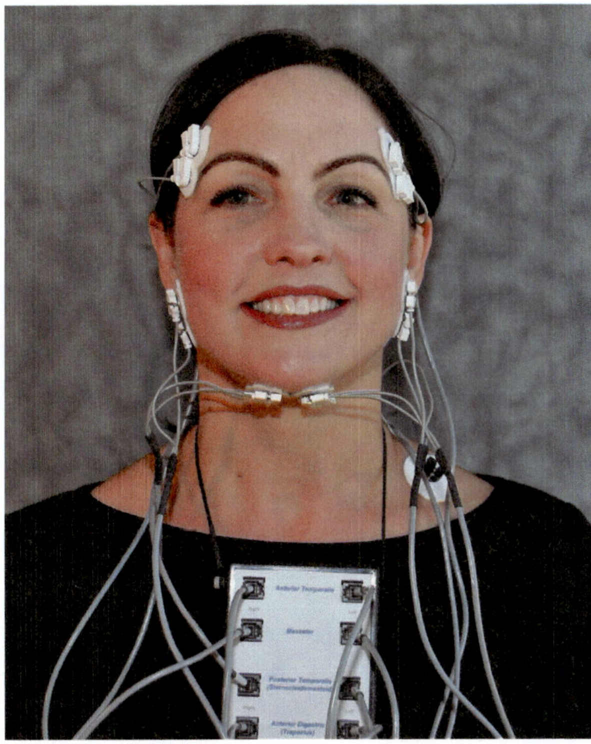

Fig. 5.5 Showing sEMG pre-amplifier connected to eight channels on patient: several muscles are being tested: Temporalis, Masseter and sub-mental

Scans, such as scan 9, are sweep mode recordings of muscle EMG output during a fixed time frame. This scan can be used to test muscles of mastication resting output (muscle tonus) but can also be used to test output during functional tasks.

Figure 5.6 shows an example of scan 9.

By changing the gain (sensibility) for EMG, it can be useful to have a better overall picture of the EMG recording. Figure 5.7 is the same scan 9 as in Fig. 5.2 but with an EMG gain set to *100 μV/division.*

As a general indication, elevated resting levels of Anterior and Posterior Temporalis usually are typical of loss of posterior support with posterior mandibular displacement (distal occlusion). In other instances, higher resting levels of this muscle are seen in pain related to one side of the face. Often seen high resting levels of the temporalis in positional Class II occlusions, in which loss of posterior support is the main cause of malocclusion. The Masseter muscle is less important than the temporalis muscle as a postural muscle, therefore, it is more important to evaluate this muscle during functional tests like in maximum voluntary contraction (MVC), (scan 11) [60]. Posterior temporalis is more related to postural problems and is frequently associated with posterior headache when resting levels are elevated. The digastric muscle is immersed with other submental muscles (platysma, mylohyoid, and suprahyoid) and therefore should be called *sub-mental musculature*. It has been noted that these sub-mental muscles may be activated during voluntary mandibular

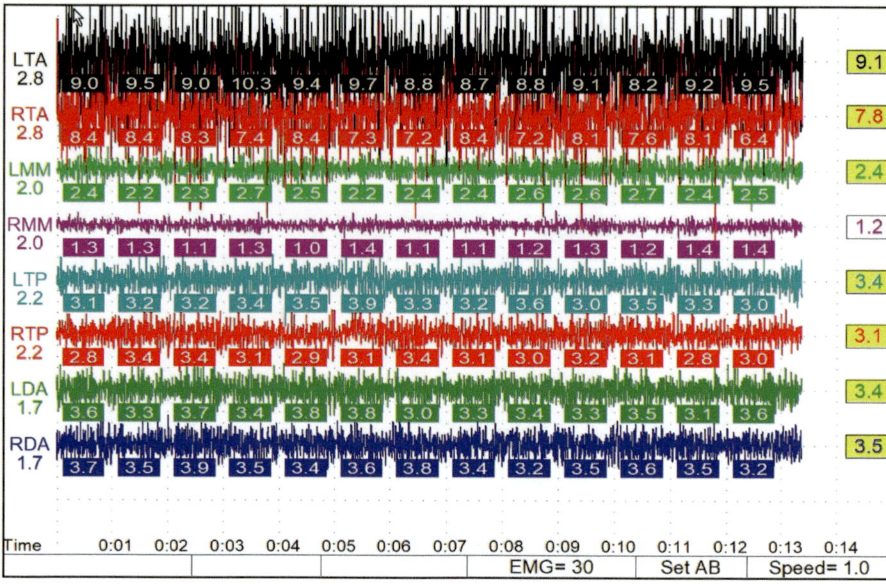

Fig. 5.6 An example of scan 9. Eight channels are used to test four muscles bilaterally. On the left is the muscle name and under it the user-adjustable average microvolt limit. On the right is the overall result. As shown, almost all muscles are higher than their normal averages except RMM. On the lower part of the screen is the time indication, every dotted square is representative of 1 s for a total of 14 s recording. Note lower right the gain for speed is set to 1.0; other gains are for EMG and muscles pre-sets. *LMM: left masseter muscle; LTA: left anterior temporalis; RMM: right masseter muscle; RTA: right anterior temporalis; LTP Left Temporalis Posterior; RTP Right Temporalis Posterior; LDA Left Digastric Anterior (sub-mental left); RDA Right Digastric Anterior (sub-mental right)*

retrusion suggesting an active participation in mandibular sagittal posture [61]. These muscles have elevated resting outputs in swallow disorders and dental open-bite individuals without lip competence. Electromyographic evaluation of these muscles is very important for the study of swallow disorders [62–66].

The sEMG recording is not a stand-alone feature of the k7® diagnostic system. sEMG can be displayed during other scan sessions giving valuable information to the practitioner, this is called *EMG monitor mode* and is a live, continuous representation of muscle electrical output. Besides testing muscle tone at rest, sEMG is used to assess the total output on functional tasks such as clench in ICP (Maximum Voluntary Contraction or MVC) and clench on cotton rolls. Figure 5.8 is an example of Scan 11 with a functional test on natural dentition and cotton rolls. Cotton rolls are placed bilaterally and centered on second bicuspid/first molar surfaces. Cotton roll test is not always applicable if teeth are missing.

Scan 11 can be carried out on practically any functional task while evaluating several muscles involved in the work. This scan is executed by applying a filter to the EMG raw output to facilitate graphic representation/interpretation. There is a precise physiological sequence of muscle activation that is of utmost importance.

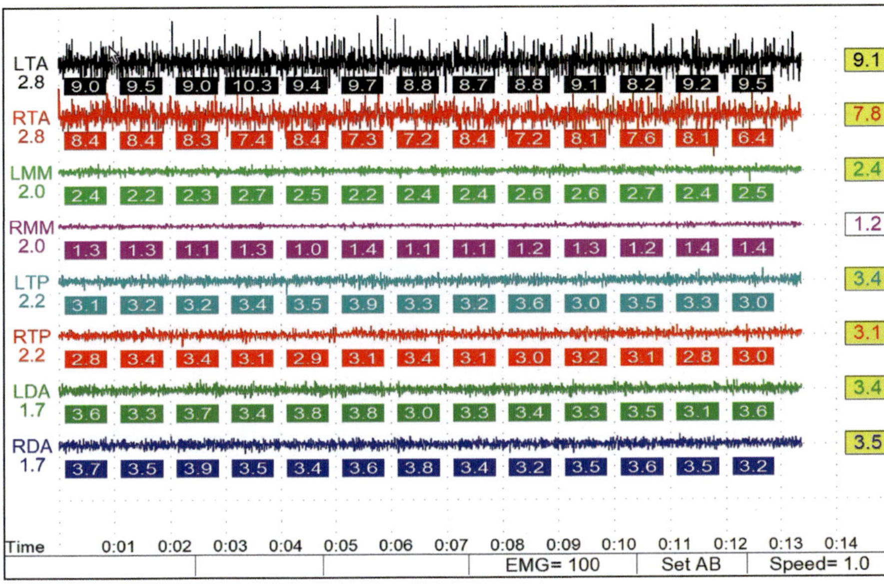

Fig. 5.7 Same EMG recording as in Fig. 5.2 but with gain set to 100 microvolts per division. *LMM* left masseter muscle, *LTA* left anterior temporalis, *RMM* right masseter muscle, *RTA* right anterior temporalis, *LTP* Left Temporalis Posterior, *RTP* Right Temporalis Posterior, *LDA* Left Digastric Anterior (sub-mental left), *RDA* Right Digastric Anterior (sub-mental right)

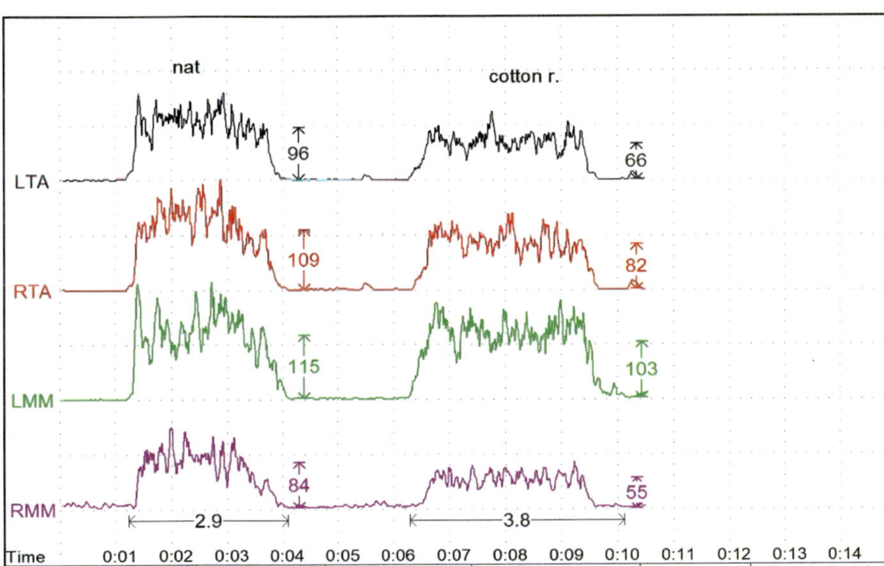

Fig. 5.8 Scan 11 in sweep mode, functional test with burst 1 MVC on left on natural dentition in ICP, and burst 2 MVC on cotton rolls. *LMM* left masseter muscle, *LTA* left anterior temporalis, *RMM* right masseter muscle; *RTA* right anterior temporalis

As mentioned before, the masseter muscles cannot be considered postural muscles in the same way as the temporalis muscles. Therefore, when the patient is at rest and then asked to close and bite hard, we can observe the sequence of activation of these two muscles. Ideally, the temporalis muscle should be activated first, followed by the masseter muscle. However, in cases where the masseter muscle is activated before the temporalis, it may be a normal response if the patient tends to place their tongue between their teeth, leading to increased inter-occlusal resistance. It is essential to note that, similar to all EMG evaluations, the total output is not the most critical feature and should be considered in a broader diagnostic context. For example, very low maximum outputs (under 50 μV) in a robust deep-bite individual could mean that the musculature is exhausted. In other circumstances, when tooth contact occurs in ICP provoking a painful reaction (e.g., pain from a cavity), sEMG output is generally very low as the patient is unable to serrate. These reactions can be seen also in TMD individuals with TMJ pain during clench in which ICP forces distal condylar entrapment. Loss of posterior support and in general, distal occlusions are somewhat characterized by a low temporal output and a mediocre masseter output during clench (Fig. 5.9). This is probably more related to chronic fatigue than to any other reason.

Figure 5.9 shows a child with TMD and a forced distal occlusion due to *front wall*. There is obviously a loss of posterior support and weak temporalis muscles

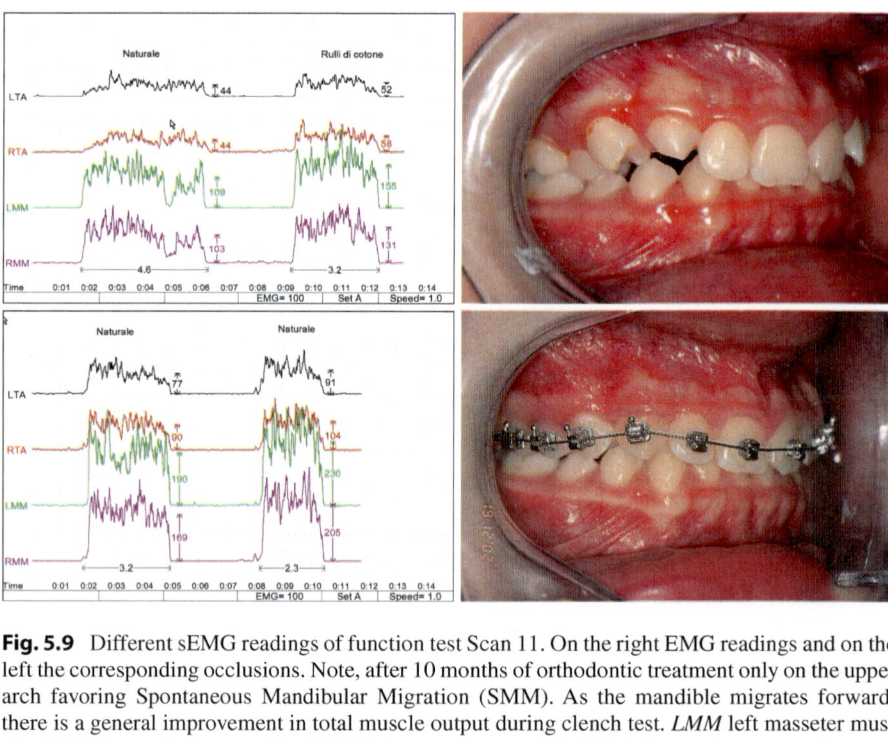

Fig. 5.9 Different sEMG readings of function test Scan 11. On the right EMG readings and on the left the corresponding occlusions. Note, after 10 months of orthodontic treatment only on the upper arch favoring Spontaneous Mandibular Migration (SMM). As the mandible migrates forward, there is a general improvement in total muscle output during clench test. *LMM* left masseter muscle, *LTA* left anterior temporalis, *RMM* right masseter muscle, *RTA* right anterior temporalis

which are exhausted in maintaining an HRP for the distal occlusion and avoiding anterior interferences as much as possible. Figure 5.10 is another example of spontaneous mandibular migration (SMM) from a forced distal occlusion. The increase in muscular performance seen only 3 months after active orthodontic treatment represents a positive neuromuscular response. sEMG final testing on scan 11 several months after occlusal settling occurs shows improvements when a proper neuromuscular occlusion is achieved. During MVC (Maximum Voluntary Contraction) test in scan 11, it is not uncommon to see high temporalis/low masseter activity in distal occlusions with conserved muscular activity.

These distal occlusion cases are characterized by a fair posterior support and a high hyperactivity of the Temporalis vs Masseters at rest (Scan 9) to avoid anterior incisal premature occlusal contacts. The bilateral activation of the temporal muscles has a retruding effect on the mandible [61]. Elevated anterior temporalis output at rest is indicative of the increased activity of the posterior temporalis too that has more horizontal fibers for mandibular retrusion. The Temporalis muscle must be considered as one functional entity and not divided in two as earlier proposed [67]. The HRP is maintained at a high cost from an energetic point of view in which the Temporalis muscles play an important role.

In Chap. 12, Fig. 12.20, is the result of scan 11 at post-treatment of a skeletal Class III case (excess freeway space, maxillary insufficiency). The Temporalis

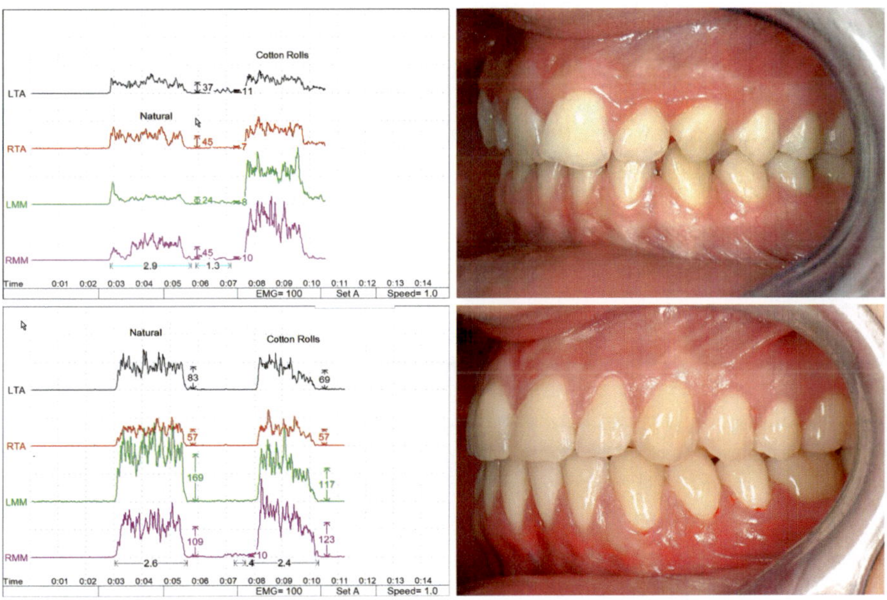

Fig. 5.10 Different sEMG readings of function test Scan 11. On the right EMG readings and on the left the corresponding occlusions. Note, before and at the end of treatment during which SMM occurred. There is a general improvement in total muscle output and balancing.; *LMM* left masseter muscle*;* *LTA* left anterior temporalis, *RMM* right masseter muscle, *RTA* right anterior temporalis

muscles finally gain an increase in function (extrusion of the posterior sectors is important and fundamental for the treatment of Class III skeletal with excess freeway space), meaning that there has been posterior extrusion and a change of the occlusal plane. Figure 12.25 in Chap. 12 shows scan 11 at follow-up of the same patient where the sEMG output is more balanced and finally adjusted showing a major increase of the Masseters over the Temporalis muscles. Even though sEMG at the end of orthodontic treatment may be specifically indicative of some occlusal/functional improvements, teeth contacts after fixed appliances are scarce, therefore there is a period of functional adjusting to a new static occlusion (that is, important for deglutition) with a constant increase of the number of occlusal contacts several months after fixed appliance therapy [68, 69]. This means that ***the ideal retention appliance should not interfere with tooth digitization***.

Scan 11 is an EMG evaluation of the static dental occlusion in relation to muscular vector directional forces and tooth contacts/anatomy. During the second part of MVC testing in scan 11, dental practitioners place cotton rolls over the dental arches. This enables them to evaluate muscle output without any tooth contact. The use of cotton rolls usually provides increased support which results in a greater output from the masseter and temporalis muscles. This could be because tooth contact, which is a factor in malocclusion, is removed from the equation. Additionally, the use of cotton rolls permits a slight but positive mandibular repositioning. However, there may be instances where muscles become exhausted and fail to produce an increase in output despite a reduction in excess freeway space, the absence of tooth contact or malocclusion.

The use of cotton rolls to eliminate tooth contact during scan 11 evaluation may reveal skeletal asymmetry discrepancies. However, the author approaches this with caution. It is important to note that a majority of the orthodontic and non-orthodontic population exhibit left/right discrepancies, either in the mandibular, maxillary, or both skeletal structures [70, 71]. These even slight asymmetries may alter muscle s-EMG output and there is some evidence that functional asymmetries might even be linked to TMD [72]. In general, everybody is somewhat asymmetric, functionally and anatomically. This means that asymmetry is a normal feature and the continuous search for a symmetric perfection is a more cosmetic matter. Symmetry is not a constant human anatomical characteristic. Animal and human internal organs are disposed of according to function rather than symmetry. Even functionally we are asymmetric: think dominant eye and right-handed control. But we identify in symmetry a characteristic of fine physical development. Attractiveness is linked to bilateral symmetry [73]. Aesthetically, all these factors are true, but not all asymmetries are perceived and measured, especially for what regards muscles of mastication. So, searching for a perfect balance during an s-EMG testing is desirable but not imperative. That is why muscle balancing should be read with an arithmetic proportion and expressed in percentages. Usually acceptable is a 15–20% difference in muscle output when left vs right is considered.

A rational clinical diagnosis for asymmetries will consider age, sex, and quantitative and functional aspects. EMG testing in asymmetries is controversial. There are two main aspects to be taken into consideration when considering asymmetry of the face, the first being the *perception of pathological face asymmetry*, and the second being *occlusal/anatomical/functional measurable asymmetry*. The two may not be linked one to the other, in the sense that there could be a perceived facial disharmony due to asymmetry without important occlusal/dento-alveolar/maxillary canting and compromised function. This is the case of aesthetic asymmetries that can be perceived either statically or/and dynamically in patients that have soft tissue deviations for the nose or chin mainly. These are aesthetic problems that are generally easy and brilliantly resolved by plastic surgeons. A different problem is when the skeletal and dental defects are the main responsible for a perceived disharmony of the face [74–77]. In addition, it is crucial for orthodontists to differentiate between two primary patient groups: growing children and adult patients. The treatment objectives differ for these two groups, as the growth potential and adaptive nature of growing children can be utilized to prevent or minimize the development of skeletal asymmetries in the future. In contrast, adult patients may require surgical interventions or, at best, dental prosthetic treatment in conjunction with mandibular repositioning. Orthodontic treatment plays a significant role in preparing severe asymmetries perceived in adult patients for pre-surgical and pre-prosthetic procedures.

Asymmetry of the Face in the Growing Child

Children presenting an asymmetry of the face should always be assessed for juvenile idiopathic arthritis [78–80] and ocular torticollis [81]. Postural inclinations of the head determine an alteration/adaptation in the masticatory system as a form of compensation for a change in head posture [82]. Facial/dental asymmetries accompany more frequent sagittal discrepancies, and the causes are skeletal (sometimes even genetic) and dento-alveolar [83–85]. When dento-alveolar asymmetry is present, usually the mandibular condyles are symmetric, but with time the orthodontically untreated young patient may develop a condylar skeletal discrepancy. Fortunately, early resolution of dental crossbite avoids severe condylar asymmetry [86–88]. When pain is present, whatever the grade of aesthetic asymmetry, a functional analysis should be carried on determining if the asymmetry could be the cause to TMD-related pain. As neuromuscular dentists, we apply a TENS to decondition the musculature and uncover the cause of the aesthetic-skeletal asymmetry. The majority, if not all asymmetries, lie in a condylar resorption/anomaly; it is very rare to identify a pure mandibular body/ramus anatomical asymmetry.

Asymmetry of the Face in Adulthood

Adults with open-bite skeletal morphology are at higher risk of bilateral condylar resorption and associated asymmetries [89]. Besides the specific morphological open-bite trait, in general, the alteration of the mandibular symmetry is generally associated with canting of the maxillary plane of occlusion. This maxillary skeletal inclination may be skeletal or dento-alveolar. So, besides the cases due to specific pathologies where the asymmetry is a result of obvious factors like trauma, diseases like hemimandibular hyperplasia or hemifacial microsomia, tumors, or similar causes, we as neuromuscular practitioners *apply TENS to decondition muscular adaptation to the skeletal asymmetry* and undercover the possible anatomical alterations that cause asymmetry. Since, as previously said, muscle insertion and origin do not change and cannot be changed by treatment, deconditioning the postural musculature uncovers the cause of skeletal discrepancy. Figure 5.11a, b shows a schematic representation of what happens to mandibular/condylar position after correct TENS application on a laterally deviated to the left adult individual with crossbite. These asymmetries are the most frequently observed in orthodontic offices and are categorized as orthodontic, pre-surgical, or pre-prosthetic, depending on the severity. Skeletal asymmetry typically originates from the condylar/fossa area, where one condyle is underdeveloped or absorbed for unspecified reasons. The occlusal plane is usually tilted toward the deviation, and a dental crossbite may be present. By applying TENS, the skeletal discrepancy can be identified by detecting the differential quantitative freeway space on the affected side. This can result in significant improvement of both aesthetic asymmetry and freeway space. Patients with skeletal asymmetry often have associated functional asymmetry, as muscle function adapts to the skeletal asymmetry. Usually, masseter hypertrophy is observed in patients with a reduction of the vertical dimension on the working side. Caution must be taken in evaluating any asymmetry of the face because there is always a remote possibility of familial or congenital masseter hypertrophy [90]. If, by applying ULF-TENS properly, there is no gain of the vertical dimension on the affected side, it is usually due to wrong ULF-TENS application for a non-identified disc interference (or any other internal derangement of the TMJ), which is a contraindication to TENS use. In other circumstances, obviously, the resulting bite

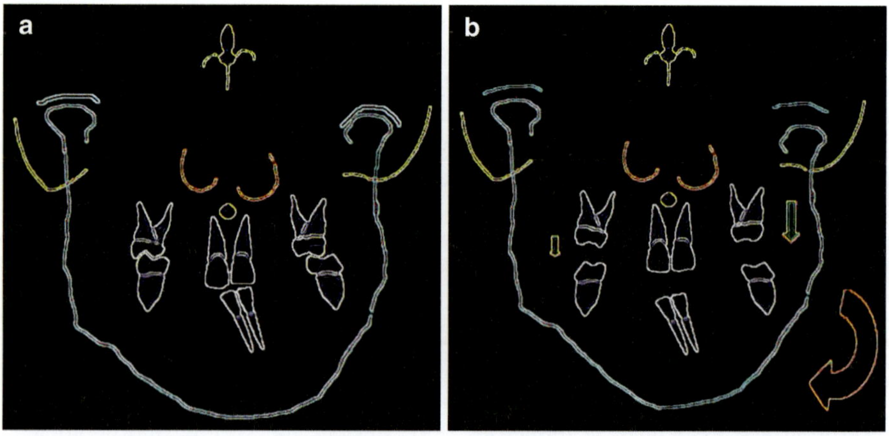

Fig. 5.11 (**a**, **b**) Resulting effect of TENS on skeletal asymmetry of the face in an adult individual before and after TENS application according to N.O. protocol

registration is ***at best*** equivalent to the missing occlusal and skeletal support needed for the correction. Therefore, when a dental correction is sufficient, orthodontics seems the correct solution, with forced extrusion mechanics of the teeth on the reduced VD side for the maxillary plane canting. This produces a vertical/sagittal condylar distraction that with time will readapt anatomically. The same can be said for prosthetic solutions, which correct the occlusal plane in a much shorter period of time. Furthermore, a neuromuscular orthotic can be immediately constructed and be utilized before any other therapeutic decision to validate the mandibular/condylar position and its function. These types of "condylar distraction" are the result of a new condylar position dictated by muscle deconditioning and or manual intervention. When orthodontics alone cannot be considered the sole therapeutic approach because the discrepancy is beyond orthodontic (prosthetic) limits, then a wise programming for surgery is necessary.

There is some bad news too for the treatment of asymmetries. If we do not consider some exceptional lifetime results regarding orthodontic/prosthetic *mild* cases of asymmetry that are stable for years, *all asymmetry treatments relapse.* Surgical treatments, orthodontic treatments, and prosthetic treatments, give very beautiful pleasing results at the end of active treatment. When analyzed at regular annual intervals, relapse increases proportionally. There are not many studies on the relapse rates, and indications seem to be between 24 and over 50% [91–93]. This means that the treatment objectives for specific asymmetry correction should be more realistic and less hypothetical. These objectives include *camouflage surgery* for expected relapse for facial asymmetry following orthopedic surgical correction, the *absence of dental crossbites* for adults, and *improvement of facial symmetry* in the growing child. The main objective of any correction of skeletal asymmetry or dento-alveolar asymmetry remains the creation of a correctly positioned maxillary plane. It may seem logical to many, but the correction of maxillary plane canting should be the first step to correction to any skeletal asymmetry.

Condylar hyperplasia is a rare condition that can be the cause of facial asymmetry and this pathology should be considered when evaluation any facial deformity [94]. This is a condition that should be diagnosed with bone scintigraphy and not confused with other pathologies like hemifacial hypertrophy, unilateral micrognathia, or laterognathia [95]. These rare conditions are most likely treated with orthognathic surgery [96]. Our main interest though, lies in the most common asymmetries that are perceived as pathological because the visual threshold of symmetry is exceeded [77], and the accompanying malocclusions are of orthodontic interest. Mandibular displacement can be the cause of facial asymmetry and there is evidence that unilateral and bilateral crossbite determines condylar asymmetry as well [86–88, 97, 98]. Treatment, correction of crossbites, should be initiated early in childhood to avoid adult condylar asymmetry [88]. Emphasis must be acknowledged to not treat maxillary plane canting with intrusion on the normal vertically developed side, but rather *favor condylar vertical distraction of the affected side.* The affected side being an anatomically reduced/altered condyle. This is because there is evidence that condylar vertical/AP distraction improves condylar surface remodeling [99–101], while compressional forces on the condyle can do the opposite with chondrocyte proliferation [102]. Furthermore, after TENS application, the bite registration can be used to build a functional appliance (especially in the growing patient), possibly the Frankel or Bionator activator, that will sustain articular position and at the same time provide condylar remodeling [103]. These functional appliances regulate and control mandibular movements favoring a symmetrical aperture/closure trajectory.

Figures 5.12, 5.13, 5.14, 5.15, 5.16, 5.17, and 5.18 show an interesting "family case" where the first treatment was surgery performed to the father of two children, the second to his eldest son with functional therapy after RPE. The third child is still very young and still a baby but already has some mandibular postural problems (see photo). The small baby postures the mandible left at rest position. Besides cases where genetic traits are the main factors in the determination of skeletal discrepancies, and of course this family case could fall in this group, there seems to be something altered in mandibular posture more linked to habit rather than anything else. Could there be a genetic trait to mandibular posture habits?

Figure 5.9 shows the intra and extraoral photos of the father before surgical and orthodontic correction. Note how the bi-pupillary plane is correct during ICP but is

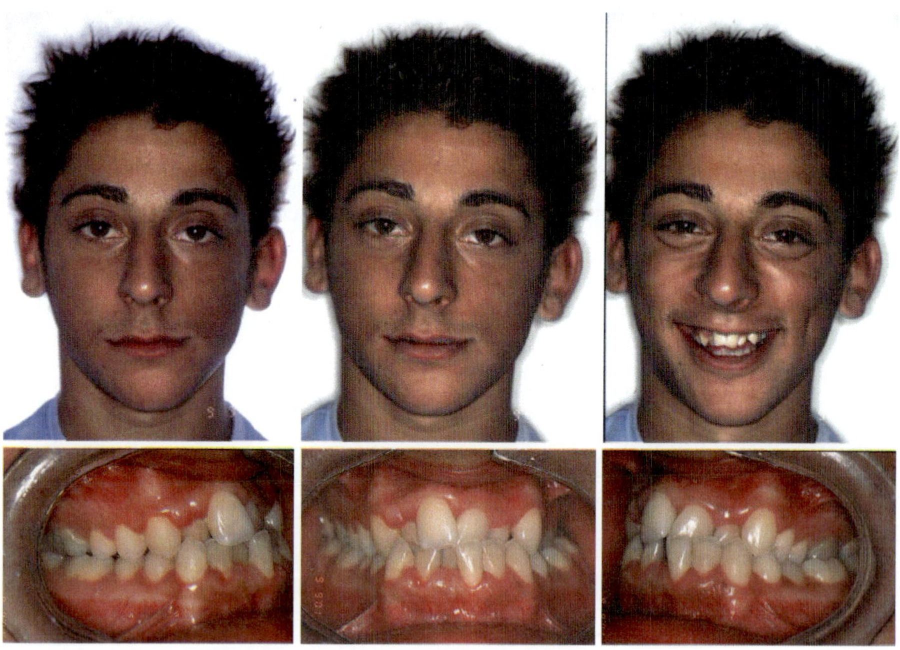

Fig. 5.12 Class III with facial asymmetry. Showing initial extraoral and intraoral photos of father before orthodontic presurgical treatment. Upper, from left to right frontal in ICP, frontal in HRP, frontal during a smile. Lower from left to right intraoral occlusion in ICP lateral left, frontal, lateral right

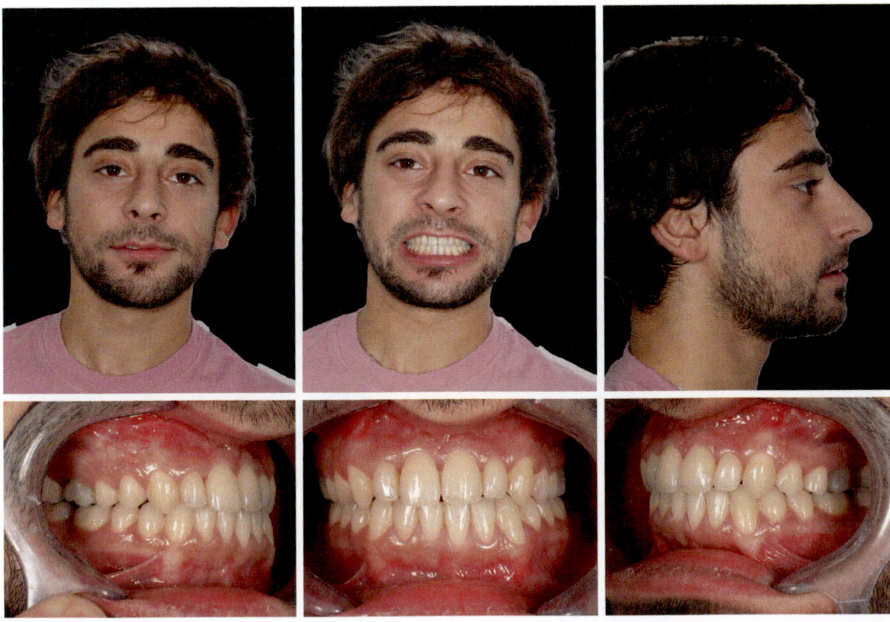

Fig. 5.13 Same case as in Fig. 5.9, Class III with facial asymmetry. Showing final extraoral and intraoral photos at 1 year after orthodontic surgical correction. Upper, from left to right frontal in ICP, frontal in CO while smiling, lateral during CO. Lower from left to right intraoral occlusion in ICP lateral left, frontal, lateral right

tilted to patient's left (affected side) as soon as teeth are not in CO (in HRP). The intraoral photos show posterior bilateral crossbite and crossbite of both lateral incisors.

Figure 5.13 shows the final case after surgical and orthodontic correction. The first part of the surgical correction was a SARPE, and the expansion obtained was the maximum possible for the RPE screw (10 mm). Bimaxillary surgery, although successful, did not correct all of the maxillary canting. Patient was satisfied with the results.

Figure 5.14 shows extra- and intraoral photos after 17 years of surgery. Unfortunately, retention was very limited, and the patient did not show up for regular check-ups. While the extraoral photos show an acceptable aesthetic result after 17 years, the intraoral photos show a relapse of the left posterior first and second molar toward crossbite (working side). We took advantage of the rare opportunity to visit the father to perform a complete K7 functional analysis the results of which are shown in Fig. 5.15.

Figure 5.15 shows the partial of a complete functional analysis of the pre-mentioned patient. With some surprise, the results look better than expected. Scan 1 shows a good opening and a good speed for the functional task. Scan 2 shows an excess of freeway space (5 mm) and a good AP movement (3.1 mm). Mandibular

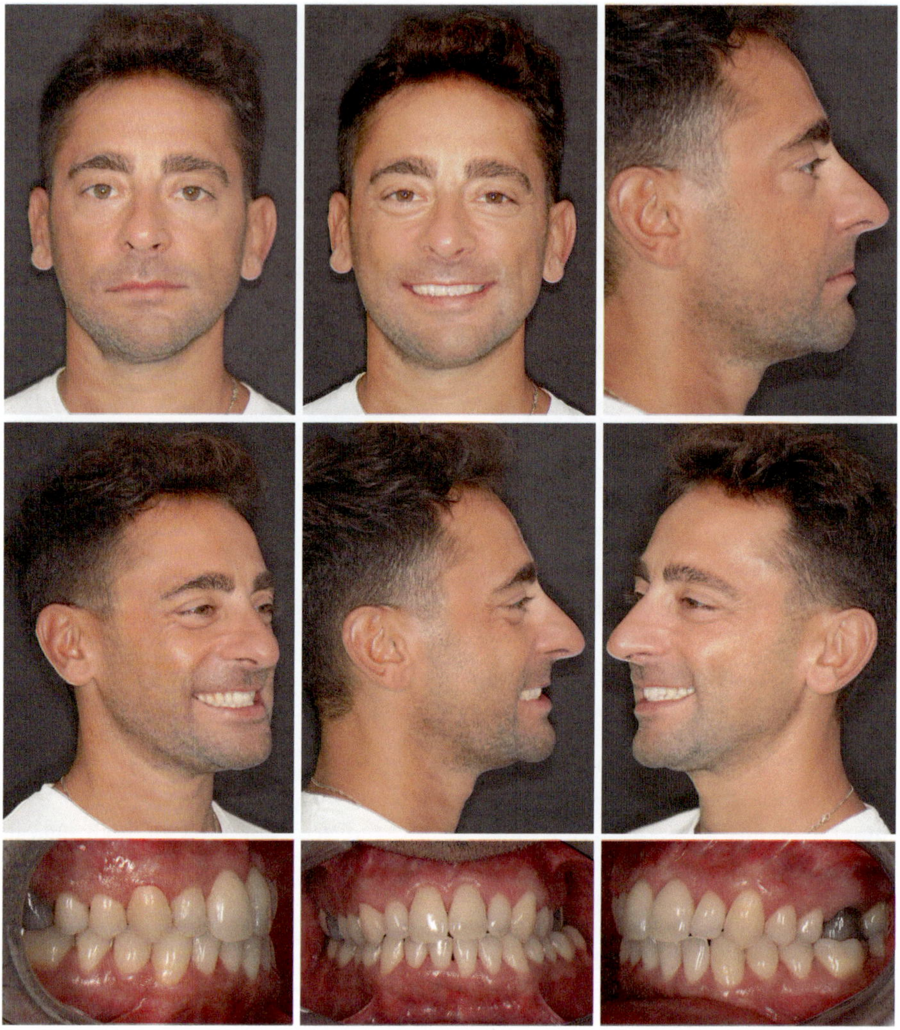

Fig. 5.14 Continued from Fig. 5.13, Class III with facial asymmetry. Showing extraoral and intraoral photos at 17 years after orthodontic pre-surgical and surgical correction. The patient applied retention for 6 months after treatment. Upper, from left to right frontal in ICP, frontal in CO while smiling, Lateral during CO. Middle from left to right, lateral right, right profile, and lateral left. Lower from left to right intraoral occlusion in ICP lateral left, frontal, lateral right

rest position is obviously to the right, at 1 mm away from the midline in CO. Scan 11 in natural maximal clench shows a good overall output of both the temporalis and masseters, with a slight cross-pattern where LMM > RMM and RTA > LTA. These results can be explained by the general tendency for systems to increase function stability over time. The masseter output on the working side is greater than that of the balancing side [104]. This is in contrast with some literature where masseter activity in MVC (Maximum Voluntary Clench) is reduced on the crossbite side and there is an increase in Anterior Temporalis output due to force

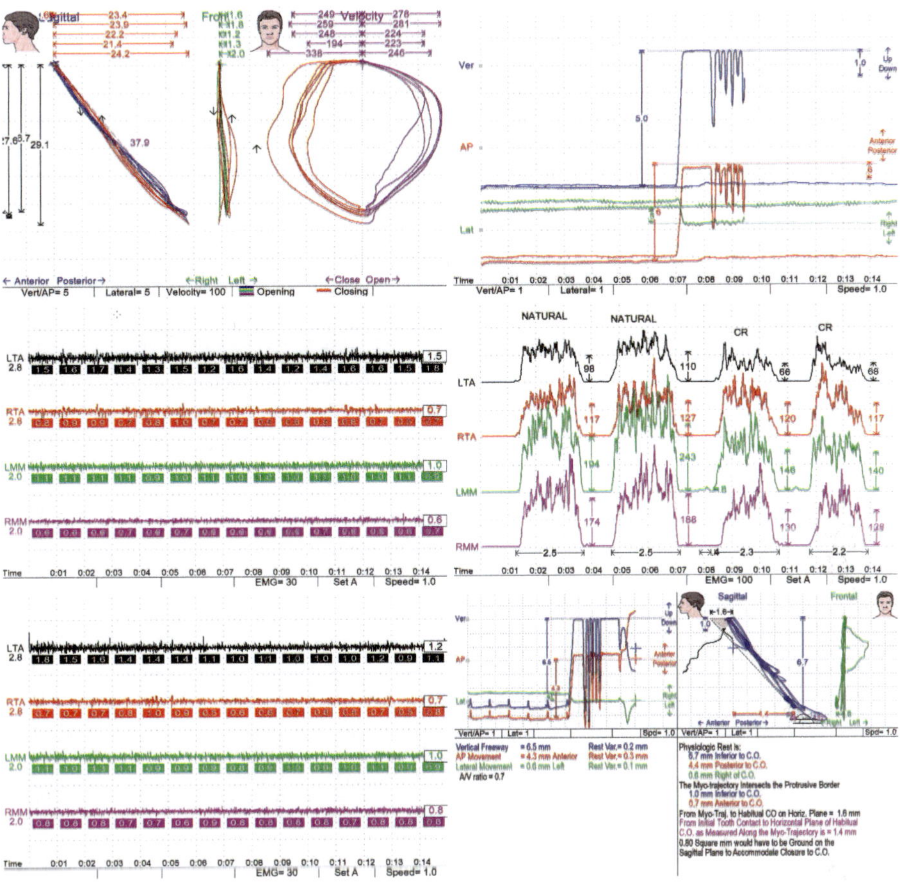

Fig. 5.15 Partial complete scan analysis of the same patient in Figs. 5.13 and 5.14, 17 years after treatment. Upper from left to right: scans 1 and 3. Middle from left to right scans 9 and 11. Lower from left to right scans 10 and 4/5

compensation [105]. In general, in ***young individuals***, the thickness of the masseter on the working side could be reduced to avoid occlusal interferences thus reducing masseter muscle function in MVC [106]. As time passes and developmental and adaptive functions compensate occlusally (muscle function initially adapts but with time is a developmental factor), an increase in function via scan 11 can be appreciated. Scan 4/5 confirms an increase in freeway space and a sagittal discrepancy of 1.6 mm on the horizontal plane of occlusion. The patient is asymptomatic and has never had any occlusal complaints. A quick analysis of the panoramic radiology assessments in the years does stimulate suspicion of a modest case of right condylar hyperplasia, even though in these cases of asymmetry, the contralateral condyle is generally stimulated to a compensating growth pattern and can increase in size (Fig. 5.16).

The young boy seen in Fig. 5.17 is the son of patient seen and described in Figs. 5.12, 5.13, and 5.14. A Class III with skeletal open bite can be a familiar issue

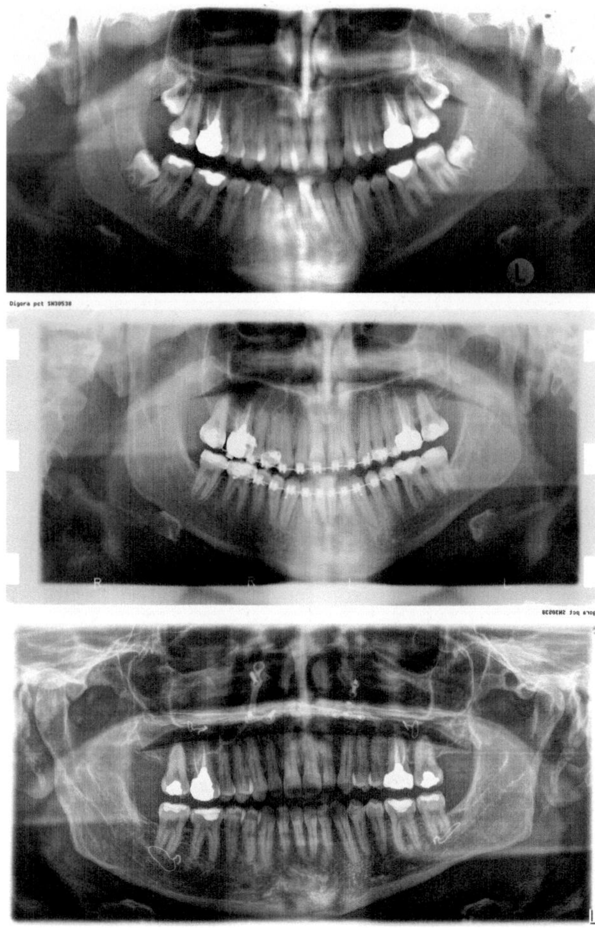

Fig. 5.16 Panoramic X-rays before, during, and at 17 years after treatment

and, as previously said, skeletal facial asymmetry is more frequent in Class III individuals [91]. There is a crossbite of the left upper incisor and left upper canine. The lateral deviation is accompanied by upper maxillary dento-alveolar canting to the affected side. By "affected side," it is intended that there is a reduction in the height and development of the left condyle. The lateral deviation to the left is the result of an altered condyle *which is a skeletal problem.* There is a reduced vertical dimension (an increase in freeway space) on the same side, and this reduction of vertical dimension is *a dental-alveolar response to a change in the functional dynamics* caused by a mono-lateral working side (left). Unfortunately, the decreased vertical dimension on one side as seen in asymmetries, determines an asymmetric function of mastication with compressional forces mainly on the working side, thus aggravating the asymmetry over time.

Figure 5.18 shows photos at age 7.5 years. Since collaboration is doubtful, a simple upper removable appliance is manufactured to guide the mandible in a more

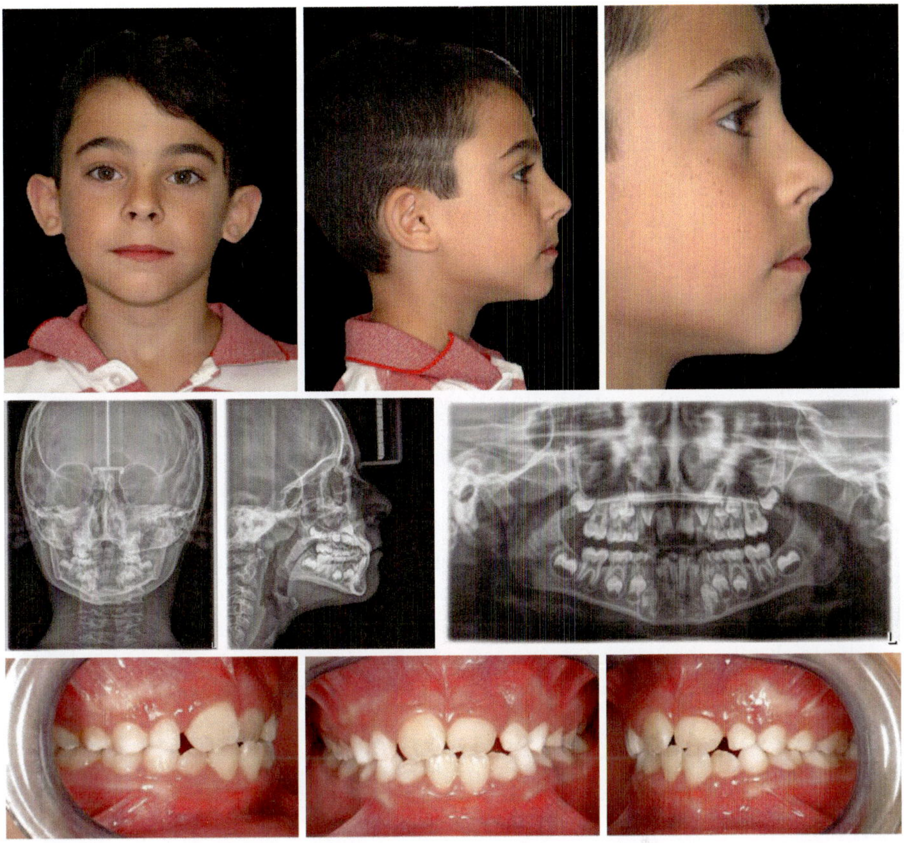

Fig. 5.17 Boy at 7.5 years age Class III open-bite with facial asymmetry. Showing initial extraoral and intraoral photos and cephalograms, panoramic X-rays before treatment. Upper, from left to right frontal in ICP, profile during CO. Middle: from left to right, PA cephalogram, lateral cephalogram, and panoramic X-rays. Lower from left to right intraoral occlusion in ICP lateral left, frontal, lateral right

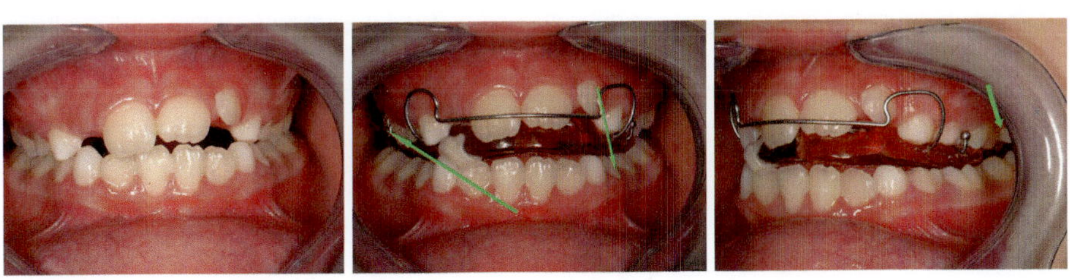

Fig. 5.18 Intraoral photos from left to right, age 7.5 years, frontal, frontal with an upper removable appliance, lateral with an upper removable appliance. See text for explanation

centered position in CO while the posterior upper left molar is left free to erupt (green arrow on the image on the right). The dento-alveolar canting of the upper arch should be corrected by permitting the extrusion of the left molar and consequently maintaining the achieved extrusion to use as the posterior vertical reference for the extrusion of the premolars. This ideal extrusion of the upper posterior sector of the affected side should rebalance and correct upper arch canting. At age 8 years, Fig. 5.19, a Bionator is constructed and a composite is added to the left superior deciduous canine. The objectives here are different and resemble functional rehabilitation techniques that aim to correct the Functional Masticatory Angle (FMA) as suggested by Planas [107, 108]. The composite increases the steepness of lateral left canine disocclusion, while selective grinding of the lower deciduous teeth on the right side, permit an increase of the angles of lateral disocclusion. The green arrows show how there is a selective grinding of the acrylic that permits upper molar extrusion while limiting lower molar extrusion on the affected side. Figure 5.20 shows intraoral photos of the same patient not wearing the Bionator. Note the correction given by the left canine reconstruction and its contact with the deciduous lower premolar. The green arrows show how the reconstruction of the left canine favors a more vertical disocclusion and how a slight grinding of the deciduous teeth on the right favors an increase of the disocclusion angle on that side. The functional changes adopted by changing the FMA favor an increase of work on the right side and diminish it on the left. There are indeed other treatment possibilities according to the Planas philosophy, like fixed acrylic or composite planes. The Bionator III

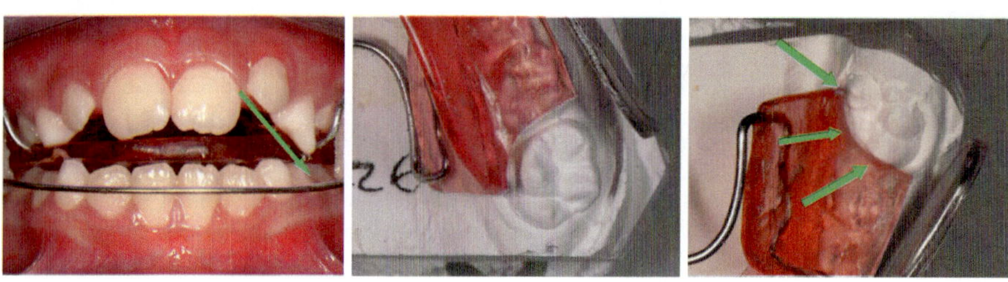

Fig. 5.19 Intraoral photos from left to right, age 8 years, frontal view with Bionator III, occlusal view of upper arch for Bionator construction, occlusal view of lower arch. See text for explanation

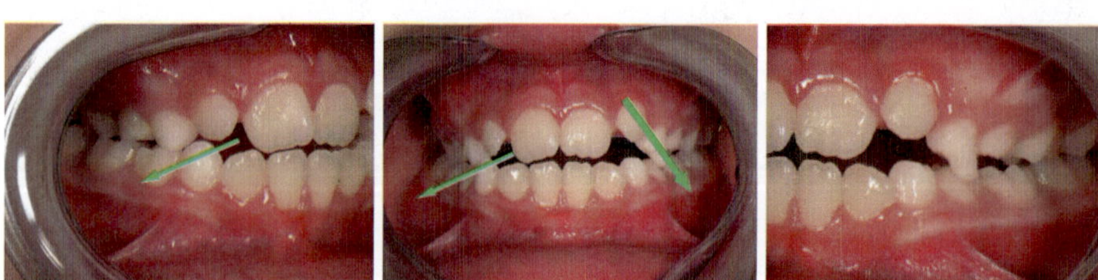

Fig. 5.20 Intraoral photos from left to right, age 8 years, from left to right, lateral right. Center, lateral left. See text for explanation

permits mandibular movements toward CO to be directed and adjusted according to functional needs. One of the characteristics of the Bionator is the acrylic behind the lower incisors that acts like a slide for the tongue that is therefore directed upward to the premaxilla and to the Coffin wiring (for appliance stabilization). There is no contact between the tongue and the lower incisors, which is usually a problem with Class III individuals because tongue posture is generally low and forward.

Figure 5.21 shows the same patient at age 9.5 years. A bonded acrylic RPE is applied with a facemask to ensure proper transverse development and sagittal improvement. The bonded acrylic is about 1 mm thicker on the posterior left molar contact (affected side). This leaves the lower right molar without acrylic contact during initial mouth closing. During slight clench, this space between acrylic and lower right molar is reduced. This determines a slight vertical condylar distraction on the affected side. One other important reason for which RPE has a positive effect on asymmetry, is that it generally determines a lowering and forward movement of the mandibular condyles [109], thus the affected side benefits greatly as the condyle moves away from the glenoid fossa to a more downward and forward position. Some authors have reported that the condylar position on the affected side is slightly higher and posterior.

At age 10.5 years another Bionator III was delivered. The functional appliance is applied on an 18-hour base to provide stabilization for the molar extrusion and to permit development of permanent teeth with selective extrusion of the affected side. Figure 5.22 shows photos taken at age 11.5 years. A general improvement in the midline and symmetry can be appreciated. The next step for the treatment of this Class III with asymmetry will be fixed appliance therapy. Now that compliance has increased with age, it is possible to assess the functional asymmetry with bioelectrical instrumentation (Fig. 5.23).

Scan 4/5 on Fig. 5.23 (bottom) shows results indicating that a vertical correction can reduce sagittal discrepancy. An asymmetric extrusion should be applied favoring the working side. PRP is slightly (0.5 mm) right to CO. Fixed appliance therapy should be applied with some left condylar distraction: the stimulation of the left condyle with the dento alveolar correction of the maxillary plane canting seem the only treatment possibility.

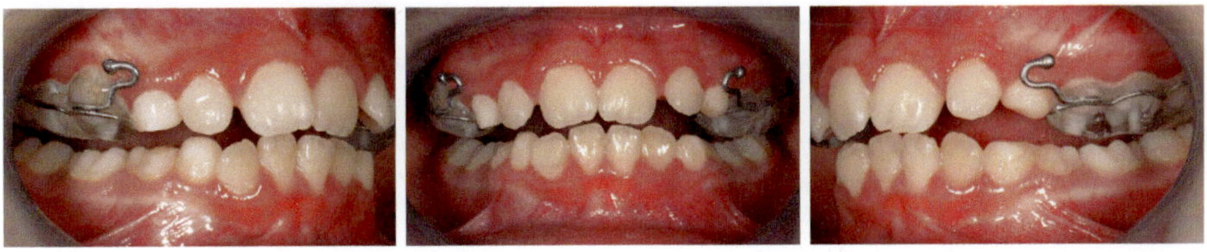

Fig. 5.21 Showing same patient at age 9.5 years. Note the pivot effect on the patient's left side created by a thicker acrylic during occlusion on bonded acrilic RPE. There is no tooth contact of the lower right first molar with the appliance at *initial contact* in CO. As bite force is increased, a vertical condilar distraction is created on the left (not shown)

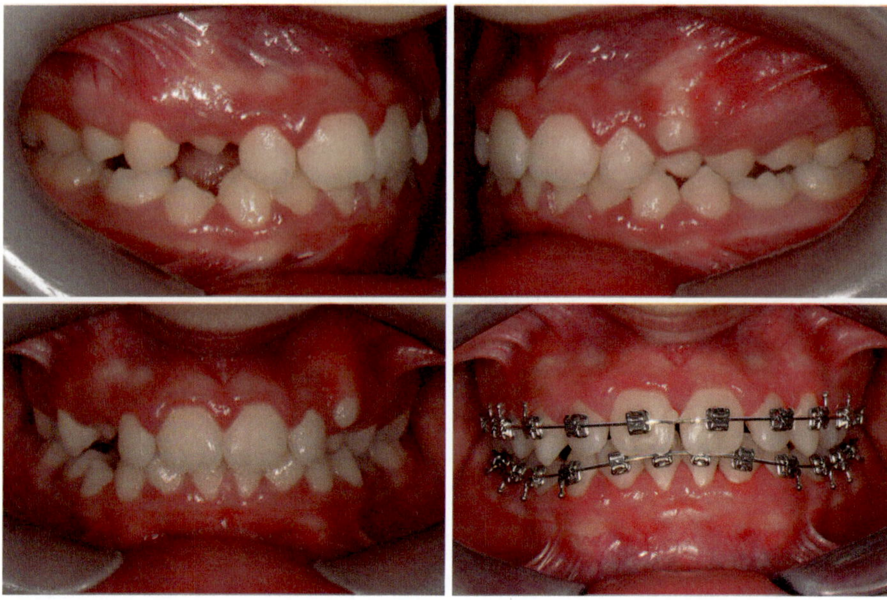

Fig. 5.22 Intraoral photos at age 11.5 years, in CO and with fixed appliance at 12 years of age

Figure 5.24 shows photos taken of the 41 months brother. This mandibular position seems a habit and there is no medical reason for this. All family has been checked by an ENT and are all well from a breathing issues. Also eye problems have been taken into account and no pathology uncovered. Nothing worth mentioning in medical history.

sEMG in maximum clench (scan 11) in morphological asymmetries can give mixed results, but in general there is a diminishedtotal output during MVC on the side of the reduced vertical dimension if a crossbite is present [110, 111]. Not all researchers agree with these results [112]. Hypothetically, other factors concur with the results of the S-EMG outputs, like AP discrepancies that cause mandibular entrapment. The cotton roll test, which excludes dental occlusion and for this reason excludes prematurities and deviating tooth contacts, generally tends to balance total muscle output. The increase in freeway space on the affected side is de facto a reduction of the occlusal support and for this reason should be responsible for a diminished muscle output relative to the unaffected side, but the *self-compensating factors and continuous exercise* due to "working side activity" tend, over time, to re-establish bite force/output of the masseters (as seen on scan 11 Fig. 5.15). For this reason, when a posterior crossbite is present on the affected side, it could be that premature tooth contacts initially reduce muscle response on that same side. In general, the adult patient usually produces higher muscle outputs during MVC on the working side.

It is important to note that functional muscular asymmetries are often present in the general population despite appearing normal, having good dental occlusion, and

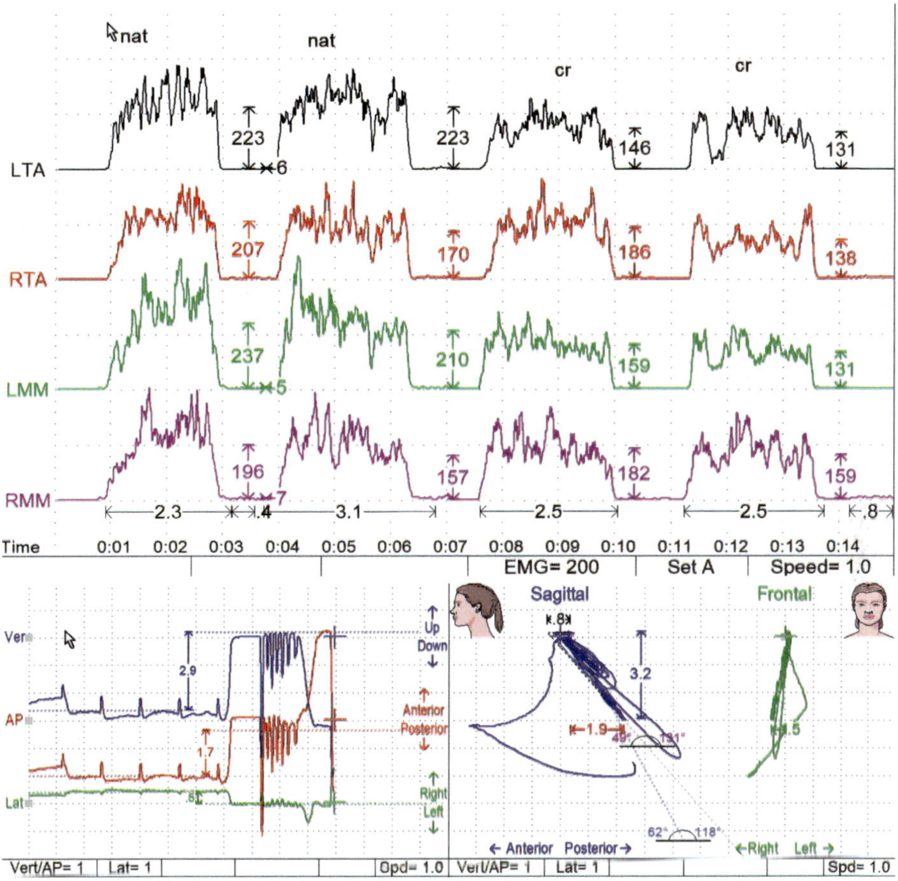

Fig. 5.23 Top: scan 11 showing MVC in occlusion and cotton rolls (second two bursts). Left masseter and left temporalis muscles have higher outputs. There is an overall high output, balanced temporalis and a good masseter response. Lower: Scan 4/5 showing that the neuromuscular trajectory is close to habitual path of closure and that the total sagittal discrepancy (0.8 mm) can be corrected by slight extrusion

facial symmetry. Therefore, the objective of treatment should focus on correcting maxillary canting by lowering the affected side where there is a loss of VD. Once the maxilla is corrected, the resulting condylar distraction of the affected side should stimulate morphological improvement of the condylar head. On the other hand, if the affected side experiences an increase in VD, it is usually due to hypocondylar activity (growth), leaving surgery as the only option available.

Sometimes visible and manually detectible, is a masseteric enlargement on the affected side in the ***adult***. The muscle shortens more on the side with reduced VD and generally it is considered a muscular hypertrophy. Surprisingly, an important case study by Newton et al. poses some interesting questions on the type of muscular enlargement. Biopsies have demonstrated muscular hyperplasia [113].

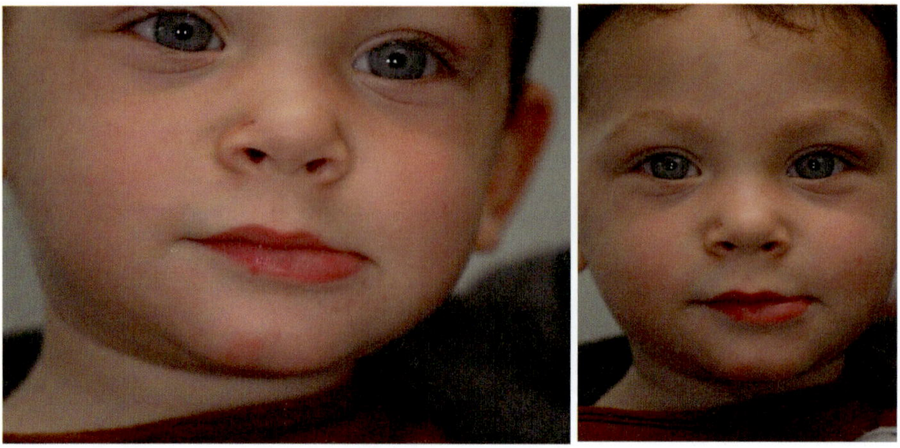

Fig. 5.24 Young brother at age 41 months with functional lateral deviation

Scan 9 evaluation of muscles at rest can show an increase in resting levels of the Posterior Temporalis (PT) on the non-affected side when compared to the affected side [114]. The PT has an important activity in lateral and retrusive movements of the mandible, and its activity is important in stabilizing the mandibular position. It could be that this functional request during chewing and swallowing elevates the resting output tone of the PT. These results are of low diagnostic value and must be framed in the general picture of patient diagnosis. Several other publications affirm the exact contrary on muscular resting outputs than the above mentioned [115, 116].

Some authors have recommended "normalizing" the sEMG during maximum voluntary contraction (MVC) because results can be affected by differences related to bioimpedance, electrode positioning, and muscle morphology [117]. Botelho et al. underline the importance of standardization (normalization) of the sEMG signal and agree with Ferrario et al. on this procedure. All these studies were conducted on healthy subjects (without missing teeth or notable skeletal asymmetries) and no control group [117, 118]. Therefore, the standardization for the sEMG could be important, but the normalization procedure done on cotton rolls during MVC is questionable. There is no general consensus on the best method for the normalization of EMG data [119]. Castroflorio et al. have demonstrated the validity and reproducibility of S-EMG during MVC and rest position [120, 121]. The use of sEMG in Neuromuscular Orthodontics and Dentistry overcomes this debate because sEMG is not a *stand-alone procedure* but part of the diagnostic technique that includes CMS. Furthermore, repetitive s-EMG assessements give overlapping outcomes when tested on the same patient on different occasions and by different operators.

As we consider relapse in asymmetry treatments, all asymmetry treatments relapse. Certainly, mild adult asymmetries treated with occlusal build-ups have a greater chance to stabilize and stimulate condylar remodelling, while orthodontic treatments have very limited success in adult treatment when attempted without maxillary plane correction or prosthetic correction.

It is important to resolve general associated issues with asymmetries, as TMD and in general TMJ pain. Cervicalgia can be present with other postural problems. Treatment objectives should be discomfort/pain improvement and a better quality of life. The reduction of the grade of severeness and the absence of initial TMJ discomfort/pain after several years of treatment are important factors and represent successful treatment objectives. Also, aesthetic acceptance years after treatment is very important. In the treatment of children and teens, the preventive aspect is the most important. Treatment at these ages represents the only way to effectively *reduce the severity of skeletal discrepancy at later ages*. Asymmetric faces do not only accompany skeletal Class I but Class II (positional and skeletal) and Class III. Therefore, sagittal discrepancies (which are generally noted by family members), are important as much as transverse discrepancies of the maxilla and the mandible (which are less noted by family members and can be identified by qualified practitioners). Prevention of more severe adult asymmetries lies in correct orthodontic procedures as well as correct orthodontic diagnostics in the child. In this regard, it is not infrequent to identify reduced condylar development (or absorption) in children that have been affected by juvenile idiopathic arthritis or similar diseases. The application of TENS as previously described, immediately increases the VD on the affected side revealing where treatment is necessary. Trauma of the mandible can also be a cause of asymmetry; even small mandibular fractures can alter the growth pattern [122]. Mono-lateral untreated crossbite determines mandibular asymmetry [88]. Functional appliances can be very useful in these cases [123–127].

Summarizing the rationale for diagnostics and treatment protocols for facial asymmetries of dental interest we can consider the following:

1. Young individuals with growth potential
   (a) Asses general pathologies that can be related to condylar development. Head posture can be determining issue in facial asymmetry and can be due to eye-related problems such as ocular torticollis [81]. Torticollis can be the result of a variety of pathologies [128]. Once excluded postural and general diseases that can affect the condyle and or the mandible, focus should be on determining the amount of discrepancy and detecting if the maxillary canting is only dento-alveolar or/and skeletal.
   (b) Setup cast models on articulator with face bow. Evaluate maxillary canting by P/A lateral cephalogram [129]. CBCT, although useful, can be avoided.
   (c) Apply TENS as by N.O. protocol for 45 min. Setup casts on articulator and TENS bite recording to evaluate correction due to muscle deconditioning.
   (d) Use this bite registration to construct functional appliances or to create any fixed or removable media for forced or spontaneous sectoral dental extrusion [79].
   (e) After correction, functional appliances should be used as retainers.
2. Adult individuals
   (a) Setup cast models on articulator with face bow. Evaluate maxillary canting and midline shift by P/A lateral cephalogram. CBCT is very useful because its use can pinpoint alterations in the anatomy of the mandible and maxilla.

In TMD cases, knowing the position and quality of the TMJ disk with MRI is imperative. Setup on the articulator should be also done with TENS bite registration. Sometimes, ULF-TENS application to relax postural mandibular musculature is not as effective as we could expect after 45 min. of application. Very useful, ULF-TENS application can be accompanied by manual vertical distraction on the affected side. Aqualizer application can be anticipated as well so that there is a prolonged and more efficacious effect of mandibular distraction.

(b) The degree of severity should be judged from an aesthetic perspective and with a functional evaluation of the masticatory system. In general, there is no exact measure to assert the grade of severeness, but aesthetically, the human eye notices any canting of the oral commissure over 3–4 mm [75] and about 4 mm of lateral deviation of the chin [130]. When possible, orthodontic, and prosthetic treatments should aim to re-establish an aesthetic acceptance and improve function of the TMJ and associated pain if present. Surgical treatment after a thorough orthodontic preparation is not an infrequent option.

(c) For nonsurgical treatments, very useful is a mandibular repositioning orthotic with a therapeutic mandibular position. Midline references for correct mandibular repositioning are the upper and lower frenulum as indicated by Silvestrini [131]. This transitory reversible treatment option is a good way to evaluate patient acceptance. Lower arch orthotics do not correct maxillary occlusal plane canting but compensate it. The orthotics aiming at temporary reversable compensation of the occlusal plane should be constructed on the upper arch. Once patient acceptance is confirmed the orthotic can be suspended, build-ups and general prosthetics should always correct maxillary plane as first step.

Even though infrequent, condylar hyperactivity should also be addressed. The reason lies in the differential diagnosis between hemimandibular hyperplasia with bone mass growth and hemimandibular hyperplasia with bone elongation. A third type is a hybrid form [132]. The affected side in these cases shows an increase in the vertical dimension, with occlusal canting and even possible loss of tooth contact in CO. There is no literature on EMG studies sufficient to be cited. Surgery is indicated only after bone scintigraphy shows end of growth in the adult. High condylectomy is usually performed accompanying other maxillary and mandibular surgical corrections.

Finally, on why treatment of asymmetry relapses so frequently, there are only a handful of hypotheses. Even the smallest differential residue of dento-alveolar or skeletal maxillary canting after treatment will determine a differential in VD to one side. Occlusal forces and swallow will always increase work toward the minimum VD side.

Since the minimum VD side will represent the working side, this aggravates the anatomically altered maxillary canting by an increased functional reaction. Furthermore, hypothetically, relapse could be the result adaptive functional pathways that the CNS has created as an *accommodation* to the pretreated asymmetry that is not completely cancelled with treatment. For example, could an adaptive swallow pattern and tongue posture to asymmetry be a cause for relapse after treatment? [133]. As previously mentioned, literature reports that what we previously believed to be a masseter hypertrophy of the affected side could indeed be hyperplasia. This could change our perspective on the treatment of asymmetries.

Surface EMG utilized on the Myotronics K7 System, as said, consists of eight channels making this system capable of evaluating the musculature of muscles that are linked to the stomatognathic system, but reside in other anatomical districts. These muscles gain importance from a more postural point of view. Testing the sternocleidomastoid or the trapezius muscles is done by many practitioners.

Surface EMG records an *average* of the muscle output and is influenced by tissue fat and resistance. The variability of surface EMG recording depends on electrode quality, placement, and bioelectrical equipment in general. When the quality of the materials used is good and there is a consensus on the procedures, the results are easily reproducible. These factors do not jeopardize the s-EMG results that can be compared in their variability to other results from other well-accepted instrumental analyses.

References

1. Johnson M, Martinson M. Efficacy of electrical nerve stimulation for chronic musculoskeletal pain: a meta-analysis of randomized controlled trials. Pain. 2007;130(1-2):157–65.
2. Anderson SI, et al. Chronic transcutaneous electrical stimulation of calf muscles improves functional capacity without inducing systemic inflammation in claudicants. Eur J Vasc Endovasc Surg. 2004;27(2):201–9.
3. Denegar CR, et al. Influence of transcutaneous electrical nerve stimulation on pain, range of motion, and serum cortisol concentration in females experiencing delayed onset muscle soreness. J Orthop Sports Phys Ther. 1989;11(3):100–3.
4. Lazarou L, et al. Effects of intensity of transcutaneous electrical nerve stimulation (TENS) on pressure pain threshold and blood pressure in healthy humans: a randomized, double-blind, placebo-controlled trial. Clin J Pain. 2009;25(9):773–80.
5. Mummolo SDP, et al. Ultra-low-frequency transcutaneous electric nerve stimulation (ULF-TENS) in subjects with craniofacial pain: a retrospective study. Cranio. 2018:1–6.
6. Wessberg GA, et al. Transcutaneous electrical stimulation as an adjunct in the management of myofascial pain-dysfunction syndrome. J Prosthet Dent. 1981;45(3):307–14.
7. Cooper BC, Kleinberg I. Establishment of a temporomandibular physiological state with neuromuscular orthosis treatment affects reduction of TMD symptoms in 313 patients. Cranio. 2008;26(2):104–17.
8. Cooper BC. The role of bioelectronic instrumentation in the documentation and management of temporomandibular disorders. Oral Surg Oral Med Oral Pathol Oral Radiol Endod. 1997;83(1):91–100.

9. Chipaila N, et al. The effects of ULF-TENS stimulation on gnathology: the state of the art. Cranio. 2014;32(2):118–30.
10. Fagade OO, Obilade TO. Therapeutic effect of TENS on post-IMF trismus and pain. Afr J Med Med Sci. 2003;32(4):391–4.
11. Ferreira AP, et al. Short-term transcutaneous electrical nerve stimulation reduces pain and improves the masticatory muscle activity in temporomandibular disorder patients: a randomized controlled trial. J Appl Oral Sci. 2017;25(2):112–20.
12. Shanavas M, et al. Transcutaneous electrical nerve stimulation therapy: an adjuvant pain controlling modality in TMD patients—a clinical study. Dent Res J (Isfahan). 2014;11(6):676–9.
13. Kamyszek G, et al. Electromyographic evidence of reduced muscle activity when ULF-TENS is applied to the Vth and VIIth cranial nerves. Cranio. 2001;19(3):162–8.
14. Monaco A, et al. Effects of transcutaneous electrical nervous stimulation on electromyographic and kinesiographic activity of patients with temporomandibular disorders: a placebo-controlled study. J Electromyogr Kinesiol. 2012;22(3):463–8.
15. Bazzotti L. Electromyography tension and frequency spectrum analysis at rest of some masticatory muscles, before and after TENS. Electromyogr Clin Neurophysiol. 1997;37(6):365–78.
16. Frucht S, Jonas I, Kappert HF. Muscle relaxation by transcutaneous electric nerve stimulation (TENS) in bruxism. An electromyographic study. Fortschr Kieferorthop. 1995;56(5):245–53.
17. Jankelson B, et al. Neural conduction of the Myo-monitor stimulus: a quantitative analysis. J Prosthet Dent. 1975;34(3):245–53.
18. Esclassan R, et al. Optimal duration of ultra low frequency-transcutaneous electrical nerve stimulation (ULF-TENS) therapy for muscular relaxation in neuromuscular occlusion: a preliminary clinical study. Cranio. 2017;35(3):175–9.
19. Grossi DB, Chaves TC. Physiotherapeutic treatment for temporomandibular disorders (TMD). Braz J Oral Sci. 2004;3(10):492–7.
20. Núñez SC, et al. Management of mouth opening in patients with temporomandibular disorders through low-level laser therapy and transcutaneous electrical neural stimulation. Photomed Laser Surg. 2006;24(1):45–9.
21. Lund JP, et al. The pain-adaptation model: a discussion of the relationship between chronic musculoskeletal pain and motor activity. Can J Physiol Pharmacol. 1991;69(5):683–94.
22. Curran SL, Carlson CR, Okeson JP. Emotional and physiologic responses to laboratory challenges: patients with temporomandibular disorders versus matched control subjects. J Orofac Pain. 1996;10(2):141–50.
23. Wilson JL. Travell and Simons': myofascial pain and dysfunction the trigger point manual, volume 1. Upper half of body, second edition. Reg Anesth Pain Med. 1999;24(4):378–9.
24. Hsieh Y-L, Yang C-C, Yang N-P. Ultra-low frequency transcutaneous electrical nerve stimulation on pain modulation in a rat model with myogenous temporomandibular dysfunction. Int J Mol Sci. 2021;22(18):9906.
25. Graff-Radford SB, et al. Effects of transcutaneous electrical nerve stimulation on myofascial pain and trigger point sensitivity. Pain. 1989;37(1):1–5.
26. Gomez CE, Christensen LV. Stimulus-response latencies of two instruments delivering transcutaneous electrical neuromuscular stimulation (TENS). J Oral Rehabil. 1991;18(1):87–94.
27. Kamali F, et al. The effect of transcutaneous electrical nerve stimulation of sympathetic ganglions and acupuncture points on distal blood flow. J Acupunct Meridian Stud. 2017;10(2):120–4.
28. Prabu R. *Neurally mediated ULF-TENS to relax Cervical and Upper Thoracic musculature as an Aid to Obtaining Improved Cervical Posture and mandibular Posture* ICCMO Antology, 2010. **XI**.
29. Eble OS, Jonas IE, Kappert HF. Transcutaneous electrical nerve stimulation (TENS): its short-term and long-term effects on the masticatory muscles. J Orofac Orthop. 2000;61(2):100–11.
30. Weinberg LA. The role of muscle deconditioning for occlusal corrective procedures. J Prosthet Dent. 1991;66(2):250–5.

31. Schindler HJ, Blaser W. T.E.N.S., a myofunctional concept for oral rehabilitation. Quintessenz. 1982;33(11):2181–91.
32. Hugger A, Hugger S, Schindler HJ. *Surface electromyography of the masticatory muscles for application in dental practice. Current evidence and future developments.* Int J Comput. Dent. 2008;11(2):81–106.
33. Monaco A, et al. Neuromuscular diagnosis in orthodontics: effects of TENS on maxillo-mandibular relationship. Eur J Paediatr Dent. 2007;8(3):143–8.
34. Thomas NR, Thomas TD, Thomas NR. The relationship between the dental occlusion, upper cervical spine and temporomandibular joints prior to and following TENS treatment in thirty six patients suffering from temporomandibular disorder. Oral Health Care. 2019;4:1–8.
35. Thomas N, Thomas T, Thomas N. The relationship between the dental occlusion, upper cervical spine and temporomandibular joints prior to and following TENS treatment in thirty six patients suffering from temporomandibular disorder. Oral Health Care. 2019:4.
36. Raman P. *Neurally mediated ULF-TENS to relax Cervical and Upper Thoracic musculature as an Aid to Obtaining Improved Cervical Posture and mandibular Posture.* Anthology IX ICCMO, 2010. **IX**.
37. Iunes D, et al. Craniocervical posture analysis in patients with temporomandibular disorder. Braz J Phys Ther. 2009;13:89–95.
38. Matheus RA, et al. The relationship between temporomandibular dysfunction and head and cervical posture. J Appl Oral Sci. 2009;17(3):204–8.
39. D'Attilio M, et al. Cervical lordosis angle measured on lateral cephalograms; findings in skeletal class II female subjects with and without TMD: a cross sectional study. Cranio. 2004;22(1):27–44.
40. Olmos SR, et al. The effect of condyle fossa relationships on head posture. Cranio. 2005;23(1):48–52.
41. Raman P, L. MICCMO. Physiologic neuromuscular dental paradigm for the diagnosis and treatment of temporomandibular disorders. CDA J. 2014;42:8.
42. Lerman MD. A revised view of the dynamics, physiology, and treatment of occlusion: a new paradigm. Cranio. 2004;22(1):50–63.
43. Lerman MD. The muscle engram: the reflex that limits conventional occlusal treatment. Cranio. 2011;29(4):297–303.
44. Cooper BC. The role of bioelectronic instruments in the management of TMD. N Y State Dent J. 1995;61(9):48–53.
45. Melis M, Di Giosia M. Applied kinesiology and dentistry—a narrative review. Cranio. 2020:1–8.
46. Schwartz SA, et al. A double-blind, randomized study to assess the validity of applied kinesiology (AK) as a diagnostic tool and as a nonlocal proximity effect. Explore (NY). 2014;10(2):99–108.
47. Cuthbert SC, Goodheart GJ Jr. On the reliability and validity of manual muscle testing: a literature review. Chiropr Osteopat. 2007;15:4–4.
48. Welch MJ, Mac Edington CD, Ritter MR. Muscular strength and temporomandibular joint repositioning. J Orthop Sports Phys Ther. 1986;7(5):236–9.
49. Julià-Sánchez S, et al. The influence of dental occlusion on dynamic balance and muscular tone. Front Physiol. 2020;10
50. Leroux E, et al. Influence of dental occlusion on the athletic performance of young elite rowers: a pilot study. Clinics (Sao Paulo, Brazil). 2018;73:e453.
51. Abdallah EF, Mehta NR, Forgione AG, Clark RE. Affecting upper extremity strength by changing maxillo-mandibular vertical dimension in deep bite subjects. Cranio. 2004;22(4):268–75. https://doi.org/10.1179/crn.2004.033. PMID: 15532310.
52. WoŸniak K, et al. Surface electromyography in orthodontics–a literature review. Med Sci Monit. 2013;19:416.

53. Filatov GN, Pinter MJ, Rich MM. Resting potential-dependent regulation of the voltage sensitivity of sodium channel gating in rat skeletal muscle in vivo. J Gen Physiol. 2005;126(2):161–72.
54. Lauriti L, et al. Influence of temporomandibular disorder on temporal and masseter muscles and occlusal contacts in adolescents: an electromyographic study. BMC Musculoskelet Disord. 2014;15(1):123.
55. Choi KH, et al. Electromyographic changes in masseter and sternocleidomastoid muscles can be applied to diagnose of temporomandibular disorders: an observational study. Integr Med Res. 2021;10(4):100732.
56. Szyszka-Sommerfeld L, et al. The diagnostic value of electromyography in identifying patients with pain-related temporomandibular disorders. Front Neurol. 2019;10
57. Klasser GD, Okeson JP. The clinical usefulness of surface electromyography in the diagnosis and treatment of temporomandibular disorders. J Am Dent Assoc. 2006;137(6):763–71.
58. Santana-Mora U, et al. Surface raw electromyography has a moderate discriminatory capacity for differentiating between healthy individuals and those with TMD: a diagnostic study. J Electromyogr Kinesiol. 2014;24(3):332–40.
59. Zieliński G, et al. Resting activity of masticatory muscles in healthy young women. 2019;4:16–23. EJMT 4(25).
60. Möller E, Sheikholeslam A, Lous I. Response of elevator activity during mastication to treatment of functional disorders. Scand J Dent Res. 1984;92(1):64–83.
61. Duthie N, Yemm R. Muscles involved in voluntary mandibular retrusion in man. J Oral Rehabil. 1982;9(2):155–9.
62. Wheeler KM, Chiara T, Sapienza CM. Surface electromyographic activity of the submental muscles during swallow and expiratory pressure threshold training tasks. Dysphagia. 2007;22(2):108–16.
63. Vaiman M, Segal S, Eviatar E. Surface electromyographic studies of swallowing in normal children, age 4-12 years. Int J Pediatr Otorhinolaryngol. 2004;68(1):65–73.
64. Vaiman M, Eviatar E, Segal S. Surface electromyographic studies of swallowing in normal subjects: a review of 440 adults. Report 1. Quantitative data: timing measures. Otolaryngol Head Neck Surg. 2004;131(4):548–55.
65. Ertekin C. Electrophysiological techniques to evaluate swallowing in central and peripheral nervous system disorders. J Clin Neurophysiol. 2015;32(4):314–23.
66. Ertekin C, Aydogdu I. Neurophysiology of swallowing. Clin Neurophysiol. 2003; 114(12):2226–44.
67. Scott BJJ, Mason AG, Cadden SW. Voluntary and reflex control of the human temporalis muscle. J Oral Rehabil. 2002;29(7):634–43.
68. Haydar B, Ciğer S, Saatçi P. Occlusal contact changes after the active phase of orthodontic treatment. Am J Orthod Dentofac Orthop. 1992;102(1):22–8.
69. Razdolsky Y, Sadowsky C, BeGole EA. Occlusal contacts following orthodontic treatment: a follow-up study. Angle Orthod. 1989;59(3):181–5. discussion 186
70. Sheats RD, et al. Prevalence of orthodontic asymmetries. Semin Orthod. 1998;4(3):138–45.
71. Bhateja NK, Fida M, Shaikh A. Frequency of dentofacial asymmetries: a cross-sectional study on orthodontic patients. J Ayub Med Coll Abbottabad. 2014;26(2):129–33.
72. Dong Y, et al. Asymmetric muscle function in patients with developmental mandibular asymmetry. J Oral Rehabil. 2008;35(1):27–36.
73. Polak M, Trivers R. The science of symmetry in biology. Trends Ecol Evol. 1994;9(4):122–4.
74. Choi KY. Analysis of facial asymmetry. Arch Craniofac Surg. 2015;16(1):1–10.
75. Chu EA, et al. Threshold of visual perception of facial asymmetry in a facial paralysis model. Arch Facial Plast Surg. 2011;13(1):14–9.
76. Huang CS, Liu XQ, Chen YR. Facial asymmetry index in normal young adults. Orthod Craniofac Res. 2013;16(2):97–104.

77. Wang TT, et al. Discriminative thresholds in facial asymmetry: a review of the literature. Aesthet Surg J. 2017;37(4):375–85.
78. Wolford LM, Cardenas L. Idiopathic condylar resorption: diagnosis, treatment protocol, and outcomes. Am J Orthod Dentofac Orthop. 1999;116(6):667–77.
79. Stoustrup P, et al. Orthopaedic splint treatment can reduce mandibular asymmetry caused by unilateral temporomandibular involvement in juvenile idiopathic arthritis. Eur J Orthod. 2013;35(2):191–8.
80. Ringold S, Cron RQ. The temporomandibular joint in juvenile idiopathic arthritis: frequently used and frequently arthritic. Pediatr Rheumatol Online J. 2009;7:11.
81. Akbari MR, et al. Facial asymmetry in ocular torticollis. J Curr Ophthalmol. 2015;27(1):4–11.
82. Silvestrini-Biavati A, et al. Clinical association between teeth malocclusions, wrong posture and ocular convergence disorders: an epidemiological investigation on primary school children. BMC Pediatr. 2013;13(1):12.
83. Haraguchi S, Takada K, Yasuda Y. Facial asymmetry in subjects with skeletal Class III deformity. Angle Orthod. 2002;72(1):28–35.
84. Alavi DG, BeGole EA, Schneider BJ. Facial and dental arch asymmetries in Class II subdivision malocclusion. Am J Orthod Dentofac Orthop. 1988;93(1):38–46.
85. Azevedo AR, et al. Evaluation of asymmetries between subjects with Class II subdivision and apparent facial asymmetry and those with normal occlusion. Am J Orthod Dentofac Orthop. 2006;129(3):376–83.
86. Kiki A, Kılıç N, Oktay H. Condylar asymmetry in bilateral posterior crossbite patients. Angle Orthod. 2007;77(1):77–81.
87. Pinto AS, et al. Morphological and positional asymmetries of young children with functional unilateral posterior crossbite. Am J Orthod Dentofac Orthop. 2001;120(5):513–20.
88. Kilic N, Kiki A, Oktay H. Condylar asymmetry in unilateral posterior crossbite patients. Am J Orthod Dentofac Orthop. 2008;133(3):382–7.
89. Tanimoto K, et al. Characteristics of the maxillofacial morphology in patients with idiopathic mandibular condylar resorption. J Clin Med. 2022;11:4.
90. Teixeira VDC, Mejia JES, Estefano A. Tratamento cirúrgico da heipertrofia benigna do masseter por abordagem intra-oral. Rev Bras Cir. 1996:165–70.
91. Severt T, Proffit W. The prevalence of facial asymmetry in the dentofacial deformities population at the University of North Carolina. Int J Adult Orthodon Orthognath Surg. 1997;12(3):171 6.
92. Yoon SY, et al. Stability and relapse of facial asymmetry following orthognathic surgery in patients with asymmetric prognathism. J Korean Soc Plast Reconstr Surg. 2003;30(6):679–84.
93. Chen Y-F, et al. Treatment outcome of bimaxillary surgery for asymmetric skeletal class II deformity. Clin Oral Investig. 2019;23(2):623–32.
94. Olate S, et al. Mandible condylar hyperplasia: a review of diagnosis and treatment protocol. Int J Clin Exp Med. 2013;6(9):727–37.
95. Gray RJM, et al. Histopathological and scintigraphic features of condylar hyperplasia. Int J Oral Maxillofac Surg. 1990;19(2):65–71.
96. Feldmann G, et al. Orthodontic and surgical treatment of unilateral condylar hyperplasia during growth—a case report. Eur J Orthod. 1991;13(2):143–8.
97. Kasimoglu Y, et al. Condylar asymmetry in different occlusion types. Cranio. 2015;33(1):10–4.
98. O'Byrn BL, et al. An evaluation of mandibular asymmetry in adults with unilateral posterior crossbite. Am J Orthod Dentofac Orthop. 1995;107(4):394–400.
99. Rabie AB, She TT, Hagg U. Functional appliance therapy accelerates and enhances condylar growth. Am J Orthod Dentofac Orthop. 2003;123(1):40–8.
100. Hagg U, et al. Condylar growth and mandibular positioning with stepwise vs maximum advancement. Am J Orthod Dentofac Orthop. 2008;134(4):525–36.
101. Xiong H, Rabie AB, Hagg U. Neovascularization and mandibular condylar bone remodeling in adult rats under mechanical strain. Front Biosci. 2005;10:74–82.

102. Teramoto M, et al. Effect of compressive forces on extracellular matrix in rat mandibular condylar cartilage. J Bone Miner Metab. 2003;21(5):276–86.
103. Shen G, Darendeliler MA. The adaptive remodeling of condylar cartilage—a transition from chondrogenesis to osteogenesis. J Dent Res. 2005;84(8):691–9.
104. Kim S-S, Lee N-K, Cha B-K. A study on the correlations between facial biotype, submento-vertex cephalometric measurements and surface EMG activity in patients with facial asymmetry. Korean J Orthod. 2006;36(3):218–27.
105. Moreno I, et al. Electromyographic comparisons between clenching, swallowing and chewing in jaw muscles with varying occlusal parameters. Med Oral Patol Oral Cir Bucal. 2008;13(3):E207-13.
106. Michelotti A, et al. Effect of occlusal interference on habitual activity of human masseter. J Dent Res. 2005;84(7):644–8.
107. Chateau MÉ et al. *Réhabilitation neuro-occlusale, RNO*. 2006: Éditions CdP.
108. Silveira S, Valerio P, Machado Júnior AJ. The law of minimum vertical dimension: evidence for improvement of dental occlusion. Eur J Dent. 2022;16(2):241–50.
109. Melgaco CA, et al. Immediate changes in condylar position after rapid maxillary expansion. Am J Orthod Dentofac Orthop. 2014;145(6):771–9.
110. Woźniak K, et al. Surface electromyography in orthodontics—a literature review. Med Sci Monit. 2013;19:416–23.
111. Piancino MG, et al. Muscular activation during reverse and non-reverse chewing cycles in unilateral posterior crossbite. Eur J Oral Sci. 2009;117(2):122–8.
112. Andrade Ada S, et al. Posterior crossbite and functional changes. *A systematic review*. Angle Orthod. 2009;79(2):380–6.
113. Newton JP, et al. Masseteric hypertrophy?: preliminary report. Br J Oral Maxillofac Surg. 1999;37(5):405–8.
114. Alarcón JA, Martín C, Palma JC. Effect of unilateral posterior crossbite on the electromyographic activity of human masticatory muscles. Am J Orthod Dentofac Orthop. 2000;118(3):328–34.
115. Troelstrup B, Moller E. Electromyography of the temporalis and masseter muscles in children with unilateral cross-bite. Scand J Dent Res. 1970;78(5):425–30.
116. Ingervall B, Thilander B. Activity of temporal and masseter muscles in children with a lateral forced bite. Angle Orthod. 1975;45(4):249–58.
117. Ferrario VF, et al. An electromyographic investigation of masticatory muscles symmetry in normo-occlusion subjects. J Oral Rehabil. 2000;27(1):33–40.
118. Botelho AL, et al. Standardization of the electromyographic signal through the maximum isometric voluntary contraction. Cranio. 2011;29(1):23–31.
119. Burden A. How should we normalize electromyograms obtained from healthy participants? What we have learned from over 25 years of research. J Electromyogr Kinesiol. 2010;20(6):1023–35.
120. Castroflorio T, et al. Reproducibility of surface EMG variables in isometric sub-maximal contractions of jaw elevator muscles. J Electromyogr Kinesiol. 2006;16(5):498–505.
121. Castroflorio T, et al. Reproducibility of surface EMG in the human masseter and anterior temporalis muscle areas. Cranio. 2005;23(2):130–7.
122. Oh Y, Oh S. Long term follow-up of children with facial asymmetry: a case report. J Korean Acad Pediatr Dent. 2018;45(3):378–85.
123. Pedersen TK, et al. Condylar condition and mandibular growth during early functional treatment of children with juvenile chronic arthritis. Eur J Orthod. 1995;17(5):385–94.
124. Silvestri A, Natali G, Iannetti G. Functional therapy in hemifacial microsomia: therapeutic protocol for growing children. J Oral Maxillofac Surg. 1996;54(3):271–8.
125. Deshayes M-J. Dentofacial Orthopedics to treat facial asymmetries before six years of age. How to balance craniofacial growth and enhance temporomandibular function. L' Orthodontie francaise. 2010;81(3):189–207.
126. Clark W, Clark WJ. Twin block functional therapy. JP Medical Ltd.; 2014.

127. Melsen B, Bjerregaard J, Bundgaard M. The effect of treatment with functional appliance on a pathologic growth pattern of the condyle. Am J Orthod Dentofac Orthop. 1986;90(6):503–12.
128. Ballock RT, Song KM. The prevalence of nonmuscular causes of torticollis in children. J Pediatr Orthop. 1996;16:4.
129. Padwa BL, Kaiser MO, Kaban LB. Occlusal cant in the frontal plane as a reflection of facial asymmetry. J Oral Maxillofac Surg. 1997;55(8):811–6. discussion 817.
130. Dong T, et al. Assessing the influence of chin asymmetry on perceived facial Esthetics with 3-dimensional images. J Oral Maxillofac Surg. 2020;78(8):1389–96.
131. Silvestrini Biavati P. Trattamento semplificato in gnatologia: il metodo Global Occlusion. Milano: Edra; 2019.
132. Obwegeser HL, Makek MS. Hemimandibular hyperplasia—hemimandibular elongation. J Maxillofac Surg. 1986;14:183–208.
133. Foletti J-M, et al. Is atypical swallowing associated with relapse in orthognathic patients? A retrospective study of 256 patients. J Oral Maxillofac Surg. 2018;76(5):1084–90.

A Simplified Protocol with the Bioelectrical Instrumentation

6

The Myotronics K7 Diagnostic System is widely regarded as the benchmark for Computerized Mandibular Scanning (CMS) due to its ability to record both quantitative and qualitative information (Fig. 6.1). Our objective is to standardize a protocol that simplifies the use of this system while maintaining the minimum information required for diagnosing most occlusal problems.

The use of a protocol offers several benefits. Firstly, it provides a checklist that aids in understanding and memorizing the correct sequence of scan execution. This is particularly beneficial for beginners who may overlook essential scans that are critical for the diagnostic picture. Secondly, a streamlined protocol reduces the volume of information required since it only necessitates the minimum number of scans needed for a basic functional analysis.

While it may be beneficial to record all orthodontic patients with CMS, not all orthodontists have the luxury of time-consuming examinations. Therefore, patient selection is critical, and the optimal diagnostic procedure is generally reserved for

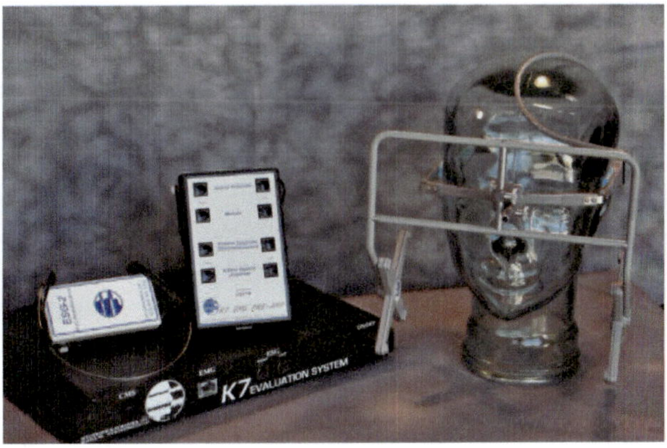

Fig. 6.1 Complete K7 evaluation system, Myotronics®, USA

F. Savastano, *Neuromuscular Orthodontics*,
https://doi.org/10.1007/978-3-031-41295-0_6

higher-risk TMD patients and adult orthodontics. For novices, it is strongly recommended that they adhere to this protocol and scan as many patients as possible within their available time.

Over time, the standardized protocol for Computerized Mandibular Scanning (CMS) will become a routine and serve as the foundation for all future evaluations. It is crucial to note that any deviation or incorrect execution, even of a single scan, can jeopardize neuromuscular orthodontic diagnostics. As the practitioner becomes more familiar with the technique, they will add scans and customize them based on specific diagnostic needs. This includes selecting and adding muscles for surface electromyography (sEMG) and incorporating additional scans as required.

The Myotronics K7 Diagnostic System provides an exceptional quantity and quality of information, and the practitioner must have the proper knowledge to adjust selection and execution accordingly. This bioelectrical instrumentation is a powerful tool to measure function and enables dynamic and static evaluation of muscle function and occlusion.

By conducting follow-ups and comparing measurements, practitioners can evaluate the quality of proper treatments and determine whether treatment objectives have been achieved. It is essential to recognize the value of consistent execution of the CMS protocol to ensure the accuracy of the diagnosis and the effectiveness of the treatment plan. In summary, adherence to the standardized protocol is crucial to the success of the CMS evaluation, and over time, practitioners will develop proficiency and expertise to tailor the protocol to their patients' specific needs.

The proposed diagnostic protocol presented herein is not confined to orthodontics but rather serves as a versatile framework for assessing occlusal function in various fields. It offers an advanced analysis that can be utilized to refine orthotic and prosthetic occlusions. The system is highly customizable and adaptable, enabling analysis of practically any muscle within the facial and neck regions, as well as beyond, using surface electromyography (s-EMG).

One of the most significant benefits of this system is the contemporaneous recording of EMG and mandibular movements. This enables a meticulous analysis of the stomatognathic system during functional tasks, thereby providing valuable insight into the complex interplay between the various components of the system. This real-time data collection allows for the identification of subtle abnormalities and imperfections that might not be otherwise detected and aids in determining the most effective interventions for addressing them.

Furthermore, the system's adaptability means that it can be employed across various disciplines and contexts, making it a valuable tool for not only orthodontics but also other related fields. It has been demonstrated to be particularly useful for fine-tuning orthotic and prosthetic occlusions, which can be challenging to achieve accurately using traditional methods. The system's ability to analyze practically any muscle in the face and neck regions, as well as beyond, provides a comprehensive assessment of the stomatognathic system, leading to more precise diagnoses and treatment plans.

Protocol Specifications

The diagnostic procedure here described, is limited to a scan description, and does explain briefly how to use the instrumentation. Further information can be retrieved from the official K7 manual.

All *diagnostic procedures* are characterized by being divided into *two parts*: before and after muscle deconditioning. *Muscle deconditioning is obtained only after 45′ minimum of TENS application with occlusal media, the Aqualizer®.*

Patient should be seated comfortably, and head posture checked according to a natural, neutral position. There has been a lot of discussion on the correct postural position for these procedures, but having a patient stand up on his feet during this examination is a complication that is not necessary.

The K7 evaluation system is composed of:

- sEMG amplifier for 8-channel electromyography.
- Electrosonograph to record TMJ noises.
- Computerized mandibular scanner.

This system plugs-in into any USB port of any Microsoft PC desktop or laptop. Mandibular movements are acquired through a sensor array that detects movements via a magnet that sticks firmly to lower incisors with a special material. The accuracy is up to 1/10 mm for mandibular movements. Since this system is highly customizable and reads movements in any direction of space, scan enumeration refers to specific pre-adjusted recordings with specific gains. All scans can be personalized with specific data output and gains setting.

Scan 1. (Sagittal/Frontal and Speed Mode) This scan analyzes an open and closed pattern. It is set to visualize sagittal and frontal movements of the mandible during opening and closing together with the analysis of speed. The patient is instructed to open and close as wide as comfily possible while increasing speed. On the right (Fig. 6.2), the speed analysis is added to this scan. The faster the speed of movement, the wider the tracing.

In general, the gains here described are 5 mm for each side of the dotted square, that is, the Vertical/Antero-Posterior and lateral are equal to 5 mm per side (Fig. 6.2). The gain selection is a magnification selection and can be changed by the operator. This would be the case of a patient that has a reduced opening and needs a magnified visualization to represent a smaller open/close pattern

One other modality of scan taking is sweep mode. This modality is a graphic representation linked to a time interval as continuous live recordings move from left to right (sweep). Sweep mode is used, as in electrocardiography to record s-EMG output data of the muscles of mastication continuously over a fixed period of time (adjustable by gain). This modality is also used to reproduce real time data of mandibular movements. Scans can be personalized to show s-EMG data and CMS movements at the same time.

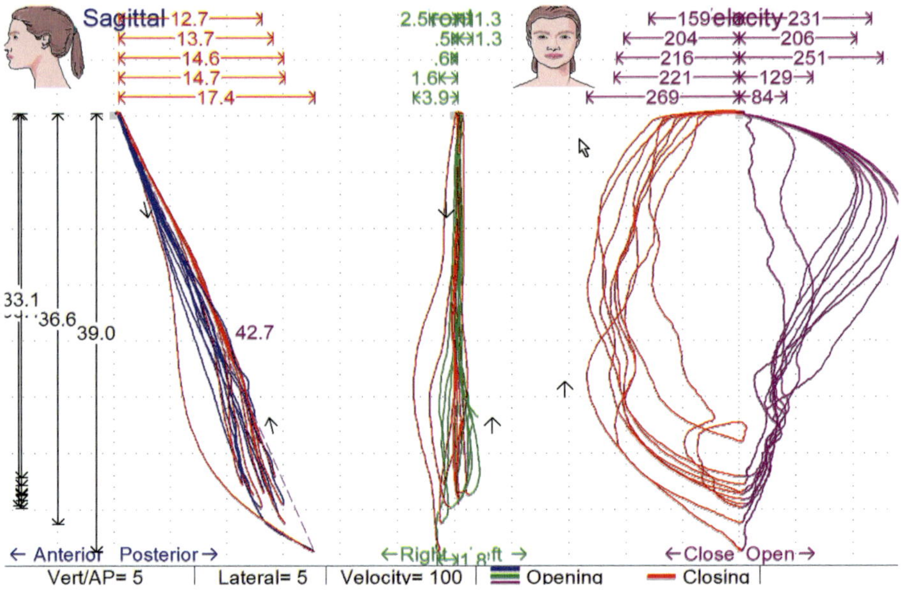

Fig. 6.2 Scan 1 of CMS with K7 evaluation system. From left to right: sagittal opening—frontal opening—velocity opening/closing diagram

Scan 3. (Freeway Space Before TENS) This scan is executed in sweep mode. It is a graphic representation with three recordings, each one for every dimension (Sagittal line, Frontal line, and Lateral line). The patient is instructed to relax, let the mandible fall due to gravity and when instructed, close to CO and then "tap-tap" to secure occlusion in ICP. This scan records the *vertical freeway space* from habitual rest position to CO. It can be visualized in non-sweep mode by changing the visualization to sagittal/frontal, like in scan 1.

Figure 6.3 shows scan 3 and the correct execution from HRP: please note that the baseline(s) should be carried at least twice on the monitor screen and overlap *to show HRP is constant*. Scan 3 cannot be completed without the "tap-tap" request to assure proper CO. Without this last execution, scan 3 is useless. The sensibility of the instrumentation is set to the highest possible magnification, 1 mm per side of the squares.

Scan 21. (Swallow Test, Sweep Mode with Filtered EMG) This scan 3 with the added filtered EMG is used to identify if the patient swallows with tongue between the teeth. The patient is asked to relax and then asked to swallow saliva and then "tap-tap" to secure CO.

Figure 6.4 shows scan 21 (scan 3+ filtered sEMG of masseters and temporalis muscles). The swallow pattern of a patient and the energy involved in the task can be best assessed through this scan, making it a critical component of patient evaluation. This scan is typically initiated by requesting the patient to perform a Voluntary Saliva Swallow (VSS) and attending a Spontaneous Saliva Swallow (SSS) for

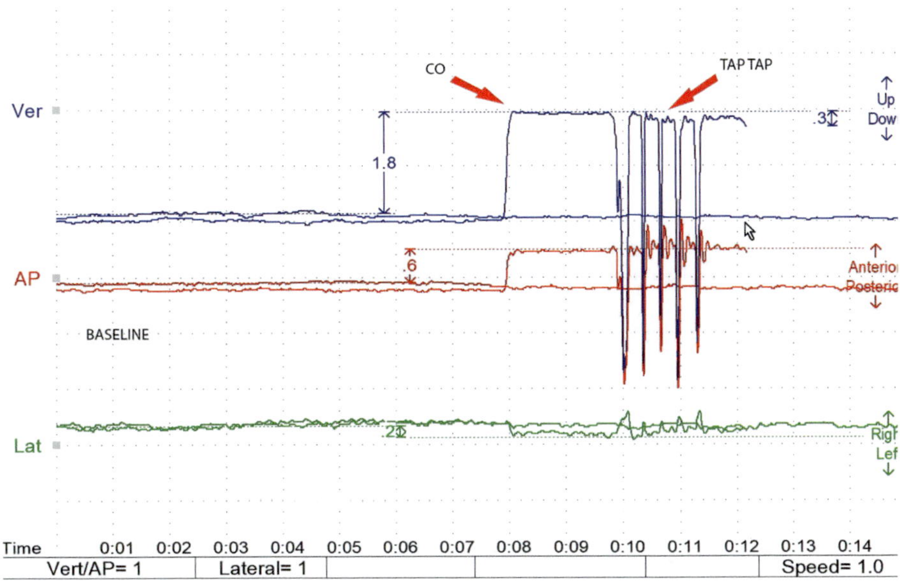

Fig. 6.3 Scan 3 of CMS with K7 evaluation system. *AP* anterior-posterior, *Lat* lateral, *Ver* vertical, *CO* centric occlusion, *TAP-TAP* repetitive closures to CO to assure ICP

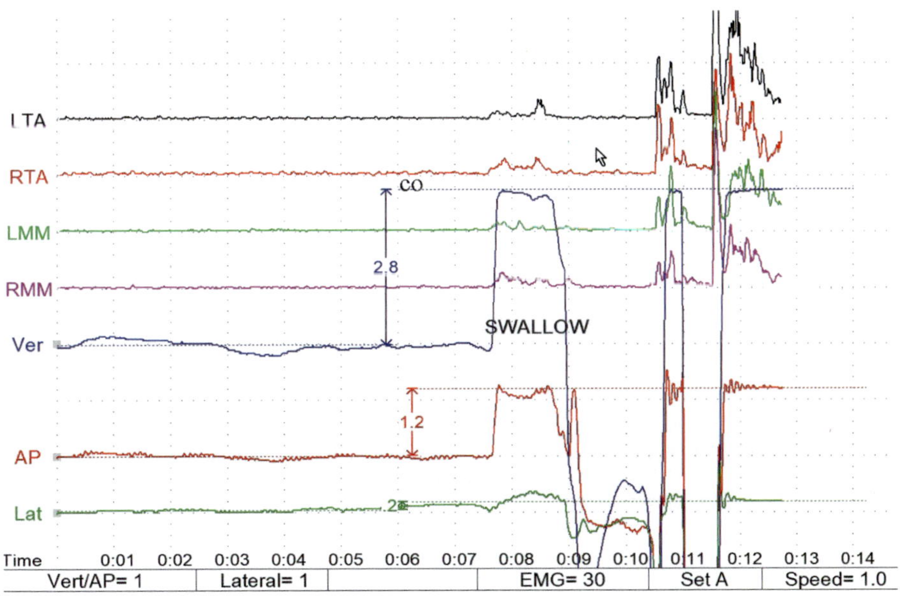

Fig. 6.4 Scan 21 of CMS with K7 evaluation system. *AP* anterior-posterior, *CO* centric occlusion, *EMG* electromyography, *Lat* lateral, *LMM* left masseter muscle, *LTA* left anterior temporalis, *RMM* right masseter muscle, *RTA* right anterior temporalis, *Vert* vertical. *Dotted line from CO = shows level of maximum intercuspation (ICP)*

accurate analysis. To ensure that the data obtained is reliable, it is recommended to record and save the scan multiple times. It is imperative to conclude the scan with a "tap-tap" procedure, which confirms the identification of centric occlusion(ICP). Without this final step, the scan would be rendered useless.

Moreover, the sensibility of the surface Electromyography (sEMG) can be adjusted to improve the identification of clinical information. By manipulating the sEMG gain, the sequence of muscle activation during swallowing can be identified with greater confidence. It is noteworthy that this scan involves recording the activity of other muscles too, such as the digastric and the posterior temporalis, peri-oral and sternocleidomastoid muscles, besides the temporalis and masseter muscles.

Figure 6.5 shows **scan 11 (EMG processed mode, MVC).** The examination of total sEMG output during maximum voluntary clench (MVC) represents a direct analysis of muscle response to malocclusion. The first burst is on natural denture and clench at maximum force in ICP. The second burst represents clench at maximum force on cotton rolls. Cotton rolls have two specific consequences on this test: first, they increase the vertical dimension, that is, they reduce freeway space. Secondly, the exclude teeth contact, that is, dental occlusion. The exclusion of dental occlusion could leave muscle function to adapt and respond only to skeletal characteristics. Even if this sounds realistic, the author is cautious on asserting such importance to this test and identifies the second burst on cotton rolls as a way of excluding teeth contact and reducing afferent periodontal proprioception to

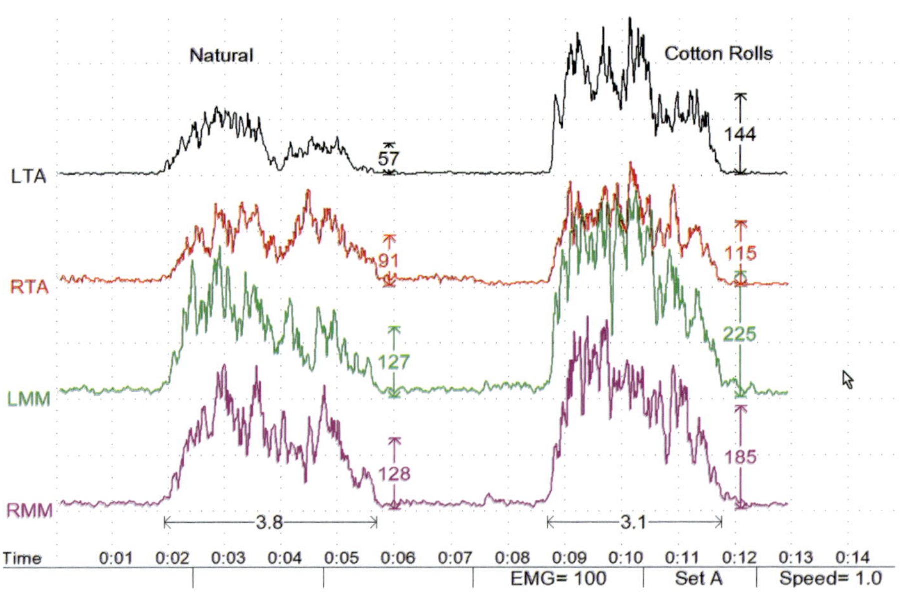

Fig. 6.5 Scan 11 of CMS with K7 evaluation system. sEMG during clench, burst 1 = natural CO natural dentition, burst 2 with cotton rolls between dental arches. *LMM* left masseter muscle, *LTA* left anterior temporalis, *RMM* right masseter muscle, *RTA* right anterior temporalis, *EMG* electromyography

CNS. Usually, the increase in the vertical due to cotton rolls will increase total output of sEMG, especially in deep bite and normo-bite individuals with increased freeway space. Sometimes there is no real gain and in general cotton roll test tends to balance muscular output. This is important information that can be clinically relevant. The difficulty in the correct execution of this test is being sure that the cotton rolls are well balanced bilaterally on the dental arches and that the patient feels comfortable with their positioning. Some practitioners see this test with cotton rolls as a way to uncover functional/anatomical asymmetries.

Figure 6.6 shows **scan 9 (EMG before tensing, muscles at rest)**. This scan is an electromyographic examination of masseter and anterior temporal muscles at habitual rest. It is useful to ask the patient to relax and to keep eyes closed. The K7 system has another two channels for each side and can evaluate eight muscles at the same time. The *basic protocol* limits the amount of information to four channels (two muscles) to make recording easier. Using all channels increases the chance of failure from lack of experience due to:

1. Increased possibility of electrode failure. More electrodes mean that skin preparation, sweat, and other external interferences have a better possibility to interfere with retrieving correct data.
2. Increased possibility of erroneous electrode positioning: while Masseter and Temporalis muscle are easy, posterior temporalis and SCM could be more complicated for example.

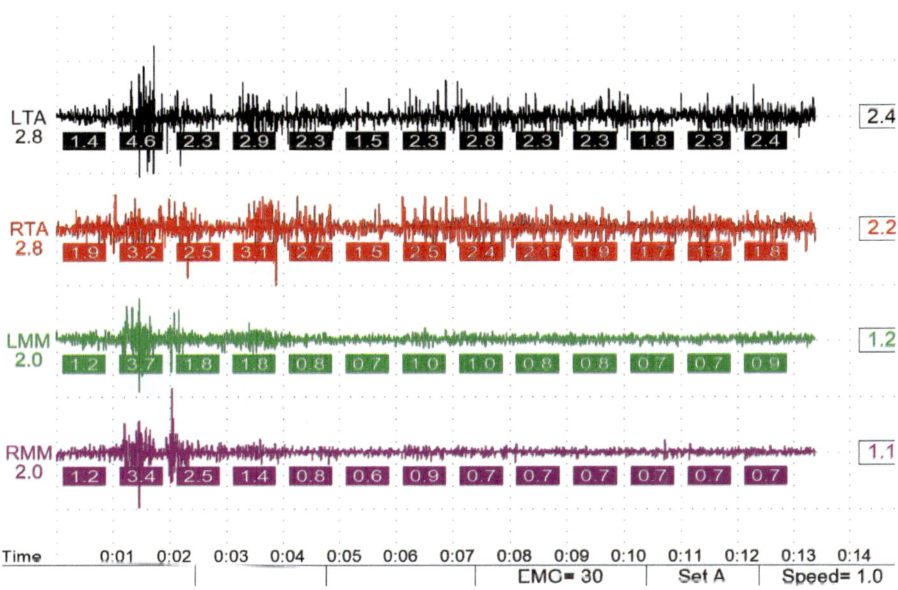

Fig. 6.6 Scan 9 of CMS with K7 evaluation system, sEMG at rest; *LMM* left masseter muscle, *LTA* left anterior temporalis, *RMM* right masseter muscle, *RTA* right anterior temporalis, *EMG* electromyography

3. For scan 10, which is a natural evolution of the muscles tested of scan 9, and that represents sEMG after deconditioning, the unexperienced practitioner may be frustrated not knowing how to identify an electrode malfunction, wire malfunction or simply not knowing how to relax a specific muscle to proceed to relaxed environment for scan 4/5 execution.

Mandatory 40 min of ULF-TENS with Aqualizer®

Figure 6.7 shows **scan 10 (EMG of masseter and anterior temporalis muscles at rest, after TENS application)**. These muscles must be ***under a minimum threshold in order to proceed with scan 4/5***. The K7 system provides the possibility of utilizing 2 more EMG channels for 4 extra muscles testing. If muscles are not relaxed after 45 min, it will be necessary to add extra tensing time.

Figure 6.8 shows **scan 4/5 (split screen with Sweep/XY tracing mode option, bite recording scan).** Note the "tap-tap" verification on horizontal plane of occlusion and ICP. Lateral canine disocclusion can be added if necessary (not shown). This split screen gives the operator the possibility to visualize the sweep mode (left), important to measure and analyze the characteristics of the spikes and visualize the AP movement. This visualization simplifies visual data in scan 5 (right). The computer, once the protrusive border is created, traces the Myotrajectory. It is important to check the Myotrajectory tracing done by the computer because

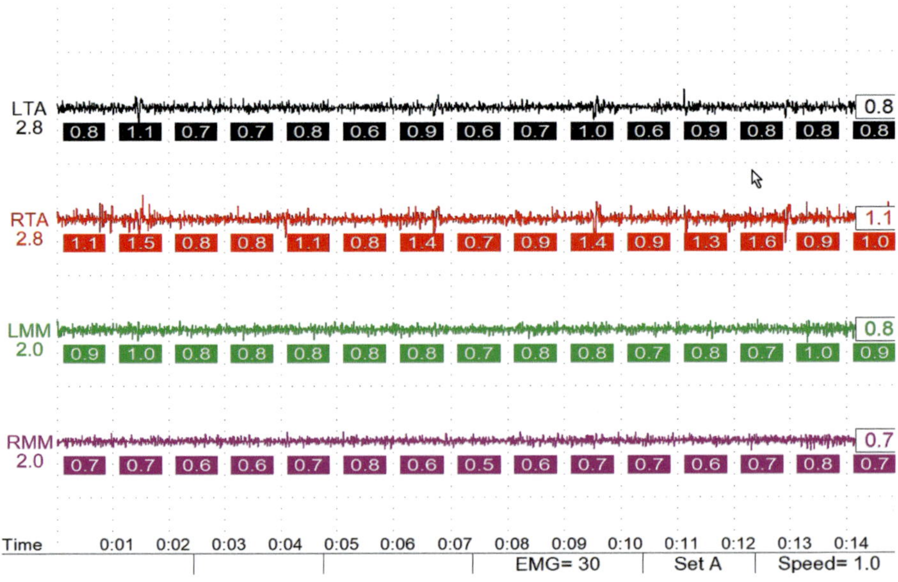

Fig. 6.7 Scan 10 of CMS with K7 evaluation system, sEMG at rest after 40 minutes of TENS application and Aqualizer®. *LMM* left masseter muscle, *LTA* left anterior temporalis, *RMM* right masseter muscle, *RTA* right anterior temporalis, *EMG* electromyography

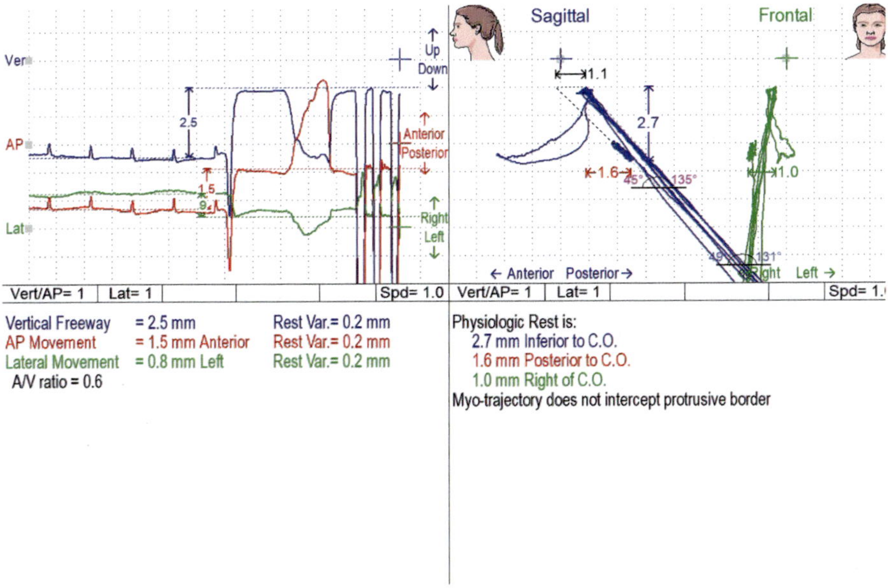

Fig. 6.8 Scan 4/5 In split screen of CMS with K7 evaluation system. *AP* anterior-posterior, *A/V* anterior/vertical ratio, *CO* centric occlusion, *Lat* lateral, *Spd* speed, *Vert* vertical

sometimes the computer cannot distinguish sensor array accidental vibrational movements. Once saved, any scan can be reproduced and redrawn at a click of the mouse. Comments and other information can be added to the scans.

This simplified protocol may not provide a comprehensive solution to all the questions that a skilled neuromuscular dentist may encounter. It is crucial to adhere to a specific diagnostic protocol when administering treatment. The author's viewpoint presented in this protocol is a culmination of over 30 years of experience in bioelectrical instrumentation and orthodontic diagnosis. Nonetheless, a skilled neuromuscular dentist should conduct multiple tests on different muscles, assess various functional tasks, evaluate specific movements, and check feedback procedures. ***It is essential to determine PRP after TENS use with interocclusal media*** before defining a diagnosis or treatment plan in neuromuscular dentistry. One of the primary challenges in neuromuscular dental diagnostics is that the correct position of the mandible (and the condyle) serves as the starting point for the diagnostic procedure, making it conceptually insurmountable.

The use of centric occlusion as the starting point for orthodontic treatment diagnostics has been a long-standing practice. Cephalometrics, clinical examination, and study models all rely on centric occlusion, which is also the starting point for non-neuromuscular diagnostics and therapy of malocclusions. However, it is important to note that all malocclusions are accompanied by a mispositioned mandible. Therefore, it is logical and more functional to consider visualizing the physiological muscular position of the mandible as the starting point for diagnostics and treatment.

Dentists worldwide are successfully treating obstructive sleep apnea (OSA) by repositioning the mandible to a lower and more anterior position, which is similar to the position determined by TENS application. Incorporating the physiological muscular position of the mandible into the diagnostic and treatment process leads to more effective outcomes for patients with malocclusions.

Options

- Descriptive analysis
- Sonography

The K7 diagnostic system helps the practitioner with a series of calculations that can be set up to show automatically. The descriptive analysis displays detailed information on the current scan. As an example, Fig. 6.9 an extra window displays extra information.

Sonography The possibility to record and analyze TMJ joint sounds is another important feature of this system. There are several scans used to record and analyze joint sounds. This is an objective recording of joint noises and should be used more frequently. Scan 15 with corresponding CMS helps the practitioner take a complete documentation of the joint sound and at what point during mandibular movement it appears.

Figure 6.10 shows an example of tracing with spectral analysis.

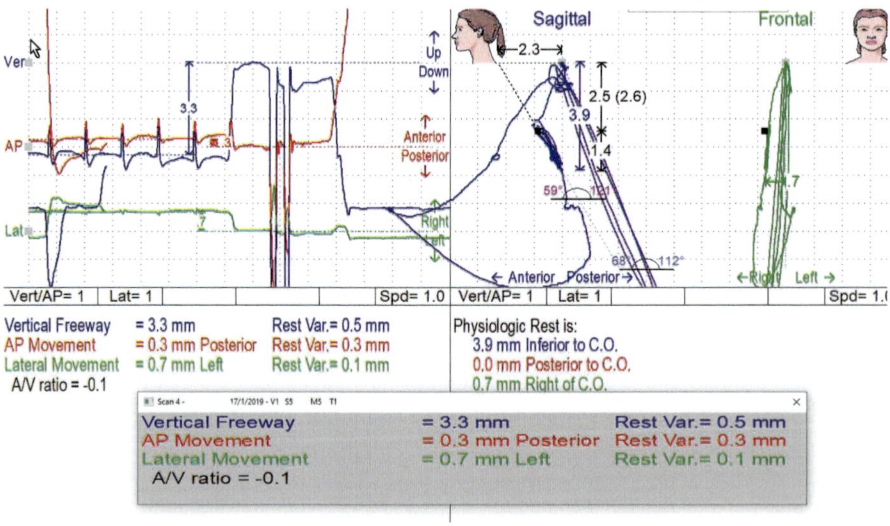

Fig. 6.9 Example of descriptive analysis for scan 4/5 split screen

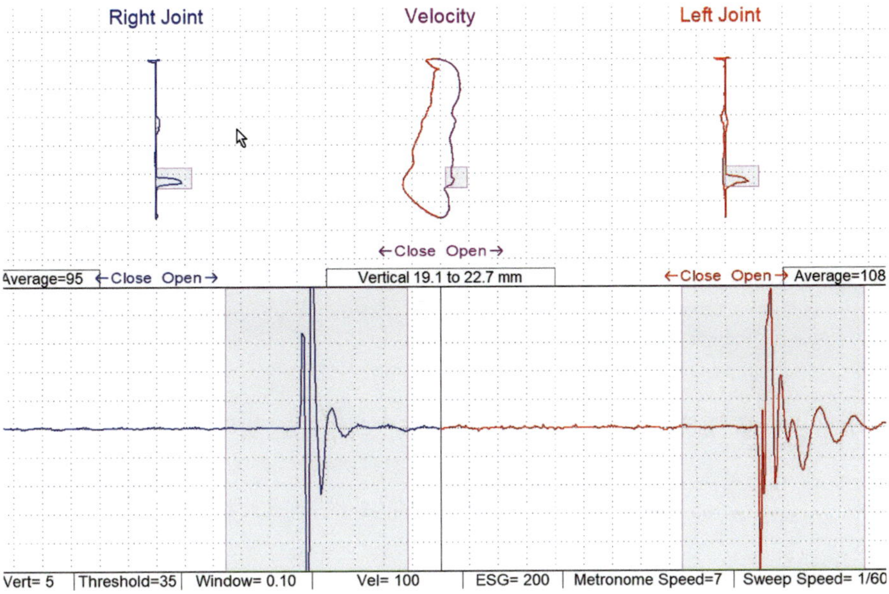

Fig. 6.10 Scan 15 with spectral analysis of joint noise

The K7 system is highly customizable. It is a great instrumentation to research with and to evaluate complex occlusal rehabilitations. CMS and the associated techniques increase our knowledge of occlusal problems. The results guide the dentist toward a physiological correction of occlusion. Since it is considered as a noninvasive diagnostic methodology, it can be easily repeated for occlusal registration and follow-ups.

This standardization of scan sequence and execution represents an important step in dialog creation among this specialty. A clear vision is easily shared because the interpretation of the results leaves no space for confusing and long-lasting discussions. For example, TENS application without occlusal media is a nonsense, even though several "neuromuscular" dentists insist on this procedure. Their scan 5 results cannot be interpreted and accepted by those who decondition with care.

Finally, this protocol focuses on Masseter and Temporalis muscles. If other patient complaints and signs are clinically observed, adding submandibular electrodes to check a swallow disorder or adding extra scans, in general, is done quite simply. The idea is that we all start comparing results and scans, to communicate properly. First step to progress is communication.

7 Schematic Kinesiographic Representation of Occlusal Dental Relationships

Orthodontists are highly trained professionals who specialize in correcting dental irregularities and malocclusions, which are misalignments of the teeth and jaws. One of the primary tools used by orthodontists to diagnose and treat such issues is the dental classification system developed by Angle, which helps them to assess the occlusion of the teeth and jaws. Additionally, orthodontists use cephalometric tracing on a lateral head X-ray to determine the skeletal type and growth direction of a patient, which can then be used to classify the patient's malocclusion as either an open-bite, deep-bite, or normo-bite. However, it is important to note that the traditional orthodontic diagnostic procedure focuses primarily on the static occlusion of the teeth and jaws, which means that it may not fully capture the complexity of a patient's dental and skeletal system. This diagnostic is linked to an analysis of the skeleton in relation to a static occlusion, or better, a static malocclusion. In order to provide a more accurate and comprehensive diagnosis, orthodontists may need to consider other factors such as the patient's soft tissue profile, facial aesthetics, and the study of dynamic occlusion.

In recent years, advancements in digital technology have enabled orthodontists to take a more holistic approach to diagnosis and treatment planning. For example, 3D imaging techniques allow orthodontists to create detailed virtual models of a patient's dental and skeletal anatomy, which can be used to simulate treatment outcomes and plan individualized treatment strategies. While the Angle dental classification and cephalometric tracing remain important tools in traditional orthodontic diagnosis, it is important for orthodontists to consider a range of factors and use advanced technology to provide a comprehensive and personalized treatment plan for each patient.

The study of the dynamic occlusion is done by Computerized Mandibular Scanning or CMS (Kinesiography). From a kinesiographic point of view, the results reported in the scans may not necessarily be characteristic of any occlusal (Angle molar class) or skeletal type. This is because our study and recordings obtained from the neuromuscular instumentation, represent a study on muscular function, may it be expressed by electromyography or a mandibular movement. This

F. Savastano, *Neuromuscular Orthodontics*,
https://doi.org/10.1007/978-3-031-41295-0_7

"physiological" mandibular rest position, which is a position unlinked to occlusion, represents a new mandibular position with a strong *reduction of accommodation*. Furthermore, *neuromuscular diagnostics* has a different starting point for any occlusal assessement, that is, the ***physiologic rest position (RP or PHP)*** and not CO as in classical orthodontics. While it is important to analyze the static occlusion (CO) because it *usually* accompanies deglutition, it is the spatial relationship between CO and RP of major interest to the neuromuscular dentist. It is not a rare finding that an occlusal Class II results in a Class I relationship after TENS deconditioning. Other skeletal/dental cephalometric measurements may differ completely from the relative spatial relationships after neuromuscular deconditioning. This is the most important finding neuromuscular dentists have been dealing with since long, and that the *specialized orthodontic community refuses to acknowledge*.

We must look forward and not focus on occlusal relationships for our diagnostic procedure. This is necessary to understand the deep implications that neuromuscular orthodontics reveals to the practitioner. As previously mentioned, the scope of neuromuscular diagnosis is the determination of the PRP and the neuromuscular trajectory. The creation of occlusion starts from here: the preliminary and fundamental step of determining mandibular rest position represents the "optimal jaw position relative to the cranium to best accommodate muscle function (and consequent TMJ function) and swallow in ICP." The orthodontist is now able to reconstruct, reassemble the occlusion to respect as close as possible, the physiologic rest position and make this rest position *coincide with the habitual rest position*. It is the ***reduction of the accommodation*** the scope of occlusal orthodontic correction. ***Ideally***, when growth is finished, centric occlusion (ICP) and Myocentric *should be coincident*. It is clear here that the author does not stand for achieving a Class I dental occlusion as the main goal for a neuromuscular orthodontic correction. It is left to the ability of the orthodontist to finish cases in Class I occlusal relationship while preserving the ideal neuromuscular mandibular posture. Not all orthodontic discrepancies can be finished with ideal Class I occlusal relationships.

CMS along with the neuromuscular protocol represents a breakthrough in current orthodontic diagnosis and treatment. Finally, we can focus on the analysis of movement and muscle function. s-EMG is ultimately being reconsidered by many clinicians. Its use is now widely accepted and there are several encouraging studies that do not justify the adverse position of some clinicians [1–4]. Objective data can be obtained during functional tasks, and these measurements can be repeated and confirmed by other practitioners. This is not true for subjective data, like muscle palpation for tenderness or clinical verification of a swallow disorder: the results are linked to the personal skills, expertise, and sensibility of the operator.

Now that we understand the premises of Neuromuscular Orthodontics, the classification of malocclusion must be changed to describe a *functional* relationship between the dental arches. The skeletal classification must remain not in cephalometric terms, but mostly as an *expression of the skeletal characteristics of the individual in respect to the general population,* for age, sex, and race; an example could be the identification of a skeletal Class III discrepancy whereas the mandible for age, sex, and race is placed at the 90th percentile and the cranial base length to the 50th [5–8]. This discrepancy between the two skeletal bases is then judged to describe the skeletal morphological features that participate in the definition of the typology of malocclusion. The Gaussian curve is still used in medicine to try to identify what is normal and what might not be [9].

The examples that are now described, are deliberately shown without a skeletal pattern, and are described based on the sole occlusal relationship in ICP. This is done to better understand the implications of muscular deconditioning on the relationship of the occlusal bases. CO is the reference point to better describe the possible outcomes after reducing accommodation. This is a straightforward way to visually describe the various possibilities of mandibular re-positioning after deconditioning that cannot be seen when analyzing CO. The reader will understand the multiple consequences that a neuromuscular diagnosis can have on diagnostics and orthodontic therapy by comparing the results of the mandibular position sagitally and vertically in respect of Centric Occlusion. The neuromuscular paradigm has changed the definition of malocclusion. The terminology like "mandibular entrapment" and "front wall" are common among neuromuscular dentists. Now is the time to say that a perfect Class I occlusion in a Class I occlusal skeletal frame can be functionally maloccluded, in the sense that malocclusion is the result of a failing dynamic occlusion. Case presentations that are distributed all over social media have very little significance, if not cosmetic, for the neuromuscular orthodontist. The demand for quality treatments as well as TMD treatments, has pushed demand to a higher standard of orthodontic diagnosis and treatment.

Occlusal Class I

Figures 7.1 and 7.2 show the possible scenarios of Scan 5 in a Class I occlusal patient. Tracing a vertical line from CO (V line) will facilitate the interpretation of Scan 5 results. HRP and its spike are colored in orange. The "habitual trajectory" passes through CO. The HRP represents an accommodative posture to occlusion. After deconditioning with TENS and Aqualizer as previously described, the possibilities of new PRP are schematically represented in different colors according to an orthodontic prognostic factor in relation to Class I occlusion. Measurements and magnification are purposely omitted to simplify scan interpretation. This is

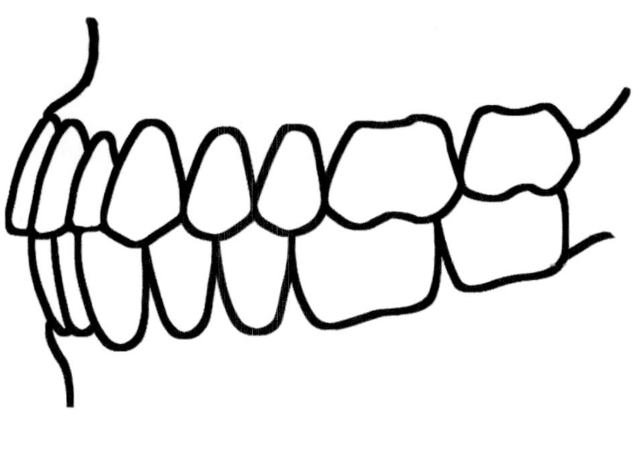

Fig. 7.1 Class I relationship

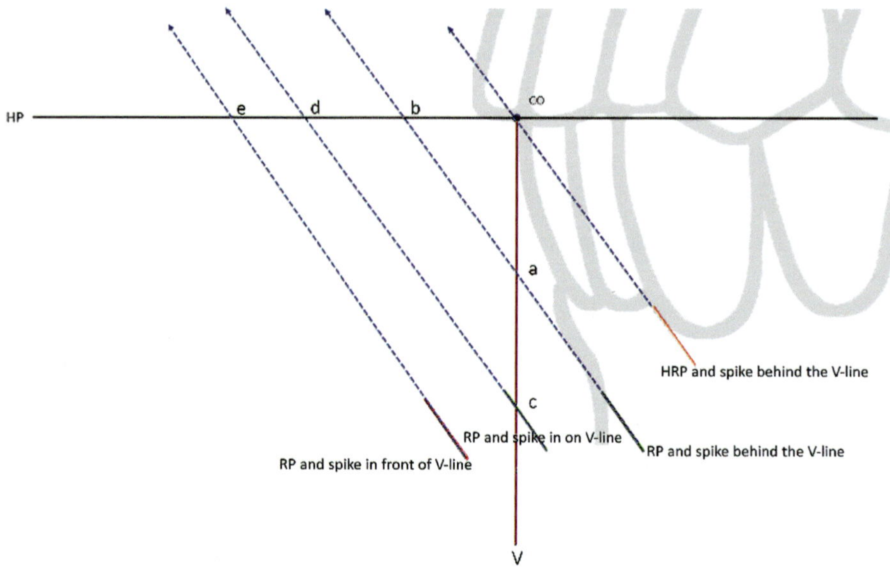

Fig. 7.2 Schematic representation of scan 5 after 45′ of TENS application with Aqualizer® in Class I occlusal relationship. Dotted blue line = neuromuscular trajectory (nt); CO = (Centric Occlusion); V = vertical from CO (V-line); a and c = nt intercepts V; b,d,e = nt intercepts horizontal plane of occlusion (HP). In red, green = TENS spikes after 45′. In orange *simulation* of closure movement from HRP. *HRP* Habitual Rest Position, *RP* Rest Position/physiologic rest position. *CO* Centric Occlusion

schematically a representation to outline the possible changes in RP after ULF-TENS application. ORANGE = Habitual (Rest Position and Spike before TENS 45′), GREEN = (orthodontic) correction possible, RED = Neuromuscular Orthodontic correction not possible. Please note that for descriptive reasons the orange spike represents a habitual rest position and spike an habitual trajectory to CO. During TENS application and some time during this process, it can be possible that the orange spike coincides or is close to the deconditioned one. A remote possibility sometimes seen in very good neuromuscular occlusions.

1. Example GREEN with a and b point. This is typical for a Class I occlusion with excess freeway space. As an example, we could have a vertical of 4 mm and an AP discrepancy on the HP (Horizontal Plane of occlusion) of about 1.5 mm. This occlusion should be defined as a mandibular entrapment in centric occlusion. The a point is at about half of the vertical discrepancy, on the Myotrajectory, and represents our ideal Myocentric. An extrusion of the upper arch of 2 mm would lower the HP and preserve a Class I occlusion. Therapy: bite registration at “a” point is delivered as a Bionator to extrude dentition about 2 mm to lower HP. Schematically, *a Class I occlusion can be maintained if the resulting centric is on the V line.*

When considering the more advanced c-d line Myotrajectory and RP, the prognostic factor is still positive (GREEN SPIKE) although some difficulties arise. If we consider a freeway space of about 4.5 mm, a solution could be to record a Myocentric as close as possible to point c on the Myotrajectory. Freeway space could be left to a minimum of 1 mm. The increased difficulty is, therefore, given by the necessity to advance the upper arch (could be a correction of upper torque or to any degree upper anterior expansion) because our ideal myocentric with a 2-mm. or more calculated freeway space on the neuromuscular trajectory would be in front of the V line. The extrusion necessary will be increased in respect of the previous example up to about 3.5 mm. (4.5-3.5=1mm.). The more extrusion is obtained orthodontically, the less AP correction (advancement/torque/expansion) is needed.

The physiologic rest position (RP) with red lined spike and Myotrajectory passing HP in "e" is of course without an orthodontic solution. In the absence of a marked skeletal Class III patient, it should be questioned how postural problems do affect the mandibular rest position. CMS is executed with the patient sitting comfortably in a chair and maintaining a natural head posture. The more head tilts forward, the more advanced RP (and HRP). This is a very common problem when taking scans: scan 5 after deconditioning should be executed with the same head posture the patient has at start of analysis. Patients sometime relax and slide to a more sacral bone sitting and tilt their head forward. This said, the AP discrepancy is excessive for the red spike example for a neuromuscular orthodontic correction even at best vertical control. Only surgical repositioning of the upper maxilla would give the orthodontist the possibility of achieving a Myocentric as a final result of treatment. It is left to the neuromuscular orthodontist the decision where to establish a limit of acceptance of the centric at the end of treatment. Between the green line spike c-d and the red passing to e on HP, there are numerous possibilities that can be of course borderline cases and not necessarily surgical.

Example Case

Clearly a Class III skeletal and Class I occlusal young girl, October 2004, age 12 years. Figure 7.3 shows intraoral photos taken at age 12 years. Note there is no space for upper canines. Lower arch is narrow, but most important sign is the lingual inclination of the lower incisors. This lingual tipping is the dental compensation to muscular and skeletal needs. It was decided to take a complete diagnostic scan to evaluate quantitively the mandibular entrapment.

Before any orthodontic procedure, a complete diagnostic scan was performed. Figure 7.4 shows scan 5 after 45' TENS application. Complete scans and clinical cases will be discussed further on.

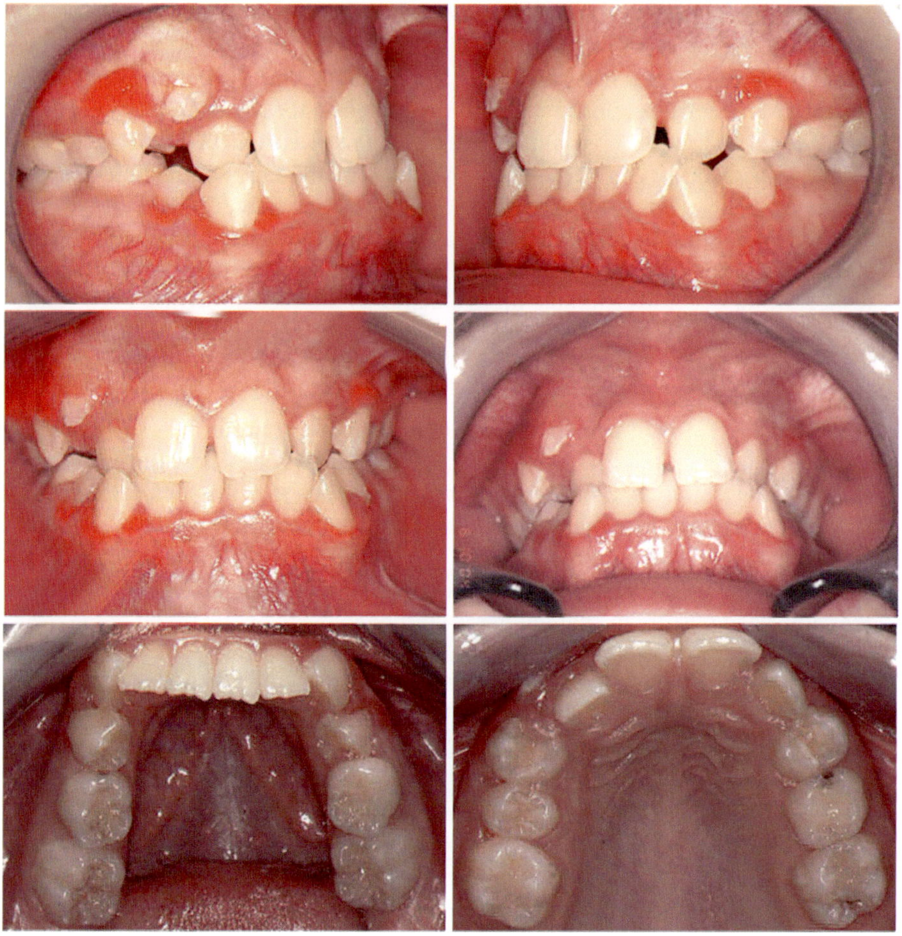

Fig. 7.3 Intraoral photos of a 12-year- old female patient. Note that the upper arch has no room for both canines. The lower arch shows a great deal of dental compensation with tip back of lower incisors

Photo 2b, surprisingly, shows that the lower incisor lingual tipping has compensated all the sagittal requirements and most probably saved TMJ function. The muscular action and skeletal nature of the mandible have forced a compensation of the lower front incisors to avoid articular damage. The neuromuscular trajectory intercepts the HP almost overlapping the habitual path of closure. This indicates that the orthodontic outcome is favorable, especially for the extra freeway space available.

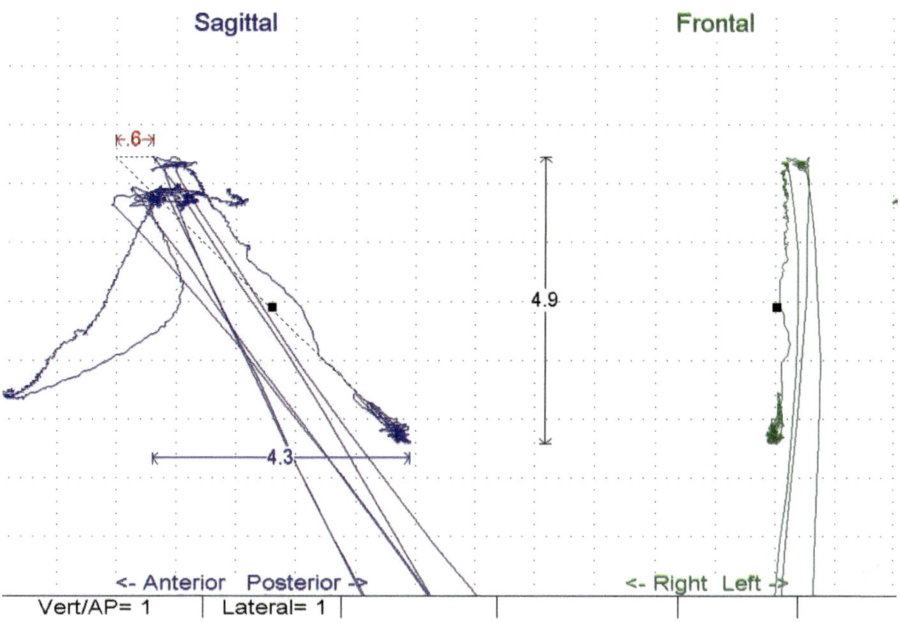

Fig. 7.4 Scan 5 after 45' TENS application with Aqualizer. Excessive force upon closure can show vibration of CO due to sensor array movement

Occlusal Class III

Figures 7.5 and 7.6 show the possible scenarios of Scan 5 in a Class III occlusal patient. The HRP and habitual trajectory with orange colored spike represents a usual context in a Class III occlusion independent from reverse or normal overjet. Scan 5 results can be surprising. The first example with green spike on the right of the image is described have a neuromuscular trajectory intersecting the HP *behind* CO. This is usually described in orthodontics as a pseudo-Class III where occlusal interferences make the mandible slide to a Class III occlusion in ICP. All results that remain behind CO (as described in this case) are positive prognostic factors that sustain an orthodontic correction. Usually, there is a slight excess of freeway space that delivers to the orthodontist an extra weapon for the occlusal correction. If the reverse overjet is not severe (alternatively it would be generally accepted that only surgical correction can resolve the skeletal and occlusal discrepancy), the Myotrajectory f-g with green spike would have a positive prognostic outcome. Indeed, it would be linked to the amount of freeway space; the more freeway space, the easier it would be to achieve the CO (a new Myocentric) behind the V line. In fact, extrusion mechanics in Class III occlusions reduces or even corrects negative OJ (for example, face mask use extrudes upper dentition). In this example of the f-g line, an extrusion of about 2 mm

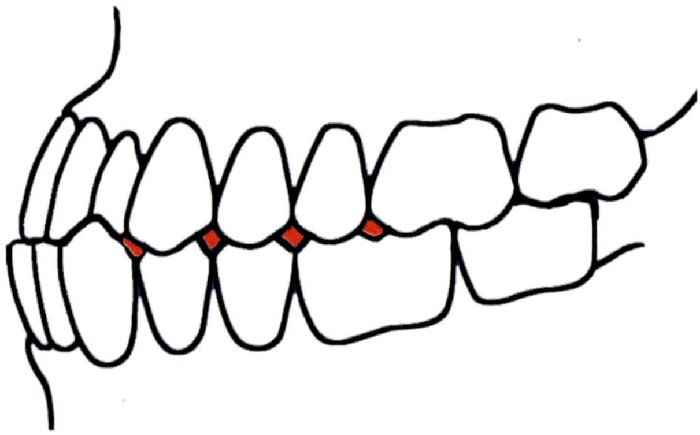

Fig. 7.5 Class III dental relationship

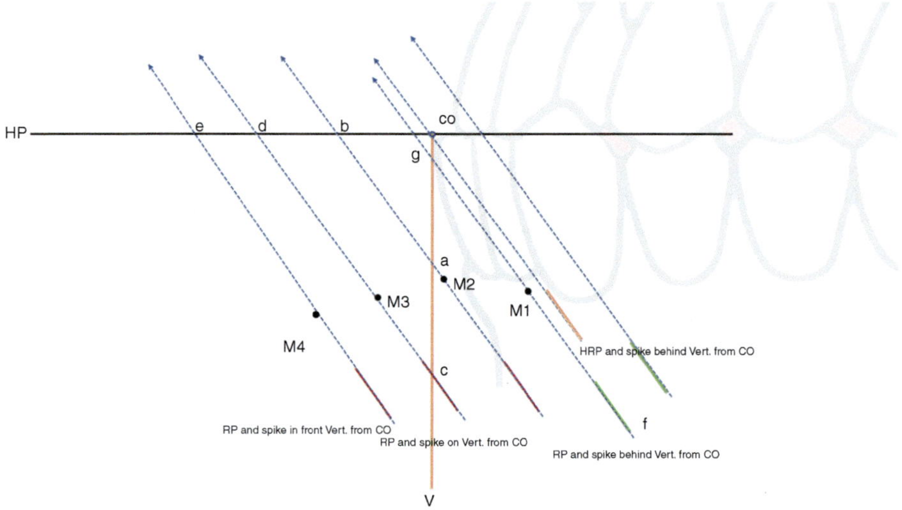

Fig. 7.6 Schematic representation of scan 5 after 45′ of TENS application with Aqualizer® in Class III occlusal relationship. Dotted blue line = neuromuscular trajectory (nt); CO = (Centric Occlusion); V = vertical from CO (V-line); a and c = nt intercepts V; b,d,e = nt intercepts horizontal plane of occlusion (HP). M1-M2-M3-M4: Myocentric (calculated). In red, green = TENS spikes. In orange habitual movement to CO

could bring the CO behind the V line on the Myotrajectory with a sccessful orthodontic treatment; this new position of the CO ***is*** the new Myocentric (M1) that we want to deliver as our treatment objective. M1, if seen as a pure sagittal perspective, now represents a Class I occlusion. The main objective in occlusal discrepancies that present a Class III occlusion, is to gain a CO on the neuromuscular trajectory that is *behind* the V line. This is because the V line represents the sagittal relation and position of ICP. For this reason, a-b, c-d, and any recording in front of c-d will have negative prognostic outcomes even with correction of freeway space (M2-M3-M4). M2, is behind the vertical V line, but the effort for this treatment could not be sufficient in obtaining an ideal occlusion and reversing completely the OJ. *The quantity of sagittal correction of the Myocentric obtained by extrusion, represents the correction of the OJ. Whatever residual OJ is corrected by upper maxillary advancement that (is in general dentoalveolar).* The Myocentric should be calculated in proximity of the TENS spike, leaving only a minimal freeway space to obtain the maximal increase in positive OJ. *Face mask* application can correct AP discrepancy with great limitation (1–2 degrees increase of SNA and according to age) while its major action relies on posterior extrusion via maxillary rotation [10–13]. As said, the M2 point could be identified very close to RP instead of the usual 2–3 mm or more calculated for excess freeway space. It is difficult to extrude more than 4–5 mm, especially on growing patients (this is because if the mandibular growth pattern is somewhat skeletal deepbite, this *produces* freeway space). M1-M2-M3 and M4 are at circa the same horizontal placement, that is in other words, at the same extrusion potential. Since Class III treatments react positively to face mask therapy, especially when applied during RPE, the RPE procedures does have some drawbacks. Applying RPE always reduces freeway space, but can also favor anterior condylar repositioning [14]. Class III, in general, does not have a posterior condylar displacement unless manifest mandibular entrapment is present [15].

Example Case

Class III occlusion with crossbite upper left canine with lower first premolar, and lower left canine with upper lateral. Lower incisors are tipped lingually, compensating some of the skeletal discrepancy. Patient is young, male, and entering growth spurt. He is a typical case of child TMD, with TMJ clicking on aperture (Fig. 7.7).

Scan 5 shows that the sagittal discrepancy on HP is circa 1 mm (Fig. 7.8). The rest position behind the V line is a favorable outcome as described in Fig. 7.6, f-g line. Treatment objectives include RPE with facemask and reduction of OB.

The main objective for this treatment is to preserve TMJ function and to reduce accommodation. To correct lower incisor lingual tipping it is necessary to create sufficient OJ with RPE and facemask therapy. Mandibular growth must also be taken in consideration in treatment planning. Mandibular Freedom (MF) should be checked regularly after treatment and OB kept to minimum to avoid posterior occlusion by end of growth. Class III occlusion can be the final occlusal result as shown in this case (Fig. 7.9).

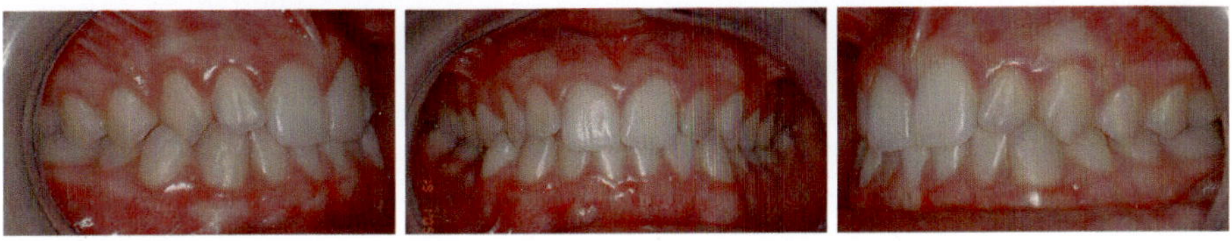

Fig. 7.7 Class III occlusion in developing Class III skeletal growth. Patient age 11 years

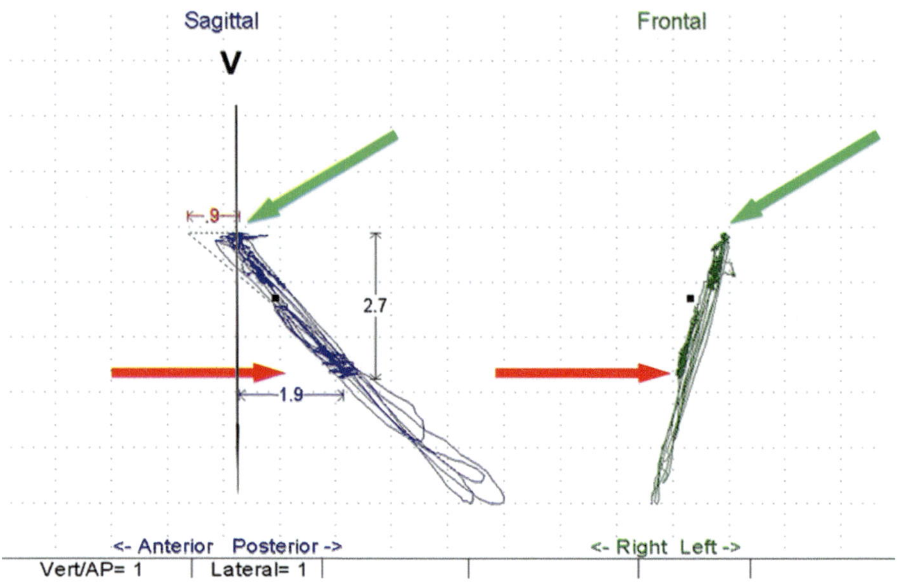

Fig. 7.8 Pretreatment Scan 5. Red arrows = RP, Green arrows = CO

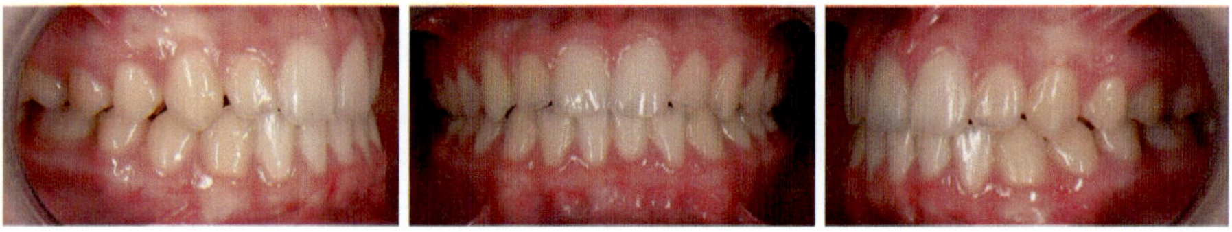

Fig. 7.9 Final occlusion in Class III Angle

After treatment CMS of scan 5 shows that the neuromuscular trajectory and the habitual path of closure are somewhat overlapping. Patient is asymptomatic Fig. 7.10.

Lateral cephalograms are taken before and after treatment and show an increase in breathing capacity, an increase in mandibular length, and an increase of cephalometric indicators of skeletal Class III (Fig. 7.11).

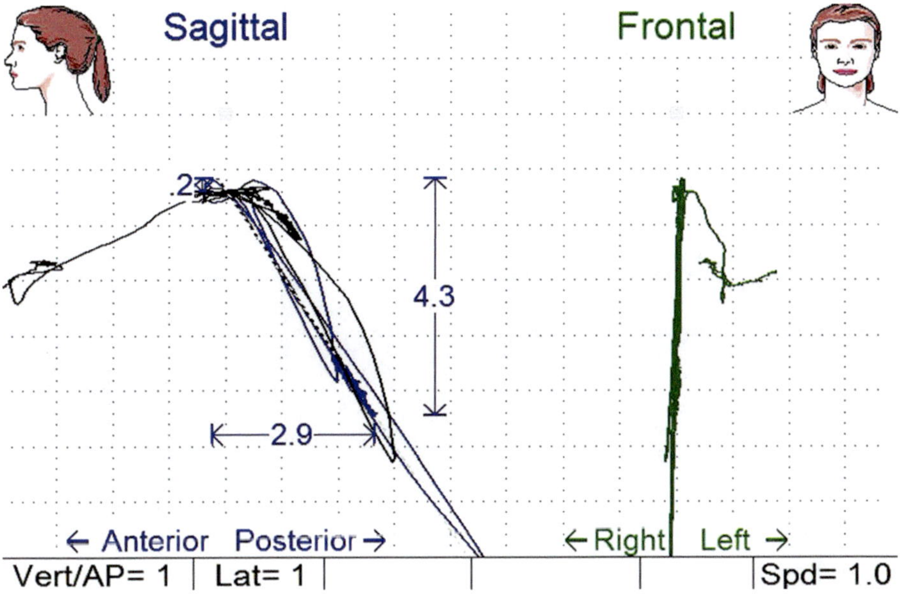

Fig. 7.10 Post-treatment scan 5 showing correction of AP discrepancy and correction of lateral HRP deviation

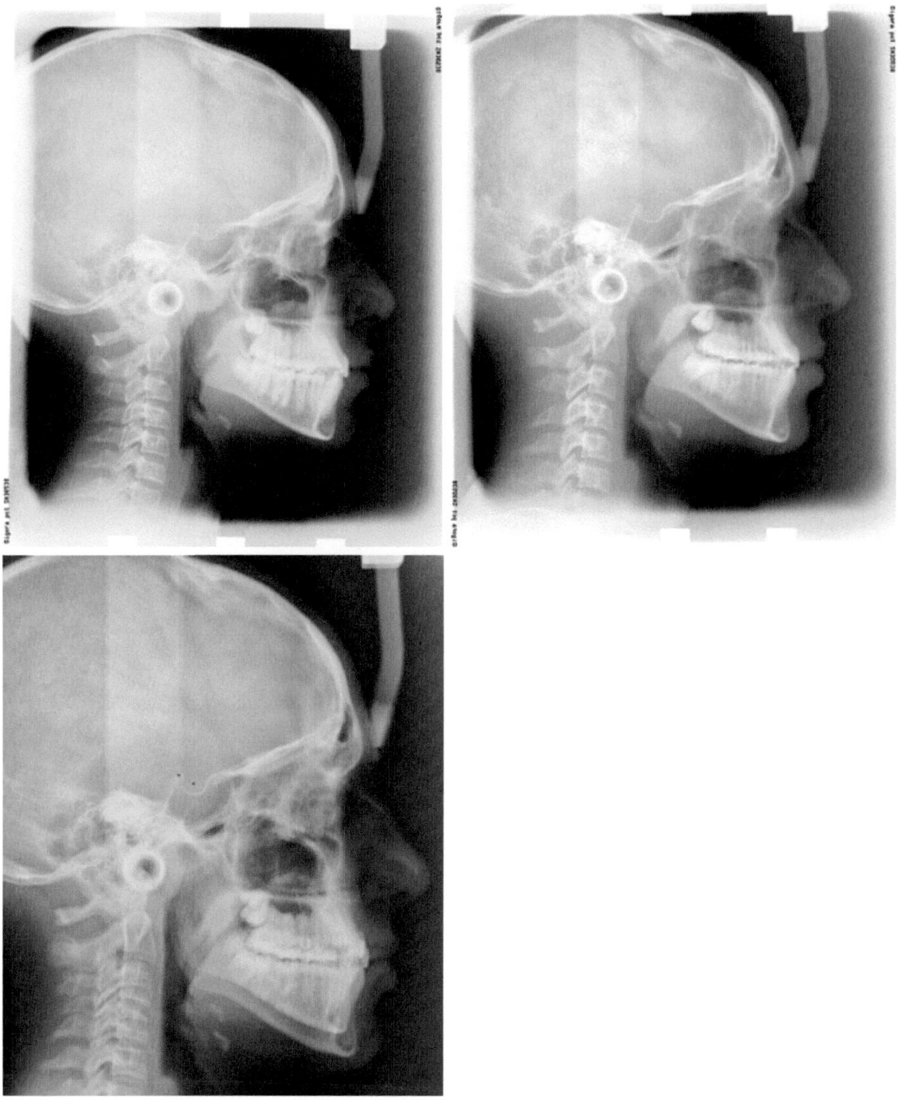

Fig. 7.11 Lateral cephalograms before and after treatment (TOP), There is an increase in lateral aspect of breathing capacity. A radiographic superimposition S-N shows increase of lower third and mandibular advancement (BOTTOM)

Occlusal Class II

Figure 7.12 show a schematic representation of Class II occlusion and 7.13 the possible scenarios of Scan 5 in a Class II occlusal patient.

One uncommon scenario would be f-g line after TENS deconditioning. Usually accompanied by 1–2 mm maximum freeway space after deconditioning, there appears to be no possible solution but that of upper distalization/maxillary impaction. The kinesiographic and neuromuscular objectives in Class II occlusions is a *forward* positioning of CO in respect of the V line. When this is not possible, upper

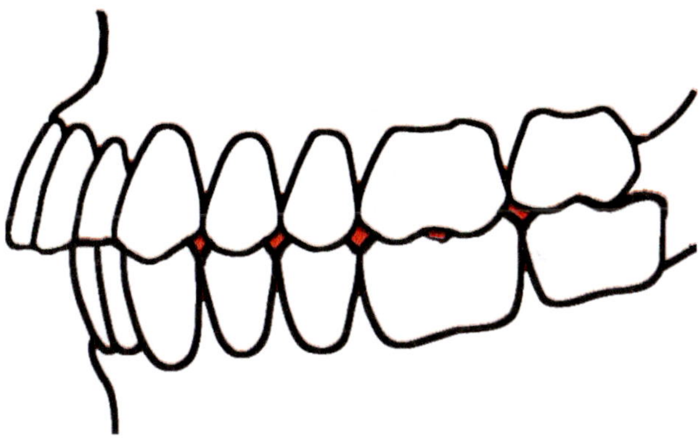

Fig. 7.12 Class II dental relationship

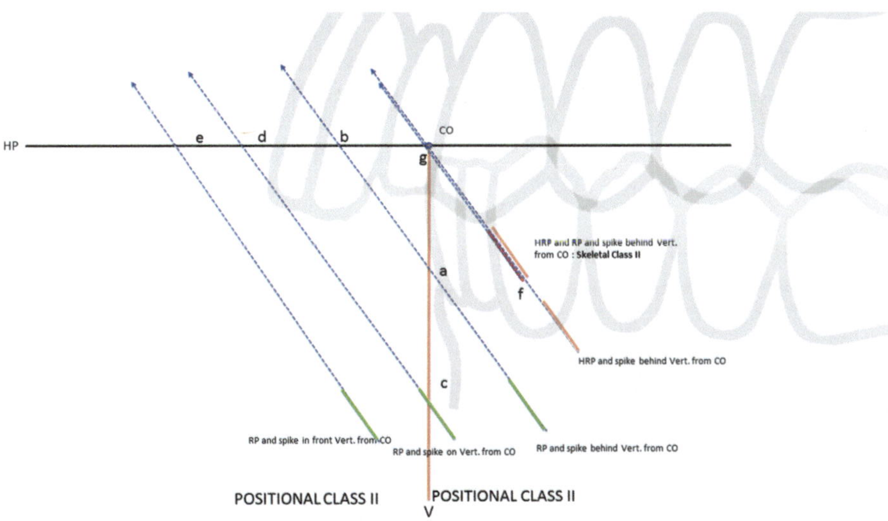

Fig. 7.13 Schematic representation of scan 5 after 45′ of TENS application with Aqualizer® in Class II dental relationship. Dotted blue line = neuromuscular trajectory (nt); CO = (Centric Occlusion); V = vertical from CO (V-line); a and c = nt intercepts V; b,d,e = nt intercepts horizontal plane of occlusion (HP). In red and green = TENS spikes. In orange simulation of mandibular habitual trajectory

distalization represents an orthodontic compensation that *mimics* a more forward positioning of the mandible in relation to the maxilla. What really happens is that there is a retraction of the V line and CO. The author classifies these cases as skeletal Class II. A skeletal Class II is a discrepancy accompanied by a smaller than normal mandible for age, sex, and race vs cranial base measurements [8, 16–18]. As you can see, the f-g line accompanies a small freeway space. Skeletal Class II discrepancies tend to a skeletal open-bite morphology.

The Myotrajectory passing through a and b points is a quite common finding in growing patients with a mild Class II occlusion and mild excess of OJ. Mandibular repositioning and extrusion alone cannot solve these cases from an orthodontic ***dental occlusion*** point of view (reduction of OJ and a Class I occlusion). While repositioning and extruding (lowering the HP) will result in a Myocentric occlusion, the relationship of the dental arches *will remain in a Class II fashion (point a).* It is necessary to understand that, as previously said, the efficacy of extrusion with the recorded Myocentric does not reduce AP discrepancy completely (it is necessary to establish a Myocentric between points a and b). When recording with bite registration, the malocclusion becomes visually represented. Extrusion is required on more posterior segments (posterior support loss of Class II). *Mandibular growth* plays a major role during the correction of these mild Class II cases. Points b, d, and e represent on the horizontal plane of occlusion three points that are functionally accepted because of the neuromuscular trajectory. Without considering the recording of vertical freeway space from a kinesiographic point of view, all three positions result in unrealistic occlusions *if posterior vertical freeway space is not corrected.* In other words, the correction of positional Class II is accomplished by creating an occlusal plane that can accommodate fine repositioning of the mandible, in a more forward position.Without posterior occlusal support, CO is always physiologically positioned at its lowest available VD of the occlusion [19]. In fact, when bite recording favors a more forward position, there is usually a major increase of freeway space in the posterior sectors. It is in this space that the orthodontist decides where and how to position the occlusal plane.

The c-d line and all RP in front of V line represent the ideal tracings functional orthodontists desire. The sagittal correction in mm for the new centric will represent the mm needed for OJ correction. The positive outlook is easily established by the fact that the Myocentric is *always* in front of V line, thus reducing drastically the OJ. The correction of this positional malocclusion requires calculating the Myocentric on an ideal vertical line to establish a Class I relationship with the upper arch, leaving a fixed vertical extrusion requirement for an ideal OB and OJ (Fig. 7.14). The aggressive reduction of freeway space (extrusion) and upper maxillary expansion together with the anterior repositioning of the mandible contribute to dramatic facial improvements. These positional Class II cases represent the ideal relationship between the jaws for functional/neuromuscular orthodontic treatments. Fortunately, they represent most of all Class II malocclusions, while skeletal Class II the minority. It is important to note that when OJ is severe and there is a complete whole tooth Class II occlusion, the anterior protrusive border does not necessarily represent the posterior border of the upper incisors. Anterior disocclusion may be

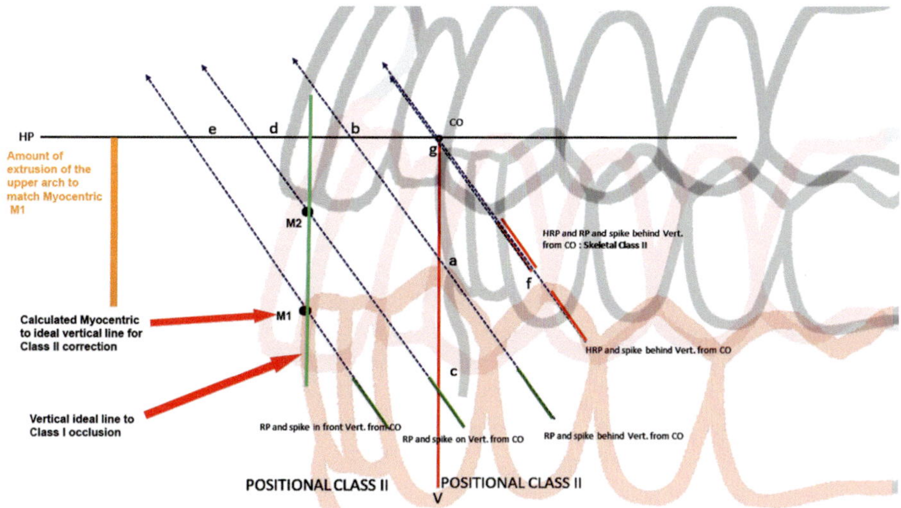

Fig. 7.14 Showing schematic representation of a Class II tracing in sagittal view with calculated Myocentric for Class II OJ correction. Note the M1 Myocentric is calculated on the Myotrajectory to point e and on ideal vertical line (green) for Class correction and reduction of OJ (In light red drawing). The vertical measurement from M1 to RP is the vertical freeway space (not described). For example, the amount of extrusion needed for Myocentric in M1 is shown in orange. In case of a Myotrajectory passing through the a-b line with a small increase in OJ, the Myocentric can be calculated on the V line in point a without correction of OJ and class I occlusion. Another example that is equally valid is Myotrajectory passing in c-d line in which the Myocentric is calculated in M2. The HP is always lowered by teeth extrusion

represented by other teeth, like premolars. This is obviously the case in Class II occlusions with severe OJ and increased torque of the upper incisors.

Figure 7.15 shows an infrequent scenario of a skeletal Class II and the ideal camouflage treatment. The intrusion of the upper maxillary dentition determines a higher level of HP (in red). Since Class II skeletal morphology is characterized by a smaller mandibular length and height in respect of the cranial measurements, intrusion of the upper arch by orthopedic treatment favors a more anterior positioning of the mandible due to a rotation around its hinge axis during closure. This treatment procedure generally increases freeway space which is scarce or absent. The cervical strain is reduced because the head extension is no longer needed to avoid posterior tooth contact during HRP.

There are several appliances that deliver a good orthopedic effect on the upper arch for this type of treatment. The Teuscher appliance [20], although conceived for treatment of both positional and skeletal Class II, changes through the selective activation of specific directional forces the outcome in hyperdivergent Class II [21]. Personal experience from the author suggests that the activation of circa 10–15° of the external short bow *below the occlusal plane* translates into a reduction of distal movement of the molar and an increase of intrusive forces in the posterior sectors,

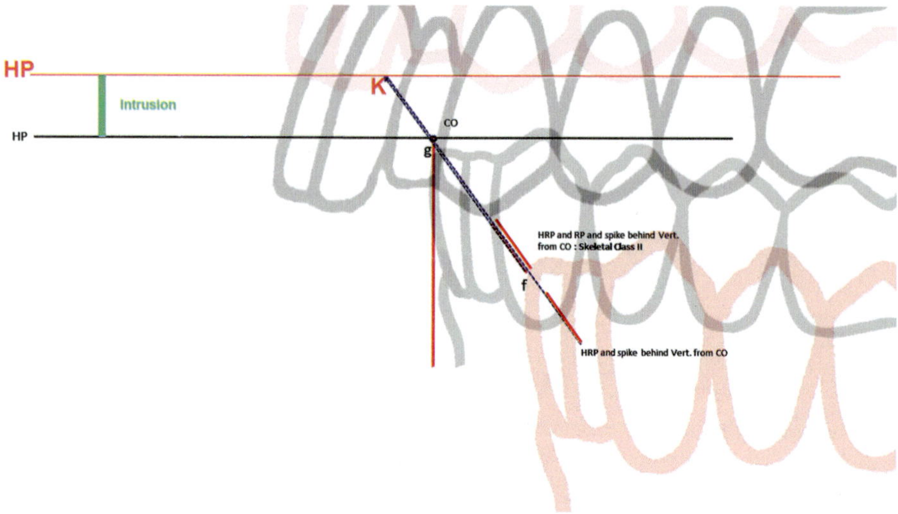

Fig. 7.15 Schematic representation of Class II skeletal treatment. In red are the reference lines to understand rotation on hinge axis during closure when upper intrusion is done on maxillary arch with orthopedic appliances. In green the amount of intrusion needed

thus favoring anterior mandibular reposition. Furthermore, the most important correction for skeletal Class II open-bite should be a reduction of steepness of the posterior occlusal plane [22–24].

These schematic representations are synthetic and help understand what the results can be after neuromuscular deconditioning. Regardless of the kinesiographic results, it is imperative to perform a visual analysis of the static dental occlusion. While teeth may not always be aligned, their position is influenced by various factors, including muscular needs, functional movements, and the pressure of tissues and muscles during rest position. Therefore, evaluating the swallow is crucial for obvious reasons. Any malocclusion observed is likely the result of compensatory measures taken by the teeth to protect the temporomandibular joint (TMJ) and maintain stomatognathic functions. Over time, teeth act as passive elements that adapt to the changing needs of the muscles by adjusting their position and being gradually abraded. Class II occlusions with and without excess OJ usually show lower arch incisal tooth wear due to incisal guidance contact, probably occurring during nighttime [25]. Tooth wear patterns do give hints on the dynamic tooth contact during deglutition in occlusion (in ICP). This reflects a normal functional task, but tooth wear patterns must be also the result of interferences typical for specific malocclusions and its tooth arrangement, as in Class II division 2 [26]. Dental attrition is associated with parafunctions, dietary habits, and some general health conditions too. In the mixed dentition it can be a normal finding due to mandibular sagittal growth [27].

The following points represent a summary of considerations on the schematic representation of dynamic occlusion in Kinesiography:

1. Freeway space in CMS is represented as a vertical measurement

   Freeway space is represented as the vertical measurement as the mandibular teeth come to contact in ICP from RP to the Horizontal Plane of Occlusion (HP).

   RP to CO is represented vertically and is a valid quantitative measurement for diagnostics. Obviously, the vertical spacings between the dental arches vary at different points of occlusion, CMS cannot easily identify, after TENS deconditioning, which teeth come in contact first during closure to CO or if there is a simultaneous contact of the occlusal platform. This vertical measurement is only needed for a *quantitative* measurement of one dimension of freeway space. Freeway space is different vertically in all sectors of the occlusion. This vertical measurement is usually referred to in neuromuscular jargon as freeway space, but all Neuromuscular dentists know that freeway space is 3D. This measurement is useful because it is a fast indication to know if there is enough space for prosthetic correction, orthotic or neuromuscular extrusion.

   When executing scan 5, the vertical recording is limited to the magnet position from PRP to ICP and cannot reflect the movement of the posterior sectors to occlusion. This also means that you cannot visualize a mandibular torquing to ICP because there is only one magnet and not 3 to define an occlusal mandibular plane movement. Mandibular torquing cannot be visualized as a movement to ICP with CMS. This is one of the main reasons bite recording is necessary.
2. The HP represents an ideal horizontal plane, it is not the real plane of occlusion

   The HP refers to a plane calculated across the CO point. It is drawn *horizontally* and should be *parallel to the floor*.

   Occlusal plane cannot be flat but curved as per the curve of Spee. There is no way of measuring or representing this curve with CMS only. When recording a Myocentric bite, most probably there will be a wide gap in the posterior sectors of interocclusal space. The HP cannot represent a true occlusal plane but it is the closest way of repeating a reference plane in respect of the maxillary position. This demonstrates how important correct sensor array alignment and natural head posture are important for proper diagnosis.
3. CMS shows a physiological mandibular trajectory with TENS on which the MyoCentric is calculated by the practitioner

   Our ideal treatment objective is having the habitual and physiological mandibular trajectories overlap. CMS indicates clearly where the direction of treatment should be brought to. The Myocentric is calculated on the physiologic mandibular trajectory, the Myotrajectory. The Myotrajectory is the prolongation of the TENS spike to the HP and represents an involuntary movement. CMS shows the PRP and HRP too. For treatments with functional appliances such as the Bionator, checking the Bionator so it is constructed correctly on RP is mandatory if you have a K7 system.

The calculus of the MyoCentric is essential when finalizing an orthotic or full mouth rehabilitation. Here the MyoCentric is the treatment objective together with other physiological and gnathological dynamic variables. In Neuromuscular Orthodontics it is important to know where the MyoCentric lies, but treatment objectives must be more realistic and achievable. For this reason, the Myotrajectory is of greater importance for the orthodontist.

4. The V line is a reference line perpendicular to HP

   Why is the V line important? Because it represents the ideal line on which the HP lowers as extrusion is carried on. If dentition is extruded all together, simultaneously, the HP of occlusion lowers perpendicular to the V line. Since the HP is set to be parallel to the floor, the V line is set at 90° from it. The occlusal plane, which is determined by the upper arch, is not extruded entirely but is adjusted based on the specific orthodontic correction needed. It is crucial to understand the implications of the occlusal plane inclination when attempting to correct a Class II malocclusion, as extrusion alone may not be sufficient.

   When the second molars in the lower arch are tipped forward and slightly extruded, such as in cases of a steep posterior mandibular plane, mandibular repositioning cannot be accomplished without first addressing any posterior interferences that obstruct mandibular movement. In addition to reducing the excessive curve of Spee, it is important to tip back the lower second molars whenever possible and carry out total lower arch distalization to decrease lower incisal flaring. This approach also results in anterior condylar repositioning, further improving the overall occlusion.

5. The determination of the MyoCentric varies according to different growth patterns

   Morphology plays an important role in all occlusions. The calculus for the Myocentric is not based on the ideal freeway space, but rather on orthodontic treatment objectives. When bite recording the Myocentric for functional appliances in the growing child with excess freeway space, the Myocentric should coincide with the PRP. For adult treatments establishing a Myocentric on the Myotrajectory may be sufficient. A physiologic freeway space exceeding 2 mm may be a realistic objective in adult deep bite morphology. Every time there is an increase in freeway space when calculating the Myocentric, there is a forward positioning of the new centric.

   There can be cases in which morphology and function result in 10 or more millimeters of freeway space. It is not logical to create an 8.5-mm orthotics nor is it possible to extrude 8.5 mm with orthodontic therapy. Build-ups too would create very long teeth that would not be accepted aesthetically. There cannot be a logical dental correction of that type of freeway space which is the result of skeletal and alveolar alterations. So in a growth pattern characterized by excessive freeway space in very high numbers, the calculus of the Myocentric should be linked to an ideal freeway space >3 mm.

6. The Myotrajectory is determined by the TENS spike

   Only the TENS spike can be used to calculate the physiological muscular trajectory to HP (Myotrajectory). This spike can have a different angulation in

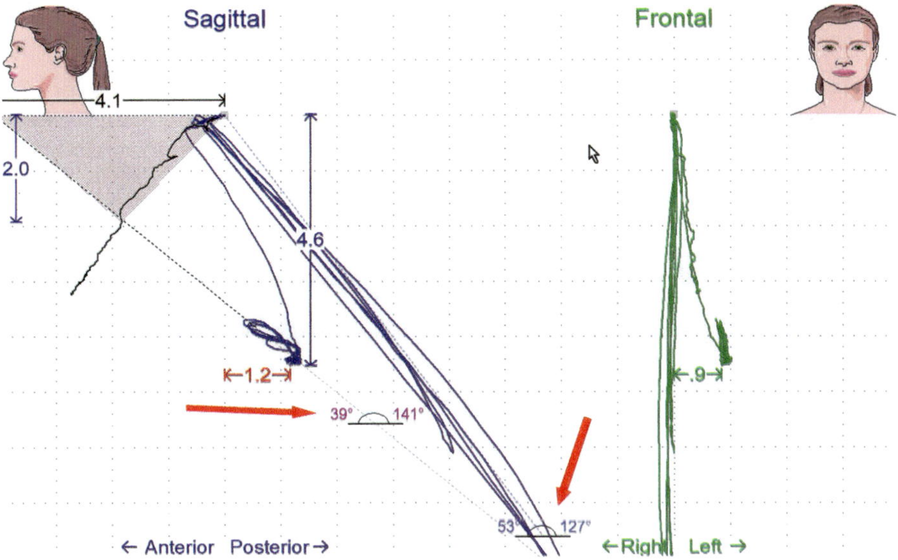

Fig. 7.16 Showing angular calculation of projected Myotrajectory and habitual trajectory to HP

respect of the angulation of the habitual path of closure, projected on HP. The K7 Diagnostic system calculates these angles as shown in Fig. 7.16.

The HP is always *the* reference plane to calculate these angles. Figure 7.16 shows a change in angular projection between habitual and after TENS path of closure. The change in this angular reading and calculus from K7 system given to the TENS spike movement is always different from that determined from the habitual path of closure. The quantitative evaluation of the discrepancy between the two measurements is another index that should be added to evaluate the severity and effort for mandibular accommodation. It is always very important to check head posture and sensor array alignment to true horizontal before proceeding with scan 5.

References

1. Smaglyuk LV, Liakhovska AV. EMG-characteristic of masticatory muscles in patients with class II malocclusion and temporomandibular disorders. Wiad Lek. 2019;72(5 cz 2):1043–7.
2. Nishi SE, Basri R, Alam MK. Uses of electromyography in dentistry: an overview with meta-analysis. Eur J Dent. 2016;10(3):419–25.
3. Wozniak K, et al. Surface electromyography in orthodontics—a literature review. Med Sci Monit. 2013;19:416–23.
4. Hugger S, et al. Clinical relevance of surface EMG of the masticatory muscles. (part 1): resting activity, maximal and submaximal voluntary contraction, symmetry of EMG activity. Int J Comput Dent. 2012;15(4):297–314.
5. Sanggarnjanavanich S, et al. Cranial-base morphology in adults with skeletal class III malocclusion. Am J Orthod Dentofac Orthop. 2014;146(1):82–91.

6. Neha. Sizing the shape: understanding morphometrics. J Clin Diagn Res. 2015;9(1):ZC21-6.
7. Chang HP, et al. Cranial-base morphology in children with class III malocclusion. Kaohsiung J Med Sci. 2005;21(4):159–65.
8. Bailey KL, Taylor RW. Mesh diagram cephalometric norms for Americans of African descent. Am J Orthod Dentofac Orthop. 1998;114(2):218–23.
9. Żytkowski A, et al. Anatomical normality and variability: historical perspective and methodological considerations. Transl Res Anat. 2021;23:100105.
10. Kapust AJ, Sinclair PM, Turley PK. Cephalometric effects of face mask/expansion therapy in Class III children: a comparison of three age groups. Am J Orthod Dentofac Orthop. 1998;113(2):204–12.
11. Gallagher RW, Miranda F, Buschang PH. Maxillary protraction: treatment and posttreatment effects. Am J Orthod Dentofac Orthop. 1998;113(6):612–9.
12. Jamilian A, et al. Methodological quality and outcome of systematic reviews reporting on orthopaedic treatment for class III malocclusion: overview of systematic reviews. J Orthod. 2016;43(2):102–20.
13. Vaida LL, et al. Correction of Class III malocclusions through morphological changes of the maxilla using the protraction face mask by three different therapeutic approaches. Romanian J Morphol Embryol. 2019;60(2):605–15.
14. Melgaco CA, et al. Immediate changes in condylar position after rapid maxillary expansion. Am J Orthod Dentofac Orthop. 2014;145(6):771–9.
15. Rivero-Millán P, et al. Comparison of condylar position in normal occlusion, Class II division 1, Class II division 2 and Class III malocclusions using CBCT imaging. J Clin Exp Dent. 2021;13(12):e1216–26.
16. Singh IJ, Savara BS. Norms of size and annual increments of seven anatomical measures of maxillae in girls from three to sixteen years of age. Angle Orthod. 1966;36(4):312–24.
17. McNamara JA. A method of cephalometric evaluation. Am J Orthod. 1984;86(6):449–69.
18. Miyajima K, et al. Craniofacial structure of Japanese and European-American adults with normal occlusions and well-balanced faces. Am J Orthod Dentofac Orthop. 1996;110(4):431–8.
19. Planas P. The Planas law for minimum vertical dimension. Rev Esp Parad. 1968;6(4):215–47.
20. Teuscher U. A growth-related concept for skeletal class II treatment. Am J Orthod. 1978;74(3):258–75.
21. Jorge M, et al. Biomechanical effects of Teuscher activator in hyperdivergent class II malocclusion treatment: a finite element analysis. J Clin Exp Dent. 2021;13(11):e1124.
22. Savastano G. Correction of a class II skeletal open bite: the Teuscher activator, part 1. EC Dent Sci. 2022;21(8):43–56.
23. Tanaka EM, Sato S. Longitudinal alteration of the occlusal plane and development of different dentoskeletal frames during growth. Am J Orthod Dentofac Orthop. 2008;134(5):602. e1-11; discussion 602-3
24. Fushima K, et al. Significance of the cant of the posterior occlusal plane in class II division 1 malocclusions. Eur J Orthod. 1996;18(1):27–40.
25. Janson G, et al. Tooth-wear patterns in subjects with Class II division 1 malocclusion and normal occlusion. Am J Orthod Dentofac Orthop. 2010;137(1):14.e1-7. discussion 14-5
26. Agnani S, et al. Tooth wear patterns in subjects with class II division 1 and class II division 2 malocclusion. Int J Adolesc Med Health. 2021;33:4.
27. Isidro S, Ono Y, Takagi Y. Craniofacial growth changes and dental attrition in the primary dentition. Pediatr Dent J. 2012;22(1):43–9.

8 The Ideal Function Is Linked to Ideal Swallow

Swallowing, also known as deglutition, is a crucial function of the stomatognathic system and plays a vital role in sustaining life. The process of swallowing involves taking food from the mouth, breaking it into smaller pieces, mixing it with saliva, and transporting it to the esophagus through a combination of voluntary and reflexive movements. Any deviation from the normal swallowing pattern can result in malocclusion [1]. Persistent oral dysfunctions can cause malocclusion, and it is generally accepted that there is no tongue dysfunction without a corresponding malocclusion. Trauma to the central nervous system that leads to central dysphagia, as well as genetic and neuromuscular diseases that cause dysphagia, can also cause malocclusion [2–4]. Malocclusion is also seen in individuals affected by intellectual disability, inborn or acquired brain disorders which are tongue thrusters [5]. Tongue dysfunction plays a significant role in causing malocclusion. There is an ongoing discussion among experts regarding whether tongue thrust or impaired swallowing can be a primary cause to the formation of malocclusion. Some experts believe that all tongue thrusts are a result of underlying causes and can be treated through orthodontic together with Oro-Myofunctional Therapy (OMT), while others argue that some tongue dysfunctions and tongue thrusts may have a genetic origin and cannot be cured through orthodontics or OMT [6]. In simpler terms, this second group will not benefit from correcting the form alone and can be considered a primary disfunction syndrome. It is likely that external stimuli for swallowing, such as saliva build-up or the presence of food, are not enough to trigger proper tongue function without tongue thrust together with an altered tongue posture. As a result, the outlook for this type of tongue thrust is not optimistic [7, 8]. Fortunately, the most common type of tongue thrust is a secondary tongue thrust (due to malocclusion, respiratory problems and so on), which can be corrected with orthodontic and OMT treatments during an individual's growth and development. However, the classification of primary and secondary tongue disorders is not universally accepted when it comes to tongue thrust issues. While primary tongue thrust has been described in literature, the prevailing belief among OMT specialists and orthodontists is that all tongue thrusts have an underlying cause and can therefore be treated.

F. Savastano, *Neuromuscular Orthodontics*,
https://doi.org/10.1007/978-3-031-41295-0_8

While orthodontic treatment may relapse in some cases, it fails to address the possibility of a primary cause for tongue dysfunction, as literature on this subject remains limited and outdated. Some observational studies have demonstrated a familial tongue thrust pattern [8]. Probably the most crucial factor contributing to malocclusion due to tongue thrust is likely tongue posture, which exerts constant pressure on the teeth involved. Not all individuals with tongue thrust develop an anterior open bite (AOB), even if the tongue thrust still determines an alteration of normal occlusal contacts (and therefore malocclusion). However, there is limited official data, but it appears that there has been a rise in the number of malocclusions that are untreatable and linked to swallow disorders, as well as other oral dysfunctions. The reasons for this increase in Orofacial Myofunctional Disorders (OMD) are still being debated among experts.

According to the ASHA website (American Speech-Language-Hearing Association), tongue thrusting incidence is between 33% and 50.5% of various populations. The incidence increases among pre-school children and those presenting speech articulation problems. OMD, is more frequently observed (97.92%) in TMD patients. Furthermore, the ASHA website on the causes states clearly: "*No single cause of orofacial myofunctional disorders has been identified, and its causes seem to be multifactorial. Anything that causes the tongue to be misplaced at rest limits lingual reduces or impedes the ability to obtain and maintain correct oral rest postures leading to an OMD. The following factors may coexist and play a role in OMDs:*

- *Airway incompetency, due to obstructed nasal passages, either due to nasal structural obstructions* (e.g., *enlarged tonsils, adenoids, hypertrophied turbinates, and/or allergies, that do not allow for effortless inspiration and expiration) (Bueno, Grechi, Trawitzki, Anselmo-Lima, Felicio & Valera, 2015). These may result in upper airway obstruction and open mouth posture (Abreu, Rocha, Lamounier, & Guerra, 2008; Vázquez-Nava,* et al., *2006), as well as an incorrect swallow pattern and mouth breathing (Hanson & Mason, 2003).*
- *Chronic nonnutritive sucking & chewing habits past the age of 3 years of age (Sousa,* et al., *2014; Poyak, 2006; Zardetto,* et al., *2002).*
- *Orofacial muscular/structural differences that encourage tongue fronting could include: delayed neuromotor development, premature exfoliation of maxillary incisors that encourage fronting of the tongue, orofacial anomalies, and ankyloglossia.*"

Delayed Neuromotor Development? Although the exact definition of this term is unclear as it refers to a developmental issue rather than a specific disease or pathology, and as it can result from various factors such as genetic conditions, traumatic experiences, and undiagnosed central nervous system deficiencies, acknowledging a reduction in neuromotor development as a cause of changes in tongue posture (often accompanied by tongue thrust) unlocks a wider range of explanations for the failure of tongue thrust treatments after Oro-Myofunctional Therapy (OMT), orthodontic treatment, surgery, or Ear, Nose and Throat (ENT) treatments. In other words, it cannot be ruled out that a genetic, primary, or endogenous tongue dysfunction may be the underlying cause of relapse after various treatments. There are varying degrees of neuromotor underdevelopment, and generally, the assessment is performed during the first year of life [9]. Could mild cases of misdiagnosed delayed neuromotor development during the growth period be responsible for a persisting tongue thrust at a later age? If a child has challenges in coordinating the muscles of the mouth and face, could they develop compensatory patterns that persist into adulthood? These patterns probably influence how they swallow, speak, and rest their tongue. The American Psychiatric Association says that up to 6% of children in the general population have mild to moderate motor dysfunction [10, 11]. Even if not all tongue thrusts give rise to AOB, it has been noted that AOB is present in 32.3% of patients with "neurological disturbances" [12]. AOB is not the only feature present for tongue thrusters. Other malocclusions have been described such as proclination of upper and lower incisors with spacing in non-AOB, and a retrognathic mandible with severe overjet [13].

Normal Deglutition

The description of the normal swallow event is usually divided into three phases: oral, pharyngeal, and esophageal [14]. The oral phase, also known as the voluntary phase, is initiated by the conscious decision to swallow. During this phase, the tongue and other oral muscles play a role in preparing the food for swallowing.

The pharyngeal phase, on the other hand, is considered a reflex response and involves the activation of several muscles, including the pharyngeal and laryngeal muscles, to initiate the swallow. This phase lasts about 0.6–1.0 s in humans and is constant across all mammals. Finally, the esophageal phase involves the transport of the food bolus from the pharynx to the stomach. This phase is slower and simpler compared to the pharyngeal phase and is controlled by both the somatic and autonomic nervous systems. The esophageal phase can last up to 10 s or more. For ease of understanding, the swallow is often divided into two main moments: the oropharyngeal phase and the esophageal phase. Understanding the cascade of motor events involved in the swallow can help in the identification of swallowing disorders [15, 16] (Table 8.1).

Table 8.1 The oropharyngeal phase of swallow

ORAL (voluntary)	Pharyngeal (reflex response)
↓	↓
1. Voluntary 2. Press bolus to hard palate 3. Contraction lips/cheek 4. Triggers pharyngeal phase 5. Trigeminal/glossopharyngeal/vagus 6. Bolus triggers posterior pharyngeal reflex	1. Protection of airways from palate. Laryngeal elevation 2. Tongue thrusts posteriorly to push bolus through the pharynx to the esophagus 3. The upper esophageal sphincter relaxes and opens for the bolus to move to the esophagus

The intricacies of deglutition are beyond the scope of this book, but a basic understanding of the oral-pharyngeal phase and the use of electromyographic (S-EMG) analysis is critical for the neuromuscular dentist. The ability to evaluate, diagnose, and probably treat swallow disorders is crucial for maintaining oral and overall health. Central nervous system pathologies can result in severe dysphagia and impaired swallowing, and S-EMG/CMS analysis can assist in detecting early signs of tongue dysfunction. It is important for the neuromuscular dentist to actively search for and treat common swallow disorders to ensure optimal oral function. The impact of swallow disorders on body posture, gait, and balance is well documented, highlighting the significance of addressing these issues. As a result, the neuromuscular dentist should be knowledgeable in the evaluation and treatment of swallow disorders and incorporate this knowledge into their clinical practice [17–21]. Tongue posture seems to be very important on general body muscle force and muscle output too [22]. Therefore, tongue posture during various activities involving body movement is an essential factor in determining overall muscular function. It is evident that *proper tongue function plays a crucial role in the development of normal occlusion and craniofacial morphology*. The importance of considering tongue posture and function in clinical assessments cannot be overemphasized. By taking these factors into account, healthcare professionals can ensure more accurate and effective evaluations and treatments [23–26].

The use of bioelectrical instrumentation in neuromuscular dentistry provides an effective way to study swallow disorders, particularly tongue thrust. Surface electromyography (EMG) is commonly used, but the ability to evaluate swallow function through a graphical representation of mandibular movements (CMS) is equally important as it increases understanding of the swallowing process and its alterations.

From an orthodontic perspective, stability of orthodontic treatment is closely linked to swallow function. A stable and balanced occlusion cannot be achieved if the tongue, a crucial player in the process, is not functioning properly. An altered tongue posture, such as a downward, forward, or lateral position, can significantly impact dental occlusion, potentially leading to lower diastemas, anterior open-bite, or lateral open-bite.

The polygraphic scan, including surface EMG, is performed by asking the patient to swallow saliva (VSS= Voluntary Swallow of Saliva) and attempting to capture spontaneous saliva swallowing (SSS= Spontaneous Swallow of Saliva) as well. The analysis of swallow function for orthodontic assessement can be studied dividing patients in two main groups: dental open bites with incompetent lips on one side, and occlusions with spontaneous lip competence and no anterior open-bite on the other. In the first grouping are certainly included individuals without spontaneous lip competence even in absence of AOB. Upper short lip can be present in good, occluded individuals. The s-EMG analysis of the perioral musculature is not important in AOB when compared to non-AOB with lip competence. During normal deglutition, it is well-established that the perioral musculature is either inactive or only slightly activated during the swallow of saliva. However, when lip incompetence and anterior open bite are present, the perioral musculature is always activated during the swallow because lip competence is necessary to prevent food from escaping the oral cavity. The perioral musculature is also activated when the patient is asked to swallow water, as this is a necessary spontaneous reaction to prevent liquids from escaping the oral cavity. Therefore, it is essential to evaluate the onset of perioral musculature activation with both saliva or a small bolus, since the evaluation of activation with water may not be informative.

S.EMG in Normal Occlusion

- OJ normal
- No open bite
- Competent lips
- Saliva swallow

Swallowing can occur as either a deliberate or an involuntary action. The surface electromyographic (S.EMG) analysis of the perioral musculature (Orbicularis Oris) and submental muscles during the act of swallowing saliva can reveal minimal or no activation of the perioral musculature . However, if the act of swallowing is elicited with a liquid such as water, the activation of the Orbicularis Oris is immediately noticeable and may overlap the output of the submental muscles [15]. This is also observed in dental open bite malocclusions where the activation of the perioral musculature is necessary for lip seal before swallowing.

The Polygraphic scan, a part of the suggested protocol (Chap. 6), provides a basic kinesiographic and s-EMG study of deglutition by simultaneously recording the surface EMG activity of up to 4 muscles and the graphical representation of mandibular movement simultaneously. The scan should be performed several times and results saved and recorded as spontaneous swallowing of saliva (SSS) and as voluntary swallowing of saliva (VSS). Figure 8.1 shows the Polygraphic scan with a normal swallow. Patient is asked to swallow, swallows in ICP from rest position and then executes "tap-tap" command to CO. The *sequence* of muscle activation should be Temporalis followed Masseter, because as previously said, the Temporalis muscle is the most postural muscle and is the first to activate during closure from rest position. The identification of CO facilitates the identification of HP. When swallow is initiated during VSS, it is important to view that during swallow centric occlusion is naturally achieved. If not, there could be a vertical gap that between the highest vertical mandibular closure and the level of HP as given by the tap tap sequence. This vertical gap could be occupied by the tongue during swallow that occupies space between the teeth.

There are differences between spontaneous and voluntary swallows of saliva, mainly related to the level of cortical involvement. These differences can be detected by the s.EMG and a laryngeal sensor. During spontaneous swallowing, the submental muscles activate within 100 milliseconds before the activation of the laryngeal sensor, while in voluntary swallowing, the activation occurs well before the movement of the laryngeal sensor, usually over 100 milliseconds [27]. This means that a requested swallow (VSS) takes more time to accomplish than a spontaneous swallow.

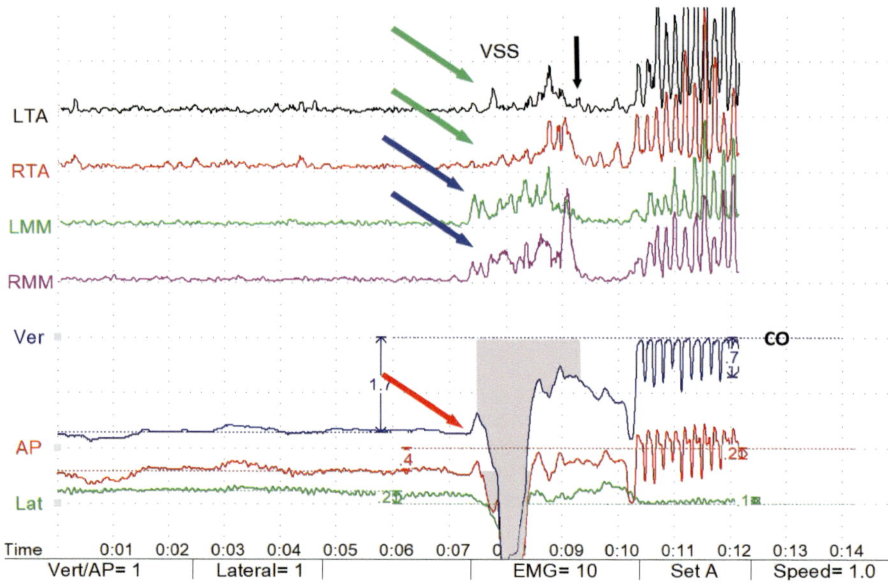

Fig. 8.1 sEMG in subject with tongue thrust. Polygraphic scan: *LTA* Left Temporalis Anterior, *RTA* Right Temporalis Anterior, *LMM* Left Masseter Muscle, *RMM* Right Masseter Muscle, *Ver*. Vertical line, *AP* Anterior/posterior line, *Lat* lateral line, *CO* Centric Occlusion. See text for explanation

To record a spontaneous swallow correctly, set the K7 system to autoclear at the end of memory during scan execution of the polygraphic setup (scan 3+ filtered EMG). Choose to limit muscle selection to Temporalis/masseter if you do not expect important swallow problems but just want to observe if the patient swallows with tongue between the teeth or not. Add more muscles like the submental (anterior digastric region), perioral (upper or lower) if you wish to gather more information. Pretend to be distracted from other than the K7 recording system to give the patient the liberty to relax and swallow spontaneously. This generally occurs because a peripheral stimulus like saliva accumulation elicits swallow. As soon as you see a swallow, press the space bar and save. Then press space bar again and have patient tap a few times in CO. Then re-save and over-write previous recording. Some authors suggest that several swallows during a 24-hour period are not performed in CO and suggest that normal swallow can include non-ICP swallow [28]. It is advisable when recording the Polygraphic scan to record VVS and SSS. Figure 8.1 shows this scan procedure with temporalis and masseter-filtered output signals. This is usually sufficient to diagnose if the patient tends to swallow with teeth together or tends to swallow with tongue between the teeth. Adding other muscles and a laryngeal sensor may be useful in the study of more complicated cases of tongue thrust or neurologic dysphagia. Fig. 8.1a shows a swallow recording of the polygraphic scan in which the patient swallows with tongue between the teeth. Note the area in gray representing the AP and Vertical space occupied by the tongue. The blue arrows show a good activation of the masseters and a poor activation of the Temporalis muscles due to the resistance of the tongue between the dental arches. The red arrow shows the initial upward movement with the beginning of a VSS. Green arrows show a scarse activation of the temposalis at initial swallow movement suggesting tongue posture is between the teeth. The Vertical blue line shows that at one point the patient lowers the mandible about 3mm. during swallow.

S.EMG in Swallow Dysfunction (S-EMG Study Hypothesis)

Figures 8.2 and 8.3 show a 10-years-old patient with a normal OJ, no open bite, with spontaneous lip competence. On Fig. 8.2 which shows an s-EMG only (not the polygraphic scan), the first burst shows a *spontaneous swallow (SSS)* in which, even though lip competence is present, there is an unexpectedstrong activation of the perioral musculature which is not justified by clinical occlusion and lip competence. Note the slight activation of the Anterior Temporalis muscles and the strong activation of the perioral musculature, red arrows (SPONT DEGL, SSS, LLO-RLO). The submental muscle activation (digastric region) shows a low output (black arrows). The activation of the perioral musculature can be interpreted as a need for lip seal (*a stronger than normal* lip seal) because the neuromuscular system *is aware of a strong forward (pathological) movement of the tongue that will appear during swallow that cannot be avoided.* Since this strong increase in perioral musculature is

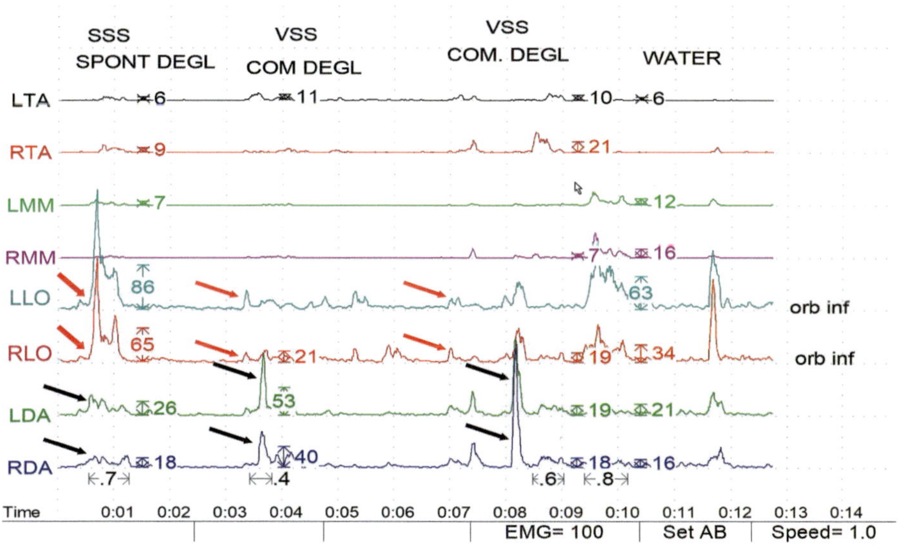

Fig. 8.2 sEMG in subject with spontaneous lip seal during a swallow sequence. *LTA* Left Temporalis Anterior, *RTA* Right Temporalis Anterior, *LMM* Left Masseter Muscle, *RMM* Right Masseter Muscle, *LLO* Left Lower Perioral muscles, *RLO* Right Lower Perioral muscles, *LDA* Left Digastricus Anterior, *RDA* Right Digastricus Anterior. Fist burst is a spontaneous swallow of saliva (SSS) followed by two bursts representing voluntary swallow of saliva (VSS), last burst is swallow with 15 ml of water

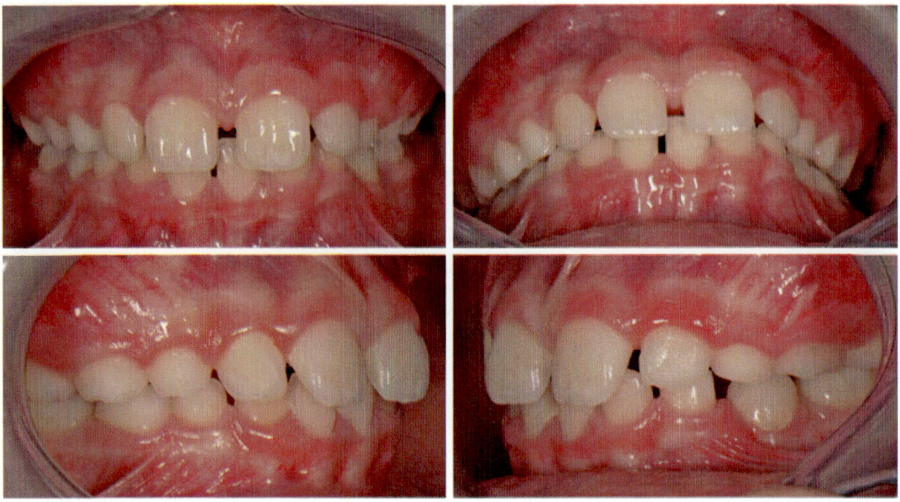

Fig. 8.3 Same patient of Fig. 8.2. Age 10 years Intra-oral occlusal photos. Note lower spacing of front incisors

generally observed during SSS, probably the subcortical swallow activation embodies a pathological altered cascade of muscular activations responsible for the anterior tongue thrust behavior.

During the second burst (COM DEGL, VSS), the patient is ready to swallow saliva voluntarily and lip seal is present as swallow is about to start in CO (CO can only be assessed clinically). Bursts 2 and 3 are further results of VSS testing. There is still present a pre-activation of the perioral muscles, just prior to the submental musculature onset, as seen during SSS, but now with a reduced output. The hypothesis suggests that the strong pre-activation of the perioral muscles in children during SSS, in the absence of any anatomical issues such as lip incompetence or anterior open bite, could be an early indication of a ***primary swallowing disorder*** with a *forward* ***tongue thrust and altered posture***. There is no clear explanation for the forward tongue posture in these cases. All ENT and speech evaluations have been carried on. The author has observed that in several cases of non-AOB primary dysfunction, there is a lower incisal spacing due to a low, forward tongue posture accompanied by anterior tongue thrust. Early detection of these primary tongue dysfunctions during the mixed dentition stage could prevent unnecessary orthodontic treatments. Instead, children could be directed to myotherapy specialists, which may provide more benefits [29]. Meanwhile, as orthodontists, we can prescribe removable swallow correction appliances that seem promising (Froggy Mouth®) [30].

Anterior open bite (AOB) in children is a major concern for the orthodontist. AOB can be present in mouth breathing individuals with severe obstruction of the respiratory tract as well as in those who have a better breathing pattern. The alteration of tongue posture and deglutition can reduce neuroplasticity [31, 32]. If these preliminary results will be confirmed in the future, the responsibility of timely intervention to help intercept cognitive impairment will fall greatly on the general health system and on the dental community.

Several authors differentiate primary tongue dysfunction from secondary tongue dysfunction[7, 8, 33, 34]. The author has formed a proper opinion in these last 30 years and agrees substantially with the results, description, and interpretation of swallow disorders as mentioned in the above literature which aknowledges primary and secondary tongue thrust.

Spacing of the lower incisors increases with age in primary tongue dysfunction without AOB. The primary dysfunction does not necessarily create an anterior open bite, but the lower incisal tipping reduces the OJ at risk of severe bone loss. Figure 8.4 shows an adult patient with a strong anterior tongue thrust and anterior lower tongue posture. This patient has never had any respiratory problems and there is no apparent reason for this tongue dysfunction. Figure 8.5 demonstrates a

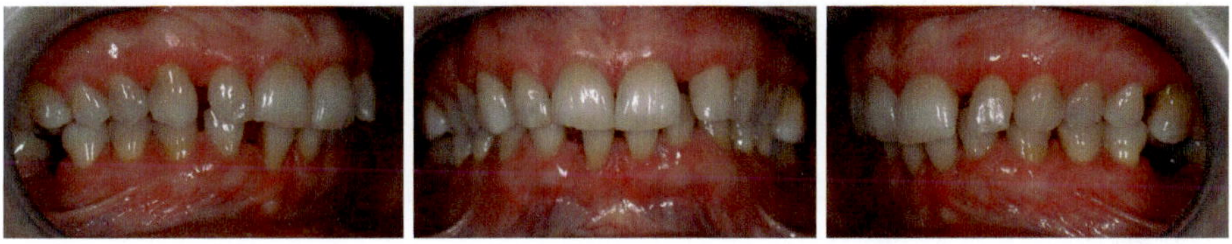

Fig. 8.4 Primary swallow disorder. Note spacing on the lower arch and reduction of OJ

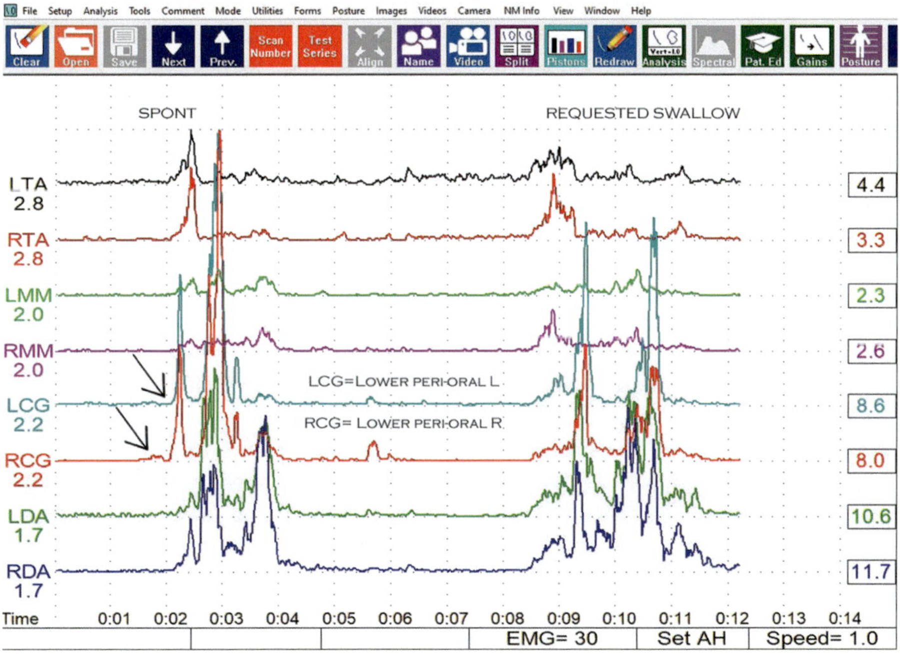

Fig. 8.5 Same patient as Fig. 8.4, Primary swallow disorder. Burst 1 spontaneous swallow (SSS), burst 2 requested swallow(VSS). *LTA* Left Temporalis Anterior, *RTA* Right Temporalis Anterior, *LMM* Left Masseter Muscle, *RMM* Right Masseter Muscle, *LCG* Left lower Perioral muscles, *RCG* Right Lower Perioral muscles, *LDA* Left Digastricus Anterior, *RDA* Right Digastricus Anterior. Note during spontaneous swallow how the lower perioral musculature activates well before the sub-mental musculature. This patient has a normal lip competence at rest

potential method for detecting swallowing disorders, which involves observing premature and unnecessary activation of the perioral muscles before the submental muscles during spontaneous swallowing.

The author has identified the spacing of the lower arch, as illustrated in Fig. 8.4, and the corresponding electromyography results, as demonstrated in Fig. 8.5, as a distinct type of primary swallowing disorder that does not involve an anterior open bite. Unfortunately, patients classified as occlusal Class II without an increased overjet who have this condition have limited treatment options. Even orthognathic surgery may not provide a long-term solution since relapse is common. Therefore, the primary purpose of using a fixed orthodontic appliance in these cases is to correct the tipping of the lower incisors and prevent their eventual loss. At present, there is no effective therapy available for these patients. While finding a solution and restoring the functional abilities of these patients is desirable, it remains a challenge to treat primary swallowing disorders.

Primary Versus Secondary Tongue Dysfunction, Hypothesis Discussion

There are various theories on the onset of primary tongue thrust. It could be a genetic problem originating from the CNS and be present at birth [8, 35]. There seems to be a permanent impediment for a normal transition to an adult swallow pattern to occur, regardless of environmental or developmental changes. In this case, primary tongue thrust is considered a pathology, distinct from an infantile swallow pattern. On the other hand, it is possible that an ongoing open bite can modify normal swallowing patterns and lead to an uncorrectable swallowing disorder. This could explain why several patients with open bite do not see lasting improvement, even after correcting their anterior open bite and vertical relationship through surgery or orthodontic treatments. This can be observed in cases where the open bite relapses and re-opens anteriorly, even after the correction of the open bite and vertical dimension with proper surgical maxillary impaction [36]. There is although, a positive outlook for those open bite individuals in which there is no primary dysfunction and in which OMT therapy is useful [37]. This simply means, that regardless of the tongue thrust diagnosis, all open-bite patients benefit from OMT treatment because it could intercept a lasting dysfunction and avoid chronicity.

It appears that our current diagnostic methods may be lacking in some regard, and the functional space for the tongue seems to be a crucial factor only in cases where primary causes are not evident. Another possibility is that the primary form of dysfunction is accompanied by a lack of oral somatosensory awareness due to a neurological central/peripheral deficiency or general CNS impairment [38–41].

Secondary tongue dysfunction refers to changes in tongue function as a response to a dental malocclusion (or breathing problems) such as an increased overjet or open bite, tongue tie, or other forms of misalignment. The presence of these conditions can impact the normal pattern of oral phase swallowing, causing the tongue to adopt a new role in preserving the swallow. In many cases, orthodontic treatment that corrects the malocclusion can determine a spontaneous correction of tongue function and improved speech.

However, some patients may require additional interventions, such as Orofacial Myofunctional Therapy (OMT), if the tongue has become accustomed to its altered function during the period of malocclusion or if there has been associated respiratory insufficiency. Even after orthodontic correction, secondary tongue thrust may persist as a habit [42]. Some of these cases that are not spontaneously corrected with orthodontic treatment and fail with OMT *could probably be undiagnosed primary tongue thrust patients* (4–10%).

The typical progression of swallowing function involves transitioning from an infantile swallow to an adult swallow starting around the age of 4 years. However, some individuals may experience a prolonged transitional stage, where they continue to display a mixture of both types of swallows past the age of 8 years old, which is considered the upper age limit for this transition. The cause of this prolonged period is still not clear, but it has been suggested that decreased maxillary development, brought on by changes in diet and an increase in respiratory issues, may play a role. Maxillary insufficiency is often linked with various forms of malocclusion, and there is limited research on the incidence of atypical swallowing in adults and children. Nevertheless, it is believed that the maturation of the maxilla-facial complex and the reduction of lymphatic tissues during adolescence may lead to fewer deglutition problems in adulthood and contribute to a later transition to an adult swallow. When a scan 21 analysis of deglutition (of saliva) reveals a swallow in Intercuspal Position (ICP) with minimal or no activation of the perioral musculature, it is considered a positive feature in adolescence and adulthood.

However, up to 40% of adults swallow without having molar contact, with their tongues positioned between their teeth at least periodically throughout the day, and do not exhibit the occlusal alterations typically associated with swallow disorders. These findings suggest that there is much more to be understood about the normal progression of swallowing function and the factors that may impact it [43, 44]. Furthermore, the link between tongue thrust and the dental open bite seems vague at times and several studies indicate that dental open-bite may be present only in 52% of tongue thrust individuals [45]. This brings us back to the individualization of primary tongue dysfunction in children where there is an abnormal tongue function and alteration of perioral activity without a dental open-bite. Tongue thrust can range in severity, with only some more severe forms being associated with a lower tongue posture and producing and maintaining a dental open bite. Other forms of tongue thrust may result in smaller changes in occlusion. The question remains to whether normal volitional deglutition should always occur in intercuspal position (ICP). Normal correct deglutition should occur in individuals with a good neuromuscular occlusion, and it is most probable that voluntary swallow should occur in ICP while SSS may not. Previous studies by Jankelson et al. have indicated that deglutition occurs in intercuspal position (ICP) most of the time. However, current scientific consensus, as indicated by Lard, is that deglutition occurs in ICP about 70% of the time [46]. It is probable that voluntary swallows (VSS) occur primarily in the intercuspal position (ICP), and when they do not, the neuromuscular adaptation to malocclusion may exceed the physiological tolerance of the stomatognathic system. In other words, when a VSS is performed with the tongue placed between the teeth, it is likely a protective reflex aimed at reducing fatigue. In cases where the neuromuscular system is unable to tolerate a swallow in the ICP due to malocclusion, it may modify the tongue function by positioning it between the dental arches. This serves as a physiological bite and reduces stress on the musculature and temporomandibular joint (TMJ) to prevent potentially harmful stimuli; but it could also be a simple energy saving mechanism reaction to malocclusion. Moreover, the tongue may occupy excess freeway space, leading to a more functional mandibular repositioning when engaged in a swallow function.

As neuromuscular dentists and orthodontists, it is our responsibility to understand the root causes of swallow disorders and take proactive measures to prevent them. In some cases, tongue dysfunctions can result from improper orthodontic and dental treatments. However, a prevalent issue in our society is maxillary insufficiency, which also contributes to an increasing number of tongue disorders. Maxillar insufficiency simply means that there is less room for the tongue. When swallow disorders are clinically and objectively diagnosed by s-EMG, the practitioner can refer the patient to other specialists for further treatment and evaluation. This is especially true for adult patients in which a primary cause of dysphagia can be related to passed CNS faults such as stroke, tumors, or other diseases of the CNS. As a result, dentists and speech specialists face a growing challenge to address these issues. Here are the key reasons for the most common mistakes made during orthodontic treatments and how they can contribute to tongue dysfunction:

1. Distalizing the upper arch.
2. Interruption of tooth contact between the dental arches during growth.
3. Orthodontic treatment without treatment of respiratory problems.
4. Orthodontic treatment without correction of parafunctions and bad habits.

Distalization of the Upper Arch

Class II *positional* occlusions are for definition Class I skeletally, in which the mandible is not freely positioned forward and down but kept distally from a variety of occlusal obstacles. Thinking ***face forward*** about growth and treatment has always seemed reasonable. The concept of promoting changes in the mandibular condyle has always been a logical approach for functionalists and it is surprising to see still such strong resistance toward functional therapy [47]. The utilization of upper arch distalization in orthodontic treatment should be restricted to situations involving skeletal or occlusal class II cases. This is particularly applicable when there's a need to address compensation of the maxillary arch due to insufficient mandibular growth that cannot be corrected by mandibular "physiological" repositioning. While it is rare to encounter a true forward position of the upper maxillary teeth and alveolus in positional Class II, upper distalization can be the preferred treatment option in such cases, in conjunction with some orthopedic mandibular repositioning. In cases of upper arch asymmetry, some hemi-arch distalization may be necessary, but in most instances, distalization of the upper arch in positional Class II malocclusions may exacerbate dysfunctional traits and worsen the malocclusion by neuromuscular standards, (and not only by those standards). Distalization of the upper arch can also potentially cause or aggravate condylar retrusion, leading to TMJ dysfunction. While some studies have investigated the effect of distalization on condylar position, they have all focused on end-of-treatment results and have not included long-term follow-ups of 10–15 years. It is worth noting that the mandible continues to grow until the age of 21 years in boys and 16 years in girls. Although it is challenging to find publications linking orthodontic treatment to TMD, any change in occlusion can impact ***condylar position***, which is known to be ***associated with TMD*** [48–60]. Determining the ideal condylar position through CBCT may not be a reliable method when there are no apparent severe positional discrepancies. This is because the method is not capable of accurately determining the disk position and cannot ensure optimal joint function during mandibular movements.

Performing a complete series of diagnostic scans on orthodontic patients who have undergone upper distalization to "correct" their Class II occlusion, usually delivers disastrous EMG testing and surprising Scan 5 results (Figs. 8.6, 8.7, and 8.8). This patient started re-treatment because of acute TMD 5 years after orthodontic treatment. Note in Fig. 8.8 the purple arrow showing a mandibular (condylar) distalization occurring at swallow. This is a dysfunctional feature common seen in patients that have undergone previous treatments with upper distalization. This

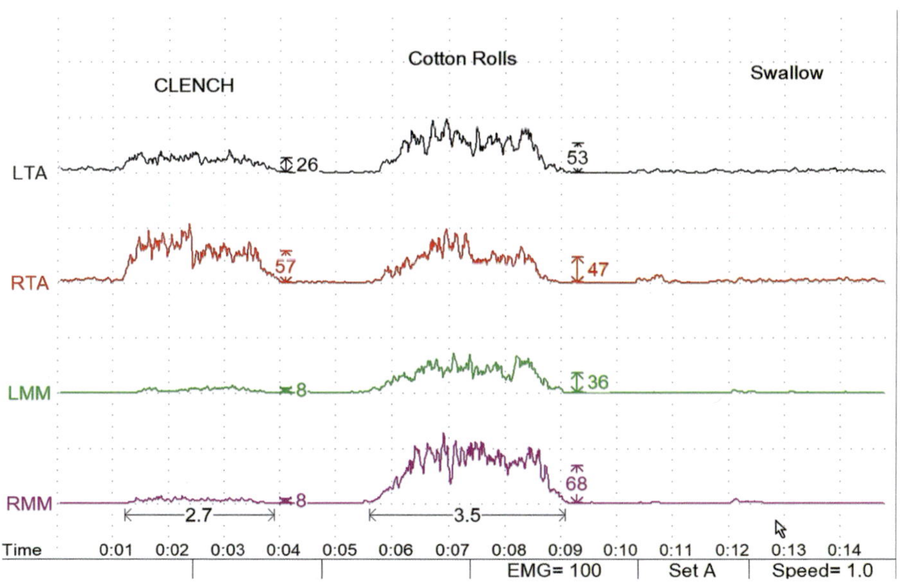

Fig. 8.6 Scan 11 shows only slight activation of LTA and RTA and practically no activation of the masseter muscles during clench in ICP, first burst. Clenching on cotton rolls increases slightly muscular activity, second burst. *LTA* Left Temporalis Anterior, *RTA* Right Temporalis Anterior, *LMM* Left Masseter Muscle, *RMM* Right Masseter Muscle

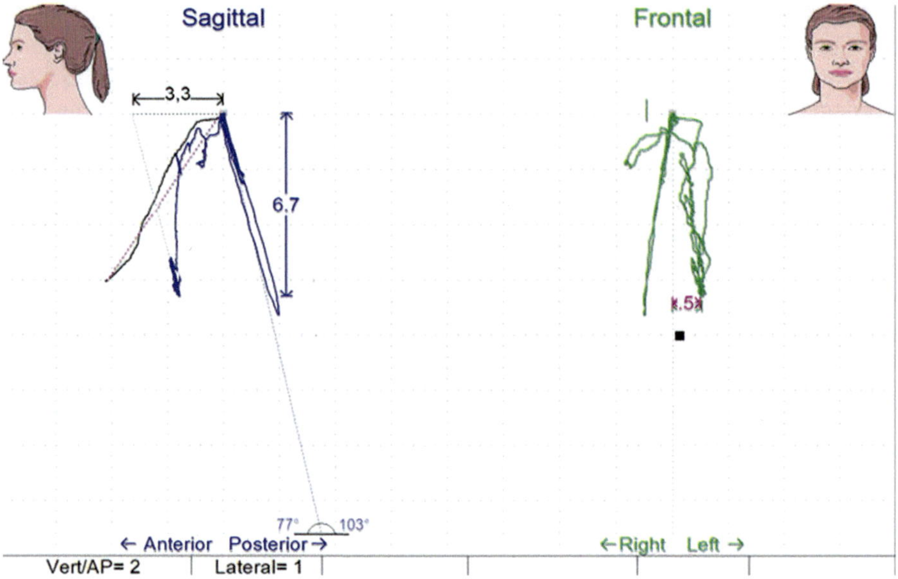

Fig. 8.7 Scan 5. Showing Sagittal discrepancy is 3.3 mm on horizontal plane of occlusion. Freeway space is about 6.7 mm

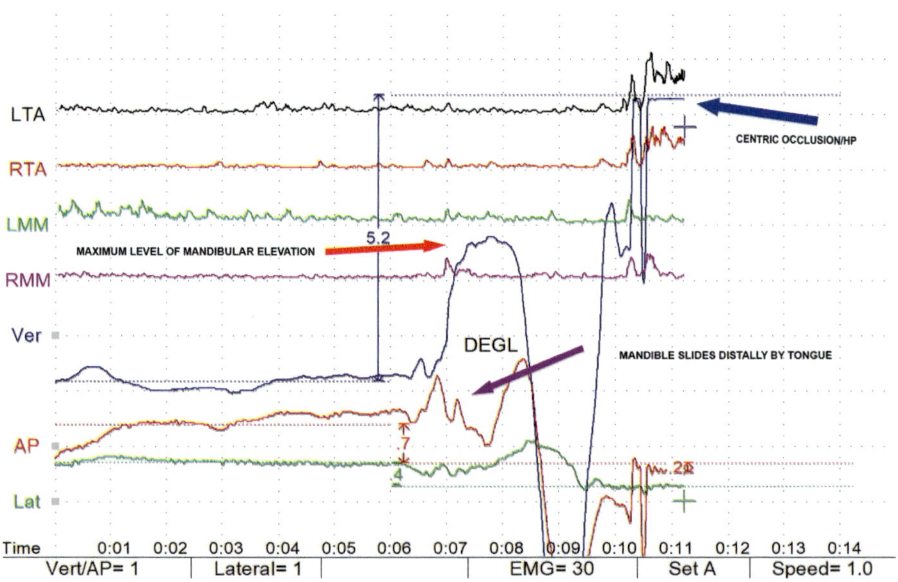

Fig. 8.8 Polygraphic scan. Patient swallows with tongue between the teeth with a maximum elevation of the mandible (red arrow) at 2.2-mm from HP of occlusion, indicated by CO and blue arrow. Purple arrow shows that during swallow, as mandible is closing attempting CO, it is pushed back from the tongue. *LTA* Left Temporalis Anterior, *RTA* Right Temporalis Anterior, *LMM* Left Masseter Muscle, *RMM* Right Masseter Muscle

continous condylar compression during swallow determines, eventually, a iatrogenic TMJ pathology.

One of the main objectives for the correction of any malocclusion should be the normalization of tongue function. Most patients that have undergone upper distalizationdo not have a correct tongue function (Fig. 8.8). This is a typical sign that the neuromuscular system is not tolerating mandibular/condylar position during swallow. When the mandible is re-postured correctly (on the neuromuscular trajectory and with sufficient posterior support), these patients tend to normalize swallow and improve EMG at rest and correct EMG swallow testing with a correct *muscular activation sequence*. Re-treatment involves the reopening of spaces and repositioning of the mandible in extraction cases. Correction of excessive distalization of the upper arch may necessitate the use of face mask therapy. Additionally, it is common to observe excessive flaring of the lower incisors. These findings may seem surprising, but some researchers have also conducted studies that reveal hidden truths. For example, it has been discovered that condylar retrusion and compression frequently occur after premolar extractions, highlighting the importance of considering the potential long-term effects of orthodontic treatments [61].

Interruption of Tooth Contact between the Dental Arches in Children and Adults: Aligner Treatment and Gummy Positioners

Whenever teeth come together, even with the slightest contact, the CNS receives a vast number of afferent signals from the periodontal ligaments, muscles, tendons, TMJ, and fascia. Oral stereognosis is a neurosensorial ability of the oral mucosae to identify, locate and distinguish objects and anatomical components within the oral cavity. The CNS relies greatly on the sensory organs to receive and elaborate afferent information to fine tune motor activity of the stomatognathic system [38]. These signals stimulate the cortex in many ways, one of which is by increasing the number of synapses [62]. This constant stimulus upload from the oral cavity is very important in the growing patient: the cortex needs continuous stimulation to increase both neurons and synapses. The brain responds by fine modulation of the stomatognathic musculature making speech and swallow possible. Feedback mechanisms and reflexes concur in making oral functions possible. *The trophic effect on these muscles avoids hypotonicity of the oral musculature.*

The afferent stimulation from the stomatognathic system to the CNS is schematically described as follows:

1. TMJ proprioception. Free nerve endings and sensory nerve organs in the disk parenchyma. This is confirmed by nociceptive afferent signals producing joint pain in temporomandibular disorders due to arthrosis or disk dislocation [63].
2. Muscle proprioception. Muscle spindles send continuous information to the CNS through the mesencephalic nucleus. This information is about muscle length (mechanoreceptive) and traumatic/excessive muscle stretch (nociceptive).

This proprioception is found in the pterygoid and other muscles of mandibular posture. Tongue somatosensory innervation is supplied by the lingual nerve (2/3rd anterior part), glossopharyngeal nerve (IX, posterior 1/3rd), and vagus nerve (X). The lingual nerve is part of the mandibular branch that derives from the trigeminal nerve(V) [64, 65].

This continuous afferent stimuli to cortex synapses and back for local trophic action, increases cognition and generates motor control response. This complex loop-like process stimulates consciousness and emotions and increases interaction with the environment [62]. You can imagine the brain needs continuous stimuli to acquire specific quality enhancements for correct brain development.

Several studies have focused on proprioception from partial or full prosthetic dentures and dental implants, proving the CNS ability to adjust when there is an anatomical loss of exteroceptors [66–68]. Obviously, proprioception is reduced by aging.

In growing children undergoing orthodontic therapy, prolonged use of gummy positioners or aligner therapies that disrupt tooth contact, alter chewing patterns, and reduce oral proprioception may result in partial or severe impairment of neuroplasticity. This hypothesis arises from the interruption of the feedback loop caused by the reduction of proprioception, which likely compromises somatosensory awareness.

Furthermore, the absence of a stable position for the mandible during voluntary swallow, because of deglutition occurring without tooth contact and *never* in ICP, can have negative consequences. It has been shown that mandibular movements during daytime activities such as mastication play a significant role in stimulating the brain, and any reduction or alteration of this stimulation may compromise general cognitive function [69–75].

(a) Over the course of my 30 years of professional experience, I have noticed a growing number of children and young adults exhibiting various degrees of intellectual disability (ID), facial hypotonicity, drowsiness, and a pronounced anterior tongue thrust with a low anterior posture. To me, it appears that oral dysfunction, and specifically tongue dysfunction, has become more prevalent and can be attributed to a combination of environmental factors. While soft, sugary foods in the diet and an increase in allergies and intolerances caused by the environment may contribute, they are only part of the problem. Impaired swallowing can also be a common response to respiratory issues. Since voluntary swallowing typically occurs in centric occlusion (ICP), any prolonged interference with mandibular stabilization could compromise correct swallow patterns. Aligner treatments, for instance, may interfere with ICP and, in turn, interfere with correct swallowing. The reduction in afferent inputs to the central nervous system can result in a drop in the efferent local trophic effect on the muscles of the stomatognathic system. As a result, these young patients appear to experience delays in maturation across all neuromuscular and neurological aspects. Furthermore, these treatments are increasingly being administered during the mixed dentition stage, making it imperative to underline the significance of this developmental phase for toddlers.

(A) Between ages 4 and 8 years there should be a shift from the infantile swallow to an adult swallow. The encephalization process that started after birth is not suddenly arrested during childhood but continues throughout growth. This process will be essential for the swallow transition from visceral to somatic and overall neurological development [76, 77]. Aligners interrupt proprioception to the CNS and are an obstacle to swallow in ICP. Furthermore, any treatment that compromises and alters a *correct swallow pattern* can be considered a possible threat to cognitive development due to the important interference of somatosensory stimulation of the cerebellum, thalamus, cingulate gyrus, and sensorimotor cortex bilaterally [78].

(b) The severity of malocclusion has been found to be correlated with oral somatosensory stereognosis, indicating that the upper and lower dental arches are interconnected and perform a single function [39–41, 79, 80]. An occlusal medium that provides an unstable mandibular position for swallowing, also leads to a reduction in stereognosis by affecting the input of sensory information to the central nervous system with a resulting decrease of subcortical stimulation. This may be perceived by the CNS system as a disturbance factor that interferes with oral proprioception, hindering muscle function. While an individual's ability to adapt to these changes in occlusion may vary, it is possible that adaptational changes in tongue posture and function may occur as a dysfunctional response to changes in oral somatosensory awareness. Patients with a low, forward tongue posture with tongue against lower and upper front incisors are typically not aware of their tongue position until instructed otherwise.

Neuroplasticity is not a trait of growing patients; it has been demonstrated that adults adapt to environmental changes also [81–84]. If so, this sudden lack of stimuli due to aligner therapy could lead to a reduction of neuroplasticity in the adult as well, and this could be linked to a reduction of cognitive abilities. Could the consequences be less severe than what (hypothetically) happens in children? The absence of a stable ICP and tooth contact due to aligner/positioner treatments is accompanied by an unstable occlusion (Centric Occlusion) during deglutition. The loss of proprioceptive feedback during mastication has been widely demonstrated to be linked to cognitive function loss in adults [85]. These treatment modalities do not respect an ideal functional ICP which is regulated by a physiological fixed mandibular position, but rather focus only on teeth alignment. During orthodontic fixed appliance therapy, any transient malocclusion allways provides a stable centric occlusion for swallow. When using functional appliances, such as the Bionator, it is important to establish a stable centric occlusion, which is the contact between the teeth when the jaw is in a stable position. This stable position is critical in starting a correct voluntary swallow sequence. Regarding aligner therapies, some newer treatments may involve extractions. However, it is generally recommended to avoid extraction therapy whenever possible. Instead, orthodontic treatments should aim to create more space for the tongue while conserving the number of teeth. This can help maintain proper cognitive function, as the tongue is crucial for proper speech, swallowing, and even breathing [86, 87].

The absence of a stable mandibular position during deglutition may hypothetically stimulate noxious feedback stimuli to the central nervous system (CNS). It is conceivable that cognitive function and swallowing may be correlated, as these two neurophysiological systems are potentially interconnected [88]. It has been well hypothesized that the ideal treatment modality that determines an increase in cerebral blood flow and an improvement in physical balance must include a stable ICP and an ideal muscular rest position of the mandible [89]. This phenomenon is evident during neuromuscular orthotic treatments, where the Myocentric is considered the most physiological centric and an ideal muscular rest position is the result of mandibular deconditioning from the original malocclusion. This is an important factor, as it provides a level of certainty to the neuromuscular system, unlike aligners and gummy positioners, which lack stable ICP feedback and create uncertainty for the neuromuscular system. All functional treatment modalities should aim to stimulate mandibular repositioning, with the perioral musculature being activated through upper and lower lip contact. Lip competence is a crucial aspect of muscular re-education toward functional correction.

While orthotic use certainly interrupts tooth to tooth contact, it provides afferent stimuli from the TMJ, muscles, fascia, and periodontal ligaments about a precise mandibular position during swallow/occlusion. This favorable neuromuscular position avoids the consequences due to muscle accommodation, such as entrapment of vascular and neural components in fascia and small orifices [90]. In addition to orthotic use, it can be speculated that the orthotic acts as a *complete prosthetic overdenture that conserves mastication, thus guaranteeing optimal cerebral blood flow, and stabilizes the centric occlusion for normal deglutition.* The conservation of the mastication process should be considered as an important factor that distinguishes orthotics, prosthetics, and fixed orthodontic appliances from other types of intraoral therapies which do not. Certainly, overdentures and orthotics may reduce oral somatosensory awareness, but the benefits justify these changes [38, 91]. The proven fact that mastication stimulates the CNS remains an important factor for neuroplasticity processes and neuromodulation in adults. All major cognitive functions are preserved and memory and learning processes are improved [92].

The idea of using an anterior bite or anterior shelf to "deprogram" occlusion and muscle memory is problematic and can result in poor electromyographic (s-EMG) results. Anterior disocclusion should only be used for a limited time and with caution. An anterior bite plane can cause uncertainty about proper positioning of the mandible during a normal swallow, leading to constant mandibular sliding of the lower incisors on the acrylic surface. This also limits the contraction of the masseter muscle, while occlusion, that should be limited by teeth contact, is now limited to the anatomy of the temporomandibular joint (TMJ). More effective methods exist to relax and deprogram the postural muscles of the stomatognathic system, like the Aqualizer® and TENS as previously described. With proper training, this procedure enables practitioners to take an accurate and "deprogrammed" bite registration based on functional needs [93].

Orthodontic Treatment without Treatment of Respiratory Problems

One of the established truths about facial development is that respiratory issues, such as nasal obstruction or adenoid/tonsil blockages, can alter a child's face and lead to the development of "Adenoid Facies." It is now recognized that not only adenoids or tonsils can cause respiratory difficulties, but any pathology of the respiratory system that requires the child to breathe through their mouth chronically can result in such issues [94–103]. The most frequent symptoms of respiratory difficulties in children are persistent mouth breathing and snoring. Sleep apnea is a common occurrence and should be promptly addressed. Even after treating respiratory issues, some children may continue to breathe through their mouth as a habit. For more than two decades, I have found mouth-sealing tape to be highly effective in re-establishing proper respiration through the nose. Mouth breathing can affect tongue positioning, causing it to drop, move down, and extend forward, which can lead to malocclusion and improper cranio-cervical posture. Children with sleep-related breathing disorders experience heightened levels of stress. These disorders are a common discovery in orthodontic practices, affecting up to 10% of patients [104]. Developmental consequences can be important, such as reduction of neurogenesis [105] and other health consequences such as cognitive defects, heart problems, diabetes, and other cerebrovascular diseases [106–110]. The importance of orthodontic treatment and correct ENT evaluation is crucial in avoiding complex OSAS treatment in adults.

The responsibility of diagnosing pediatric Obstructive Sleep Apnea Syndrome (OSAS) is gradually shifting toward dentists. As orthodontists, it is imperative that we act proactively to detect sleep-related respiratory problems in children as early as possible. Although hospital polysomnography is considered the gold standard for diagnosing OSAS in children, there are new home testing systems that can be used to screen for nocturnal apnea and hypopnea.

The WatchPAT® 300 from ®ZOLL® Itamar® is a user-friendly device that can be operated to screen OSAS in children weighing 30 kg or more. Home testing has several advantages, especially for children, as it allows them to be in a comfortable and familiar environment rather than being away from home with a parent. Additionally, there may be a shortage of hospital polysomnography services, and in rural areas, this type of diagnostic testing may not be available.

The information obtained is extensive and data can be exported for referral to a sleep specialist. The data from WatchPAT300 is proven for ages 16 and up, but the importance of screening children (30 kg. and up) remains mandatory for the practitioner. Figures 8.9, 8.10, and 8.11 show a partial of a general sleep report in a 10-year-old child. While the pAHI (average number of apnea and hypopnea events per hour of sleep) $\leq$ 5 is normal for adults, anything over 1 is considered suspect of OSAS in children. These figures show a severe sleep problem with a pAHI of 22.6. This patient was referred to an ENT and treated with adenotonsillectomy and RPE.

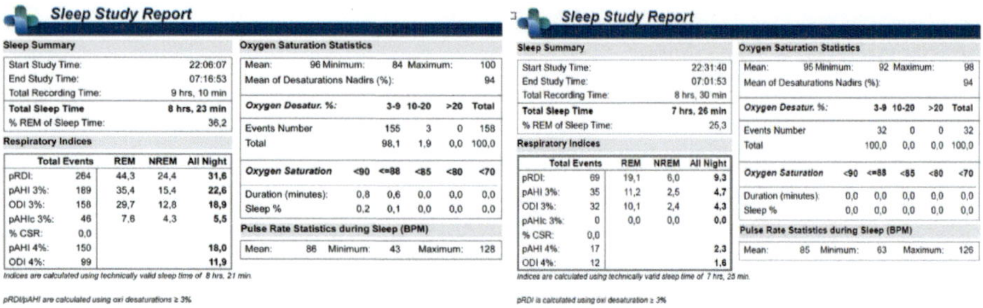

Fig. 8.9 Sleep summary report, from WatchPAT300, Itamar medical, Israel., Before and after surgery and RPE

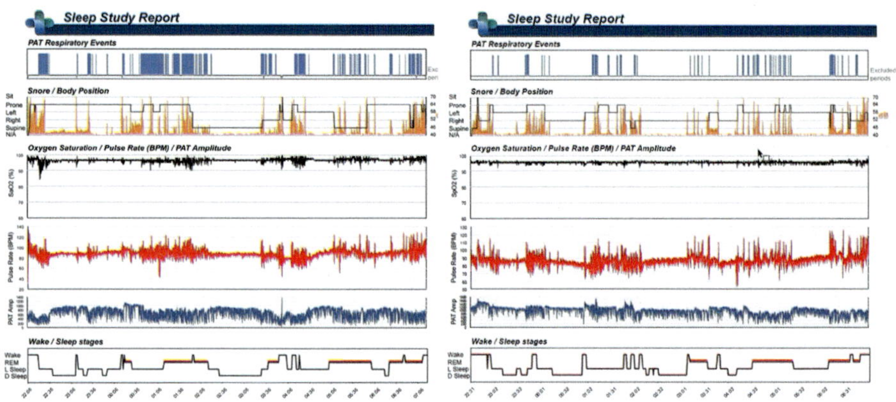

Fig. 8.10 Sleep summary report with graphics, from WatchPAT300, Itamar medical, Israel., Before and after surgery and RPE

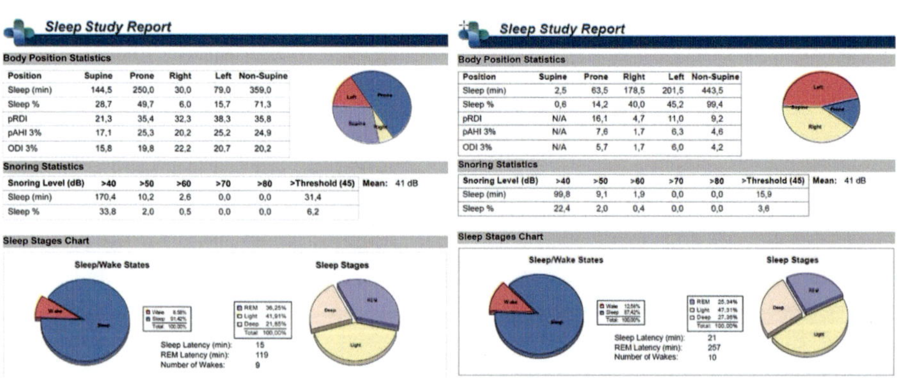

Fig. 8.11 Sleep summary report with body positions, snoring statistics, and sleep chart, from WatchPAT300, Itamar medical, Israel. Before and after surgery and RPE

The results of the effectiveness of adenotonsillectomy and RPE can be seen in Figs. 8.9, 8.10 and 8.11, in which pAHI and ODI has dropped respectively from 22.6 and 18.9 to 4.7 and 4.3. The treatment objective is oriented to lowering the pAHI and ODI level 1 and below. This may take several months after surgery where mouth taping and in general mouth breathing habits must be addressed.

Surgical and orthodontic interventions (Rapid Palatal Expansion or RPE) have proven to be highly effective in addressing various breathing impairment problems that are related to the stomatognathic system. Specifically, early intervention to correct breathing patterns and treat obstructive sleep apnea syndrome (OSAS) can result in significant functional improvements. The benefits of such interventions are particularly evident in cases where compromised swallow patterns accompany malocclusions. The gradual normalization of swallow patterns, coupled with the correction of underlying malocclusions, can lay the foundation for a complete recovery. The impact of these interventions can have a profound effect on the patient's overall quality of life. The restoration of proper breathing and swallowing functions can improve sleep quality, promote healthy digestion, and enhance overall physical and emotional well-being. It is crucial to emphasize the importance of early intervention in cases of compromised breathing and swallowing functions. With timely and appropriate treatment, patients can experience significant improvements in their stomatognathic health and overall quality of life.

Orthodontic Treatment without Correction of Parafunctions and Bad Habits

In addition to the detrimental habit of mouth breathing, there are several other habits that can contribute to the development of swallow disorders. Thumb sucking and playing certain instruments, for instance, are common habits that can impact the proper functioning of the stomatognathic system [111–117]. The cessation of these habits typically leads to a gradual and stable improvement in occlusal and oral function. Any non-functional oral behavior, such as bruxism, lip-sucking, or nail-biting, is referred to as an oral parafunction. While some of these behaviors may be unconscious, others are intentional and can contribute to swallowing disorders and phonetic issues.

These harmful habits and parafunctions are commonly observed in patients with Temporomandibular Disorder (TMD) [118–124]. This condition can cause a range of symptoms, including pain and dysfunction in the temporomandibular joint, difficulty chewing, and restricted jaw movement. The presence of parafunctional habits and swallowing disorders can exacerbate these symptoms and impede proper function of the stomatognathic system.

Effective treatment of TMD involves not only addressing the underlying condition but also identifying and addressing any accompanying parafunctional habits or swallowing disorders. The cessation of these harmful behaviors can promote healthy stomatognathic function and improve overall oral health and well-being.

References

1. D'Onofrio L. Oral dysfunction as a cause of malocclusion. Orthod Craniofac Res. 2019;22(Suppl 1):43–8.
2. Cocca S, et al. Correlation between dysphagia and malocclusion in Rett syndrome: a preliminary study. Sultan Qaboos Univ Med J. 2018;18(4):e489–93.
3. van den Engel-Hoek L, et al. Feeding and swallowing disorders in pediatric neuromuscular diseases: an overview. J Neuromuscul Dis. 2015;2:357–69.
4. Doriguêtto PVT, et al. Malocclusion in children and adolescents with down syndrome: a systematic review and meta-analysis. Int J Paediatr Dent. 2019;29(4):524–41.
5. Roane H, Ringdahl JE, Falcomata T. Clinical and organizational applications of applied behavior analysis. Academic Press; 2015.
6. Fletcher SG, Casteel RL, Bradley DP. Tongue-thrust swallow, speech articulation, and age. J Speech Hear Disord. 1961;26:201–8.
7. Subtelny JD, Subtelny JD. Malocclusion, speech, and deglutition. Am J Orthod. 48(9):685–97.
8. Tulley WJ. A critical appraisal of tongue-thrusting. Am J Orthod. 1969;55(6):640–50.
9. Gorga D, et al. Neuromotor development of preterm and full-term infants. Early Hum Dev. 1988;18(2–3):137–49.
10. Largo RH, et al. Neuromotor development from 5 to 18 years. Part 1: timed performance. Dev Med Child Neurol. 2001;43(7):436–43.
11. Largo RH, et al. Neuromotor development from 5 to 18 years. Part 2: associated movements. Dev Med Child Neurol. 2001;43(7):444–53.
12. Gershater MM. The proper perspective of open bite. Angle Orthod. 1972;42(3):263–72.
13. Jalaly T, Ahrari F, Amini F. Effect of tongue thrust swallowing on position of anterior teeth. J Dent Res Dent Clin Dent Prospects. 2009;3(3):73–7.
14. Miller AJ. Deglutition. Physiol Rev. 1982;62(1):129–84.
15. Ertekin C, Aydogdu I. Neurophysiology of swallowing. Clin Neurophysiol. 2003;114(12):2226–44.
16. Miller AJ. The neurobiology of swallowing and dysphagia. Dev Disabil Res Rev. 2008;14(2):77–86.
17. Wildenberg JC, et al. Altered connectivity of the balance processing network after tongue stimulation in balance-impaired individuals. Brain Connect. 2013;3(1):87–97.
18. Wildenberg JC, et al. Electrical tongue stimulation normalizes activity within the motion-sensitive brain network in balance-impaired subjects as revealed by group independent component analysis. Brain Connect. 2011;1(3):255–65.
19. Wildenberg JC, et al. High-resolution fMRI detects neuromodulation of individual brainstem nuclei by electrical tongue stimulation in balance-impaired individuals. NeuroImage. 2011;56(4):2129–37.
20. Wildenberg JC, et al. Sustained cortical and subcortical neuromodulation induced by electrical tongue stimulation. Brain Imaging Behav. 2010;4(3–4):199–211.
21. Bordoni B, et al. The anatomical relationships of the tongue with the body system. Cureus. 2018;10(12):e3695.
22. di Vico R, et al. The acute effect of the tongue position in the mouth on knee isokinetic test performance: a highly surprising pilot study. Muscles Ligaments Tendons J. 2014;3(4):318–23.
23. Swinehart DR. The importance of the tongue in the development of normal occlusion. Am J Orthod. 1950;36(11):813–30.
24. Posen AL. The influence of maximum perioral and tongue force on the incisor teeth. Angle Orthod. 1972;42(4):285–309.
25. Hutchinson EF, Kieser JA, Kramer B. Morphometric growth relationships of the immature human mandible and tongue. Eur J Oral Sci. 2014;122(3):181–9.
26. Sun-Hwa K. A study on the effect of the size and posture of tongue and craniofacial morphology on generalized spaced dentition. Korean J Orthod. 1996;26(5):623–36.
27. Ertekin C. Voluntary versus spontaneous swallowing in man. Dysphagia. 2011;26(2):183–92.

28. Monaco A, et al. Surface electromyography pattern of human swallowing. BMC Oral Health. 2008;8:6.
29. Svensson P, et al. Plasticity in corticomotor control of the human tongue musculature induced by tongue-task training. Exp Brain Res. 2003;152(1):42–51.
30. Quinzi V, et al. Short-term effects of a myofunctional appliance on atypical swallowing and lip strength: a prospective study. J Clin Med. 2020;9(8):2652.
31. Restrepo C, et al. Brain cortex activity in children with anterior open bite: a pilot study. Front Hum Neurosci. 2020;14
32. Arima T, et al. Corticomotor plasticity induced by tongue-task training in humans: a longitudinal fMRI study. Exp Brain Res. 2011;212(2):199–212.
33. Subtelny JD. Examination of current philosophies associated with swallowing behavior. Am J Orthod. 1965;51:161–82.
34. Subtelny JD, Sakuda M. Muscle function, oral malformation, and growth changes. Am J Orthod. 1966;52(7):495–517.
35. Ballard CF, Gwynne-Evans E. The upper respiratory musculature and orthodontics. Dent Rec (London). 1948;68(1):1–21.
36. Elhajoubi L, et al. Short and long term stability of open bite surgical treatment: a systemic review. Adv Oral Maxillofac Surg. 2021;3:100099.
37. Smithpeter J, Covell D. Relapse of anterior open bites treated with orthodontic appliances with and without orofacial myofunctional therapy. Am J Orthod Dentofac Orthop. 2010;137(5):605–14.
38. Haggard P, de Boer L. Oral somatosensory awareness. Neurosci Biobehav Rev. 2014;47:469–84.
39. Premkumar S, Avathvadi Venkatesan S, Rangachari S. Altered oral sensory perception in tongue thrusters with an anterior open bite. Eur J Orthod. 2011;33(2):139–42.
40. Koczorowski M, Woźniak W, Koczorowski R. Impairment of the oral stereognosis in the partial anterior open bite. Folia Morphol (Warsz). 2006;65(3):221–4.
41. Dahan JS, et al. Oral perception in tongue thrust and other oral habits. Am J Orthod Dentofac Orthop. 2000;118(4):385–91.
42. Tulley WJ. Some thought on prognosis and treatment planning. In: Paper presented to the 50th meeting of A.A.O., Los Angeles. 1962.
43. Subtelny JD. Oral respiration: facial maldevelopment and corrective dentofacial orthopedics. Angle Orthod. 1980;50(3):147–64.
44. Monaco A, et al. Prevalence of atypical swallowing: a kinesiographic study. Eur J Paediatr Dent. 2006;7(4):187–91.
45. Dixit UB, Shetty RM. Comparison of soft-tissue, dental, and skeletal characteristics in children with and without tongue thrusting habit. Contemp Clin Dent. 2013;4(1):2–6.
46. Lard W. Intermaxillary relationships during deglutition. J Dent Res. 1974;53(1):127–31.
47. Rabie AB, She TT, Hagg U. Functional appliance therapy accelerates and enhances condylar growth. Am J Orthod Dentofac Orthop. 2003;123(1):40–8.
48. Murakami S, et al. Longitudinal study of patients with TMJ dysfunction by tomographic examination: condylar position and clinical sign. Oral Radiol. 1993;9(1):41–7.
49. Weinberg LA. An evaluation of occlusal factors in TMJ dysfunction-pain syndrome. J Prosthet Dent. 1979;41(2):198–208.
50. Weinberg LA. Role of condylar position in TMJ dysfunction-pain syndrome. J Prosthet Dent. 1979;41(6):636–43.
51. Bean LR, Thomas CA. Significance of condylar positions in patients with temporomandibular disorders. J Am Dent Assoc. 1987;114(1):76–7.
52. Ren YF, Isberg A, Westesson PL. Condyle position in the temporomandibular joint. Comparison between asymptomatic volunteers with normal disk position and patients with disk displacement. Oral Surg Oral Med Oral Pathol Oral Radiol Endod. 1995;80(1):101–7.
53. Weinberg LA, Lager LA. Clinical report on the etiology and diagnosis of TMJ dysfunction-pain syndrome. J Prosthet Dent. 1980;44(6):642–53.

54. Weinberg LA. The role of stress, occlusion, and condyle position in TMJ dysfunction-pain. J Prosthet Dent. 1983;49(4):532–45.
55. Egermark-Eriksson I, Carlsson GE, Magnusson T. A long-term epidemiologic study of the relationship between occlusal factors and mandibular dysfunction in children and adolescents. J Dent Res. 1987;66(1):67–71.
56. Owen AH 3rd. Orthodontic/orthopedic treatment of craniomandibular pain dysfunction. Part 2: posterior condylar displacement. J Craniomandibular Pract. 1984;2(4):333–49.
57. Paknahad M, Shahidi S. Association between mandibular condylar position and clinical dysfunction index. J Craniomaxillofac Surg. 2015;43(4):432–6.
58. Shokri A, et al. Comparative assessment of condylar position in patients with temporomandibular disorder (TMD) and asymptomatic patients using cone-beam computed tomography. Dent Med Probl. 2019;56(1):81–7.
59. Imanimoghaddam M, et al. Evaluation of condylar positions in patients with temporomandibular disorders: a cone-beam computed tomographic study. Imaging Sci Dent. 2016;46(2):127–31.
60. Huang P-C, Zhang D-Q. Condylar position and condylar symmetry in patients with temporomandibular disorders. Shanghai kou qiang yi xue = Shanghai journal of stomatology. 2012;21(6):663–7.
61. Alhammadi MS, Fayed MS, Labib A. Three-dimensional assessment of condylar position and joint spaces after maxillary first premolar extraction in skeletal class II malocclusion. Orthod Craniofac Res. 2017;20(2):71–8.
62. Pimenidis MZ. The neurobiology of orthodontics. Springer; 2009.
63. Asaki S, Sekikawa M, Kim YT. Sensory innervation of temporomandibular joint disk. J Orthop Surg (Hong Kong). 2006;14(1):3–8.
64. Mu L, Sanders I. Human tongue neuroanatomy: nerve supply and motor endplates. Clin Anat. 2010;23(7):777–91.
65. Zur KB, Mu L, Sanders I. Distribution pattern of the human lingual nerve. Clin Anat. 2004;17(2):88–92.
66. Abarca M, et al. The neurophysiology of osseointegrated oral implants. A clinically underestimated aspect. J Oral Rehabil. 2006;33(3):161–9.
67. Rathee, M., et al. Oral proprioception for prevention and preservation. RESEARCH AND REVIEWS: JOURNAL OF DENTAL SCIENCES. e-ISSN:2320-7949p-ISSN:2322-0090 2014.
68. Singh V, Mattoo K. Oral stereognosis pattern in patients with dental prosthesis in the elderly population. Int J Clin Exp Physiol. 2014;1:211.
69. Teixeira FB, et al. Masticatory deficiency as a risk factor for cognitive dysfunction. Int J Med Sci. 2014;11(2):209–14.
70. Kubota K, et al. Nuclear medical PET-study in the causal relationship between mastication and brain function in human evolutionary and developmental processes. Ann Anat Anatomischer Anzeiger. 2003;185(6):565–9.
71. Fukushima-Nakayama Y, et al. Reduced mastication impairs memory function. J Dent Res. 2017;96(9):1058–66.
72. Sakamoto K, et al. Effect of mastication on human brain activity. Anti-Aging Med. 2010;7(13):153–60.
73. Sakamoto K, et al. Mastication accelerates Go/No-go decisional processing: an event-related potential study. Clin Neurophysiol. 2015;126(11):2099–107.
74. Hirano Y, et al. Effects of chewing on cognitive processing speed. Brain Cogn. 2013;81(3):376–81.
75. Momose T, et al. Effect of mastication on regional cerebral blood flow in humans examined by positron-emission tomography with ^{15}O-labelled water and magnetic resonance imaging. Arch Oral Biol. 1997;42(1):57–61.
76. Narayan RK, Verma M. Encephalization. In: Vonk J, Shackelford T, editors. Encyclopedia of animal cognition and behavior. Cham: Springer International Publishing; 2019. p. 1–3.

77. Gisel EG, Schwob H. Oral form discrimination in normal 5- to 8-year-old children: an adjunct to an eating assessment. Occup Ther J Res. 1988;8(4):195–209.
78. Malandraki GA, et al. Neural activation of swallowing and swallowing-related tasks in healthy young adults: an attempt to separate the components of deglutition. Hum Brain Mapp. 2009;30(10):3209–26.
79. Janardhanan R, et al. Evaluation of the association of oral stereognosis with malocclusion in children. Int J Clin Pediatr Dent. 2021;14(Suppl 1):S18–21.
80. Fish LC. Oral form discrimination and tongue-thrust swallowing. Int J Oral Myol. 1975;1(1):5–20.
81. Porto FHDG, et al. In vivo evidence for neuroplasticity in older adults. Brain Res Bull. 2015;114:56–61.
82. van Praag H, Kempermann G, Gage FH. Neural consequences of enviromental enrichment. Nat Rev Neurosci. 2000;1(3):191–8.
83. Guglielman E. The ageing brain: neuroplasticity and lifelong learning. eLearning Papers. 2012;29:1–7.
84. Pauwels L, Chalavi S, Swinnen SP. Aging and brain plasticity. Aging. 2018;10(8):1789–90.
85. Kubo K-Y, et al. Masticatory function and cognitive function. Okajimas Folia Anat Jpn. 2010;87(3):135–40.
86. Galindo-Moreno P, et al. The impact of tooth loss on cognitive function. Clin Oral Investig. 2021:1–8.
87. Cerutti-Kopplin D, et al. Tooth loss increases the risk of diminished cognitive function: a systematic review and meta-analysis. JDR Clin Trans Res. 2016;1(1):10–9.
88. Dehaghani SE, Doosti A, Zare M. Association between swallowing disorders and cognitive disorders in adults: a systematic review and meta-analysis. Psychogeriatrics. 2021;21(4):668–74.
89. Heit T, et al. The effect of the physiological rest position of the mandible on cerebral blood flow and physical balance: an observational study. Cranio. 2015;33(3):195–205.
90. Simons DG, S.L.T.J., *Travell & Simons' myofascial pain and dysfunction: the trigger point manual.* **1**(2nd ed.): p. 94.
91. Sessle BJ. Mechanisms of oral somatosensory and motor functions and their clinical correlates*. J Oral Rehabil. 2006;33(4):243–61.
92. Krishnamoorthy G, Narayana AI, Balkrishanan D. Mastication as a tool to prevent cognitive dysfunctions. Jpn Dent Sci Rev. 2018;54(4):169–73.
93. Lerman MD. The hydrostatic appliance: a new approach to treatment of the TMJ pain-dysfunction syndrome. J Am Dent Assoc. 1974;89(6):1343–50.
94. Al Ali A, et al. The influence of snoring, mouth breathing and apnoea on facial morphology in late childhood: a three-dimensional study. BMJ Open. 2015;5(9):e009027.
95. Nasser S, Rees PJ. Sleep apnoea: causes, consequences and treatment. Br J Clin Pract. 1992;46(1):39–43.
96. Sabuncuoglu O. Understanding the relationships between breastfeeding, malocclusion, ADHD, sleep-disordered breathing and traumatic dental injuries. Med Hypotheses. 2013;80(3):315–20.
97. Hawkins AC. Mouth breathing and its relationship to malocclusion and facial abnormalities. N M Dent J. 1969;20(1):18–21.
98. Hartsook JT. Mouth breathing as a primary etiologic factor in the production of malocclusion. J Dent Child. 1946;13(4):91–4.
99. Grippaudo C, et al. Association between oral habits, mouth breathing and malocclusion. Acta Otorhinolaryngol Ital. 2016;36(5):386–94.
100. Gois EG, et al. Influence of nonnutritive sucking habits, breathing pattern and adenoid size on the development of malocclusion. Angle Orthod. 2008;78(4):647–54.
101. Freunthaller P. Mouth breathing and malocclusion. Osterr Z Stomatol. 1975;72(9):304–8.
102. Fraga WS, et al. Mouth breathing in children and its impact in dental malocclusion: a systematic review of observational studies. Minerva Stomatol. 2018;67(3):129–38.

103. Aroucha Lyra MC, et al. Prevalence of sleep-disordered breathing and associations with malocclusion in children. J Clin Sleep Med. 2020;16(7):1007–12.
104. Orbach H, et al. Sleep-related breathing disorders in young orthodontic patients. Am J Orthod Dentofac Orthop. 2023;163(1):95–101.
105. Duman RS. Neural plasticity: consequences of stress and actions of antidepressant treatment. Dialogues Clin Neurosci. 2004;6(2):157–69.
106. Operto FF, et al. Emotional intelligence in children with severe sleep-related breathing disorders. Behav Neurol. 2019;2019:6530539.
107. Blechner M, Williamson AA. Consequences of obstructive sleep Apnea in children. Curr Probl Pediatr Adolesc Health Care. 2016;46(1):19–26.
108. Sans-Capdevila O, Gozal D. Neurobiological consequences of sleep apnea syndrome in children. Rev Neurol. 2008;47(12):659–64.
109. Bhattacharjee R, et al. Cardiovascular complications of obstructive sleep Apnea syndrome: evidence from children. Prog Cardiovasc Dis. 2009;51(5):416–33.
110. Goldbart AD, Tal A. Inflammation and sleep disordered breathing in children: a state-of-the-art review. Pediatr Pulmonol. 2008;43(12):1151–60.
111. Popovich F, Thompson GW. Thumb- and finger-sucking: its relation to malocclusion. Am J Orthod. 1973;63(2):148–55.
112. Fastlicht A. Psychological considerations about the habit of thumb sucking and its relationship to malocclusion. ADM. 1948;5(6):335–42.
113. Pang A. Relation of musical wind instruments to malocclusion. J Am Dent Assoc. 1976;92(3):565–70.
114. Herman E. Influence of musical instruments on tooth positions. Am J Orthod. 1981;80(2):145–55.
115. Herman E. Orthodontic aspects of musical instrument selection. Am J Orthod. 1974;65(5):519–30.
116. Glowacka A, et al. The impact of the long-term playing of musical instruments on the stomatognathic system—review. Adv Clin Exp Med. 2014;23(1):143–6.
117. Adeyemi TE, Otuyemi OD. The effects of playing wind musical instruments on the occlusal characteristics in a northern Nigerian population. Niger Postgrad Med J. 2019;26(3):152–7.
118. Marchesi A, et al. The correlation between temporomandibular disorders, atypical swallowing and dyslalia. Int J Oral Craniofac Sci. 2019:010–4.
119. Fassicollo CE, et al. Swallowing changes related to chronic temporomandibular disorders. Clin Oral Investig. 2019;23(8):3287–96.
120. Marim GC, et al. Tongue strength, masticatory and swallowing dysfunction in patients with chronic temporomandibular disorder. Physiol Behav. 2019;210:112616.
121. Cortese SG, Biondi AM. Relationship between dysfunctions and parafunctional oral habits, and temporomandibular disorders in children and teenagers. Archivos argentinos de pediatria. 2009;107(2):134–8.
122. Motta LJ, et al. Association between parafunctional habits and signs and symptoms of temporomandibular dysfunction among adolescents. Oral Health Prev Dent. 2013;11(1):3–7.
123. Motghare V, et al. Association between harmful oral habits and sign and symptoms of temporomandibular joint disorders among adolescents. J Clin Diagn Res. 2015;9(8):ZC45–8.
124. Fernandes G, et al. Parafunctional habits are associated cumulatively to painful temporomandibular disorders in adolescents. Braz Oral Res. 2016;30

9 Mandibular Freedom and Spontaneous Mandibular Migration (SMM)

During orthodontic training, there is significant emphasis placed on treating both the upper and lower dental arches concurrently during fixed appliance therapy. However, I rarely treat both arches simultaneously. The upper arch is a contiguous dental continuum that necessitates the lower arch to conform to the maxillary (cranial) anatomical and occlusal demands. While the etiology of malocclusion is beyond the scope of this book, it is worth noting that maxillary deficiency has become more prevalent over the last century [1, 2]. Linked to respiratory problems and changes in diet, among other environmental factors, most of the malocclusions we treat today are likely associated with strong epigenetic influences. This does not imply that there are no genetic family traits that determine facial morphology and occlusion. However, we have focused too much on attributing malocclusion and treatment outcomes to genetic factors. I was taught that 80% of facial morphology (and consequently, occlusion/malocclusion) was due to genetic factors. While I cannot speculate on the exact percentage of genetic/epigenetic factors involved, over time, I have come to believe that blaming genetic inherited and unmodifiable factors for 80% of malocclusion is excessive. Genetic factors are involved in mandibular prognathism [3] and variations of growth hormone receptor (GHR) influence mandibular ramus height [4]. A comprehensive approach would be to see important malocclusions as the result of multifactorial causes. Epigenetic factors represent an environmental change: stochasticity of gene expression is the basis for the identification of the individual "phenotype" which is the result of the combination of genetic and environmental factors. This randomness in gene expression may be a defensive biological system to adapt easier to environmental changes. It could represent an advantage or a disadvantage [5]. The "epigenetic" regulation of gene expression is widely accepted by the scientific community [6]. Probably, the most important orthodontic/dental consequential *change* of the influence of environmental factors on development of the stomatognathic system is the resulting *mandibular posture*. Mandibular posture is a physiological response to ICP. ICP is obviously the

F. Savastano, *Neuromuscular Orthodontics*,
https://doi.org/10.1007/978-3-031-41295-0_9

representation of static occlusion. Its importance is relative to deglutition. The link between swallow and dental occlusion is a unicum.

In many Class II malocclusions, the mandible is typically normal in size relative to the patient's age, sex, and race. However, maxillary deficiency can force a distal occlusion of the mandible. The resultant habitual rest position (HRP) of the mandible is necessary for proper swallowing. The reason for muscle accommodation is the need for an ergonomic HRP as a starting point for ICP during deglutition. HRP and the muscle accommodation relative to this position avoid premature tooth contact during mandibular closure to ICP. The HRP is the most optimal position for the neuromuscular system to avoid such premature tooth contacts and is the result of continuous calculations made by the central nervous system (CNS) to minimize energy expenditure in fulfilling the functional demands of the stomatognathic system. As a result of this calculus, the neuromuscular system develops muscle memory and increases muscle tone of the stomatognathic complex, while also adjusting cranio-cervical posture to maintain the optimal HRP [7]. Most malocclusions are characterized by a reduction in the size of the upper maxillary bone in all three dimensions: sagittal, transverse, and vertical. Addressing a malocclusion requires first creating a maxillary bone with appropriate proportions. However, there is often a misunderstanding of the sagittal issue, an inadequate treatment of the transverse problem and a poor treatment of the vertical correction required to address a malocclusion. The vertical correction which involves *adjusting the occlusal plane* (often referred to as posterior support), is frequently overlooked. Despite being crucial for correcting most malocclusions, the necessary vertical correction is often disregarded during most orthodontic treatments. Clearly, clockwise rotation of the occlusal plane should be avoided, and counterclockwise rotation favored [8]. In open bite tendency, the reduction of the steepness of the posterior occlusal plane and counterclockwise mechanics for the occlusal plane should be promoted. The open bite tendency is generally characterized by a steep posterior occlusal plane and this must be related to a restricted mandibular growth with mandibular backward, clockwise, rotation [9]. While the majority of Class II malocclusions often involve issues with mandibular posture, Class II open bite cases present with several distinctive skeletal and functional characteristics. Mild open bites are typically accompanied by a reduction in freeway space, which can be compensated for through cranio-cervical postural adjustments. Usually head extension is a common reaction to poor freeway space. These cases tend to be stable over time, as long as compensatory mechanisms remain effective. However, if postural compensation fails to create adequate freeway space, it could lead to mandibular growth deficiency in the ramus. Conversely, deep-bite morphology with excessive freeway space could stimulate ramus development and aggravate deep bite. Therefore, the mechanisms of growth stimulation are crucial in determining the development and progression of Class II open bites and should be considered when designing treatment plans for such cases.

Treatment of Open-bite Class II should point to creating freeway space to stimulate ramus growth. This is where orthopedic treatment is necessary for the growing child and why surgery is the only correction for the adult. There is no possibility of repositioning the mandible in absence of freeway space. Even orthopedic treatments started at a young age do not guarantee recovery of ramus growth of the mandible. Here, also genetic traits can be of obstacle to orthodontic orthopedic treatment [10, 11].

A key aspect of Neuromuscular Orthodontics is the recognition that the mandibular position observed with bite recording after full deconditioning is a way of visualizing the malocclusion. By recording a Myocentric occlusion, we establish a new physiologic position with a new centric that is in harmony with the needs of the muscles. In most of the malocclusions and temporomandibular disorders (TMD) that we treat, this involves a downward and forward adjustment of the mandible. If this is true, and we believe that this is the position our muscles would prefer setting the mandible, then this means that by eliminating the occlusal discrepancies/interferences that prevent the mandible to change HRP and ICP physiologically, we favor a ***spontaneous muscular repositioning in ICP and HRP*** of the mandible *without using any specific device or appliance*. This *Spontaneous Mandibular Migration* (SMM) has been previously described more as an occasional finding [12, 13]. Several Class II positional malocclusions are easily resolved just by eliminating these impediments. In Neuromuscular Orthodontics these obstacles or occlusal discrepancies that prevent SMM are called in neuromuscular jargon "walls." The most obvious is the *front wall* when the pre-maxilla is contracted, and the front incisors are steep and under-torqued. The upper arch is a *wall* in all its three dimensions. In general, all Class II occlusions are characterized by a narrow upper arch, and the same is said for all the neuromuscular cases in which the mandible is *recorded* in a more forward position, including Class I and III occlusal malocclusions. Upper RPE should be considered a standard routine orthodontic procedure when treating almost all malocclusions. The author is firmly convinced that the only way to properly expand the upper arch is by rapid palatal expansion (RPE) and that other techniques do not deliver the requested anatomical correction. Even RPE, when not done properly, will fail, e.g., insufficient expansion, too slow expansion, expansion with severe breathing problems, and so on. Hyper-expansion with orthodontic wires or with quad helix as well as removable appliances does not create extra bone *and causes incorrect torquing of the upper posterior segments*. This generally leads to the creation of a new *posterior wall*, rich in interferences that arise from premature contacts of the upper lingual cusps during swallow (upper loss of negative torque). Relapse of the transverse dimension and periodontal problems are very common.

Spontaneous Mandibular Migration (SMM) is intended as *down* a *forward* movement and can or cannot be symmetrical. The repositioning is always accompanied by a change in freeway space. Needless to say, SMM can only occur when there is *sufficient* freeway space. In open-bite cases without freeway space in which there is a postural compensation (head extension), a SMM can be provoked only by *creating* the missing freeway space via posterior intrusion and correction of the occlusal plane. This is more of a repositioning mechanism related to increased mandibular closure rather than a spontaneous migration. As previously described, Class II skeletal occlusions have a reduced freeway space and the application of TENS does not alter mandibular position significantly (Chap. 7).

Other walls can be identified, for example, in the lower arch. Typical is the loss of an upper second molar and the extrusion of the lower second molar with premature contact with the remaining upper segments. All these "blocks" represent obstacles to even the smallest of spontaneous mandibular repositioning possibilities. These occlusal interferences often work by *distalizing* the mandible during ICP and consequently pushing the condyle deeper back into the fossa.

Probably the most unseen wall in Class II occlusion is represented by *excess* posterior freeway space. When posterior support is missing on high numbers, no matter what other occlusal walls are corrected, the need for posterior support will be essential for SMM. The correction of Class II malocclusion is therefore in relation to the reduction of freeway space via extrusion of posterior segments and adequately correcting the occlusal plane. The Planas law on the minimum vertical dimension during swallow remains a milestone in understanding occlusion [14]. If there is a wide gap on the posterior vertical dimension, SMM will not occur because the occlusal plane, not corrected with a counterclockwise rotation from upper extrusion, will act like a posterior "slide" toward a minimal vertical occlusion, thus keeping the mandible locked posteriorily. This is important because it lets us orthodontists understand the damage we would do by treating directly sagittal discrepancies (with Class II mechanics, bite jumping and "sagittal first treatments") without correcting the posterior vertical dimension correctly. Therefore, we see bilateral open-bites as a residue of pure sagittal treatments with, for example, Twin-Block or Herbst appliances, as well as a common finding after long-term bite wearing for TMJ and sleep apnea treatments [15–21].

Example Case

Figures 9.1 and 9.2 show a young patient with TMJ clicking and bilateral joint pain and a Class II occlusion. The first step to obtaining Mandibular Freedom (MF) is removing occlusal "walls." Clinically assessed, freeway space seems scarce, so a fixed lingual bar is applied to avoid unwanted molar extrusion or movement during RPE. Note Class III occlusion after several months from upper RPE and upper fixed appliance for alignment (Fig. 9.3).

Once mandibular freedom was achieved, it was decided to scan function with K7-System in March 2016. The results are shown in Fig. 9.4. These results are considered satisfactory even if there is a rest position that is slightly right to CO (0.6 mm).

By March 2017, Fig. 9.5, both arches are aligned, and extrusion elastics ¼ 4,5 Oz. are worn bilaterally (triangle) from upper canines-lower first premolar-upper second premolar on an 18 h/day basis. This favors occlusal relationship and controls open bite tendency.

Treatment was terminated in May 2017. Figures 9.6 and 9.7 show intraoral and extraoral photos at 4 years after treatment.

At 5 years after treatment, a complete K7 functional analysis was done, and the results can be seen in Fig. 9.8.

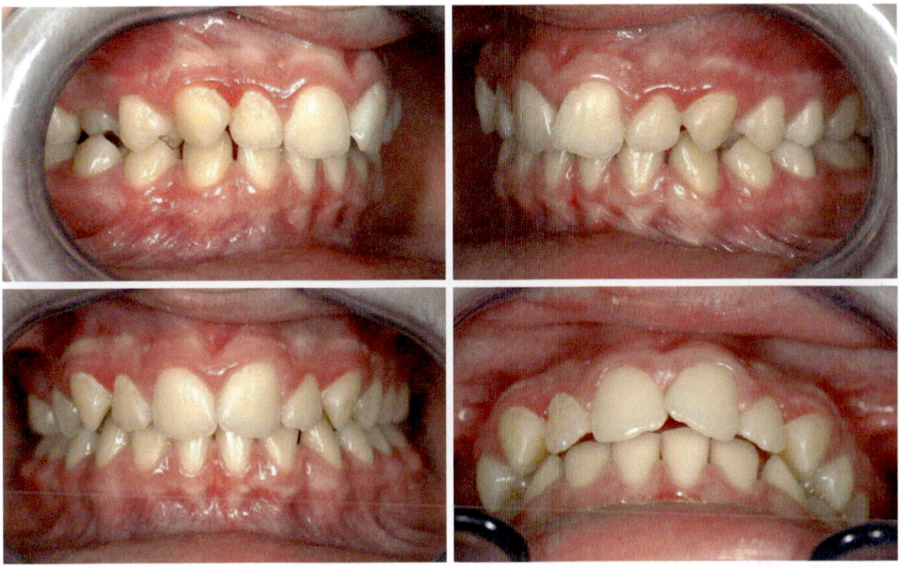

Fig. 9.1 Intraoral photo of a young boy age 11, Class II occlusion and TMJ pain, March 2014

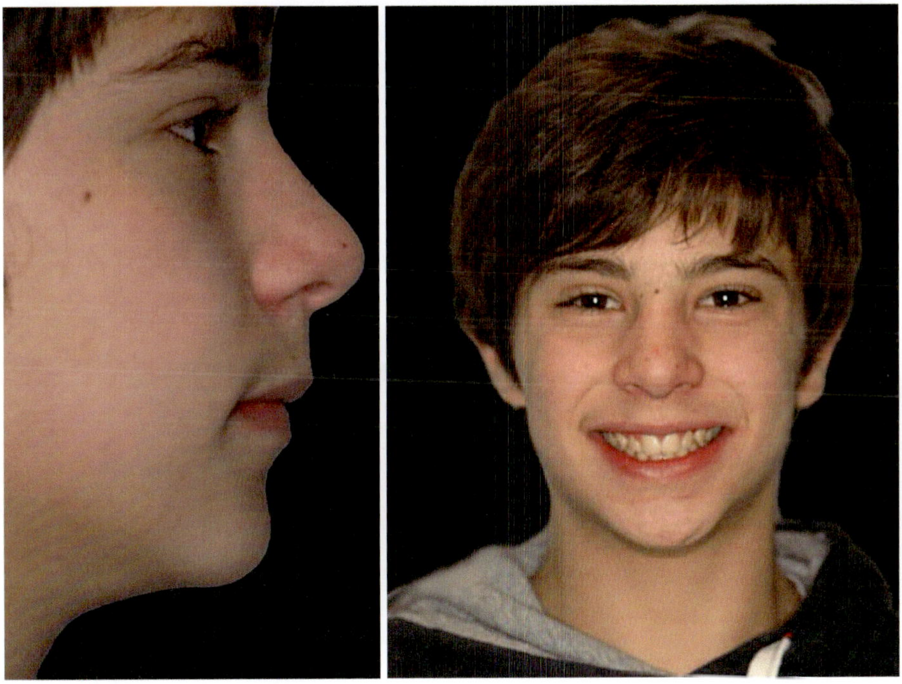

Fig. 9.2 Extraoral photos, March 2014

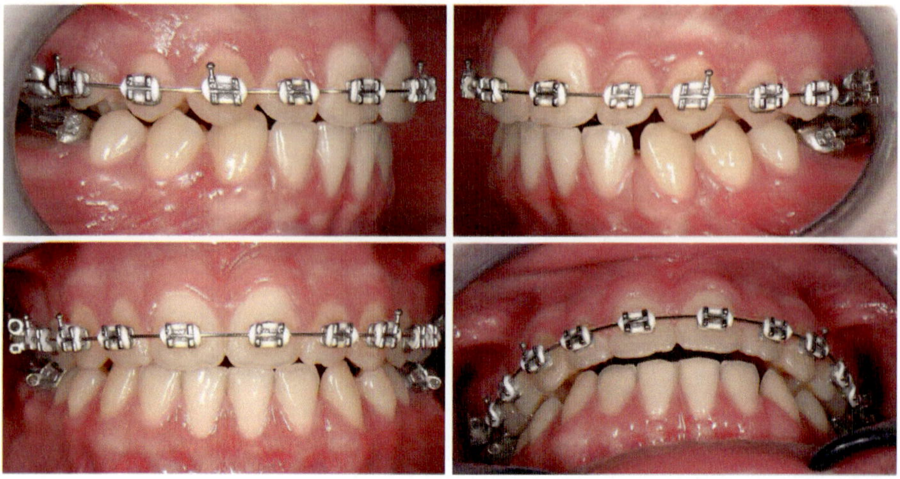

Fig. 9.3 Intraoral photos taken in December 2015. Bilateral molar Class III occlusion

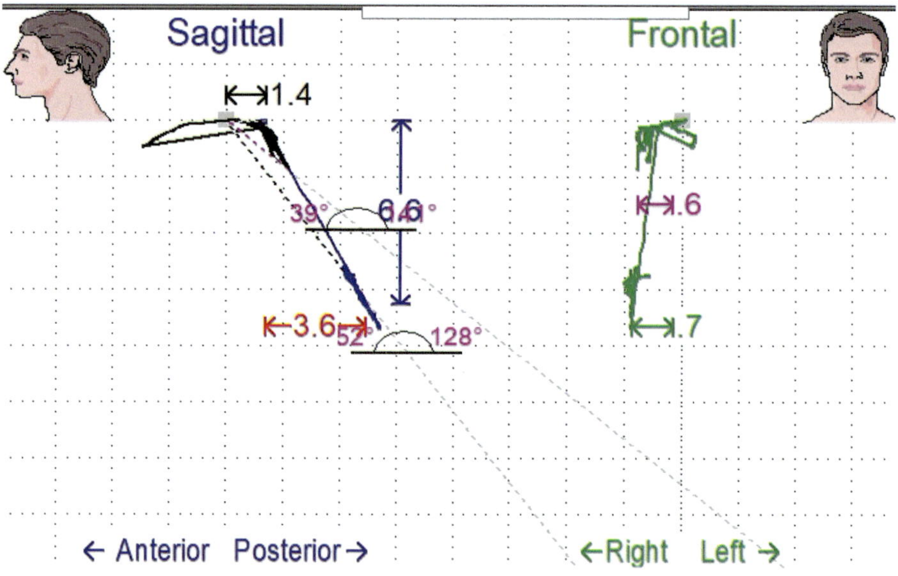

Fig. 9.4 Scan 5, March 2016 after MF and SMM: habitual and Myotrajectory are almost overlapping, 1.4 mm is the discrepancy on the HP

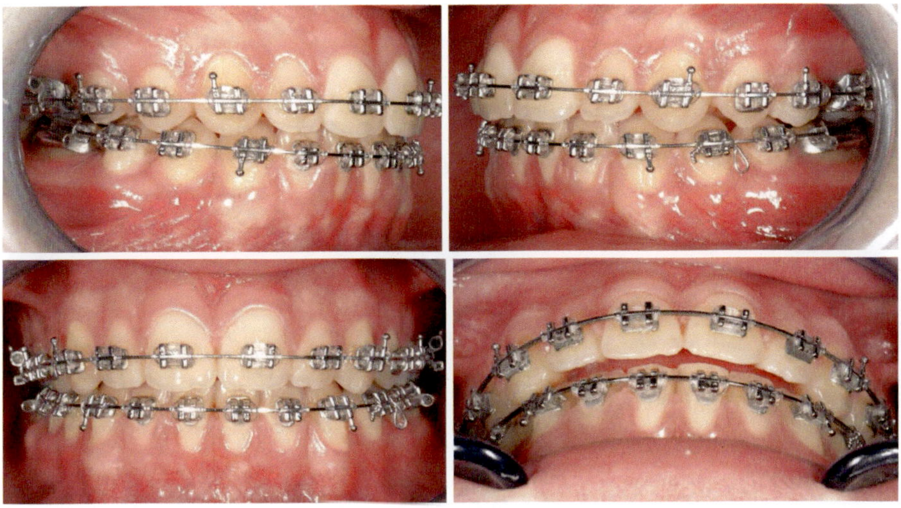

Fig. 9.5 Intraoral photos taken in March 2017, slight extrusion on premolar-canine sector, bilaterally with box elastics ¼, 4.5 Oz. (not shown)

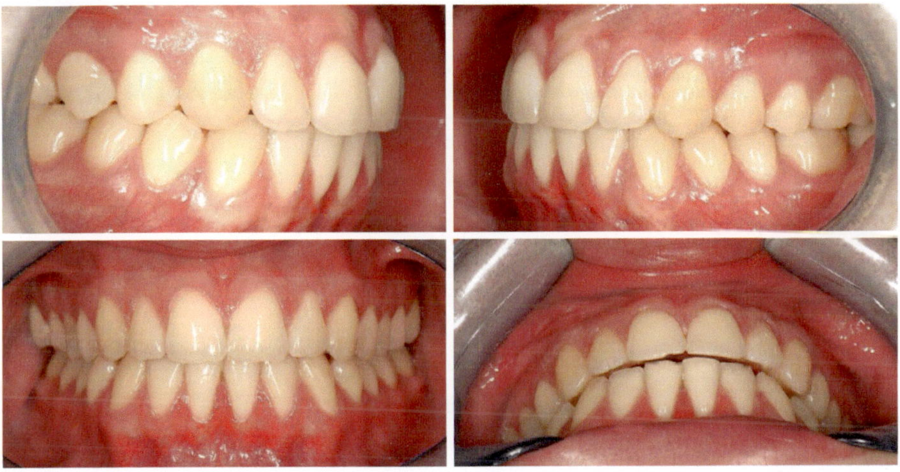

Fig. 9.6 Intraoral photos at 4 years after treatment

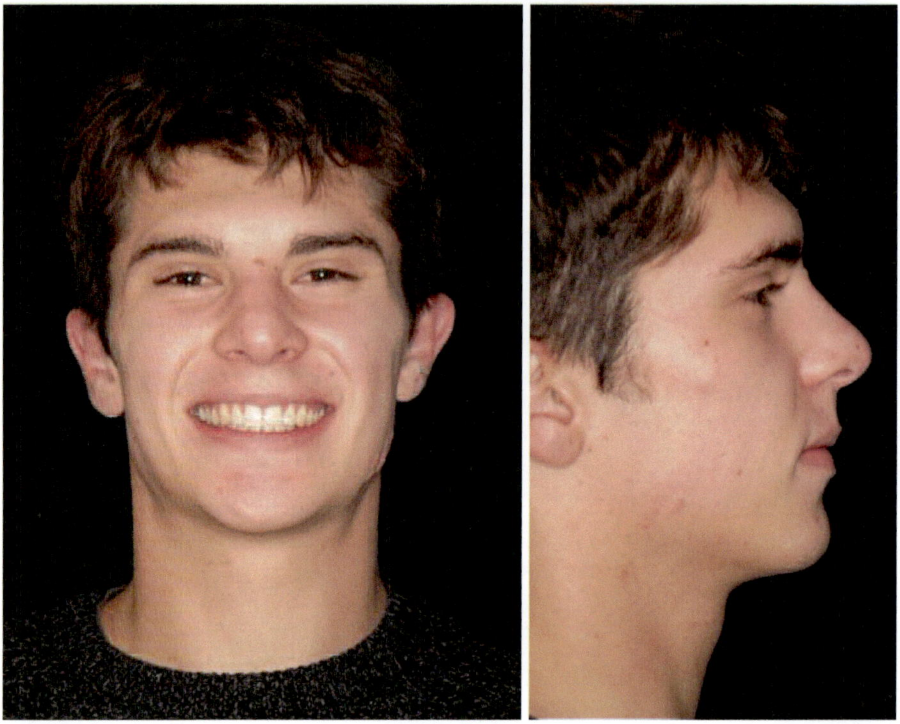

Fig. 9.7 Cont' Extraoral photos at 4 years after treatment

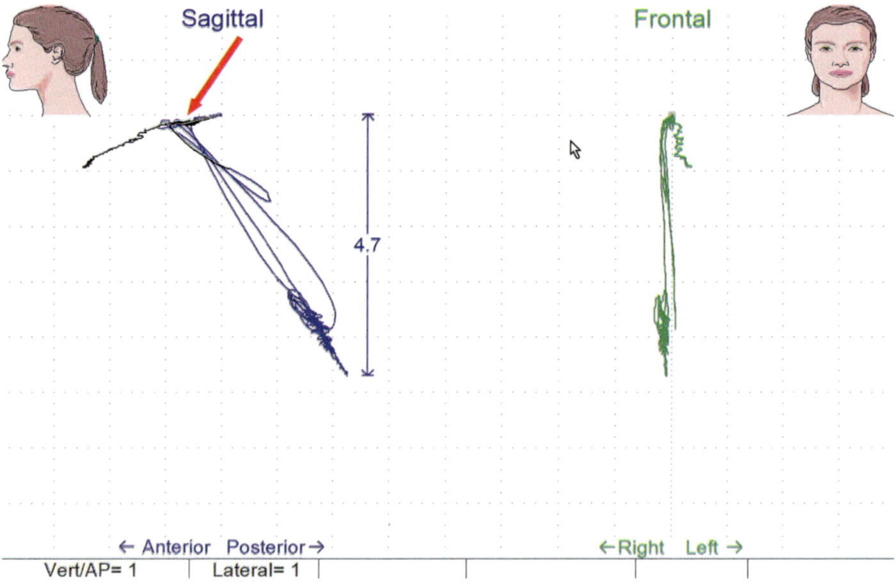

Fig. 9.8 Scan 5 in Sagittal/Frontal. Red arrow shows the position of CO

Discussion

This is a classic case of SMM. Any orthodontic treatment that would have distalized the upper arch would have created an iatrogenic TMD case. Figure 9.6 shows that it is important to check anterior wall years after treatment to avoid any relapse. Upper lip tone, habits like nail biting or instrument playing may misalign the upper incisors and create an anterior wall. TMJ clicking upon opening and TMJ pain were resolved immediately with RPE. Figure 9.8 shows scan 5 and the HRP and RP are very close and on same neuromuscular trajectory. The CMS monitoring during the coming years assures stability of orthodontic/gnathologic results. Patient was pain free since RPE procedure.

When there is a consistent increase in freeway space, a Class III occlusion may obscure a Class I skeletal and occlusal relationship. To overcome this issue, the primary objective of initial orthodontic treatment is to attain mandibular freedom (MF). Once interferences are identified and resolved, the muscles no longer need to adapt to occlusal restrictions, which effectively reduces accommodation. As a result, a new intercuspal position (ICP) and mandibular and tongue posture for deglutition may be achieved. The accommodation process is led by the CNS, which constantly elaborates on the habitual rest position (HRP) relative to ICP. Swallowing is a complex functional task that involves automatic processes, some of which may be independent of higher cortical elaboration. These subcortical automatisms must be free from any external influence due to the crucial importance of deglutition for survival. It is intriguing to compare the habitual path of closure from the habitual rest position (HRP) with that occurring during a requested (VSS) swallow from HRP (patient must relax and not swallow for at least 90 seconds). Although not detectable in all patients, this analysis can provide immediate insight into the neuromuscular demands of the stomatognathic system. Figure 9.9 shows this analysis in a Class III TMD patient with mandibular entrapment.

Mandibular freedom (MF) is achieved by eliminating with orthodontics, all clinically visible and/or detectible walls using diagnostics from bioelectric instrumentation. Mandibular tracking is useful in uncovering muscle accommodation dynamics

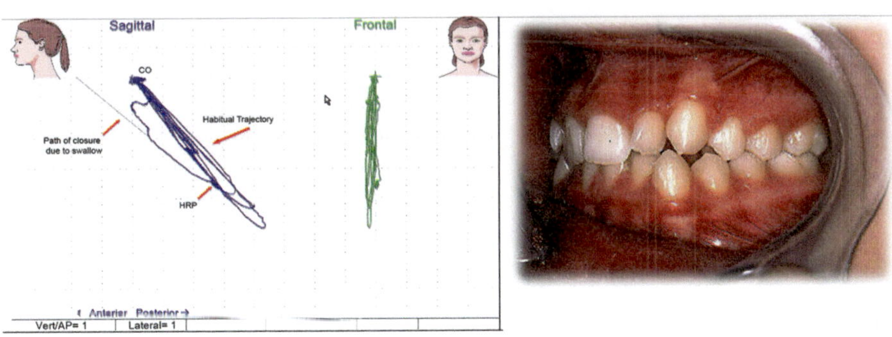

Fig. 9.9 On the left: showing swallow path of closure (dotted line) from HRP (Habitual Rest Position). Habitual trajectory to closure in CO is from "tap tap" movement to CO. On the right showing mandibular entrapment by front wall. Note how forward is the path of closure during voluntary swallow in respect of the habitual path of closure from HRP (2mm.)

leading to malocclusion. However, MF does not guarantee successful SMM due to the multistep process involved in identifying and eliminating all major walls, which can require significant effort. Additionally, Class II occlusions may present the challenge of excess freeway space, a “wall” not easily measurable clinically and only detectable through TENS diagnostics. Nevertheless, an accurate analysis of denture abrasion surfaces can provide valuable clues for identifying hidden walls by revealing the dynamics of muscle requests during swallow (daytime and nighttime) and night bruxing. Figure 9.10 shows the sagittal/frontal dynamic occlusion occurring during VSS or Voluntary Swallow of Saliva. The abrasion surfaces that can be seen in Class II individuals with increased OJ are not the result of any protrusion effort of anterior guidance but rather an occlusal guidance during closure with VSS and SSS. MF is always necessary to preserve TMJ health, even if treatment results in a Class III occlusion.

RPE is a fast way to achieve MF, but it should be fine tuned to facilitate SMM. Although some overcorrection is typically necessary, it is desirable to obtain a clean fossa/cusp corridor after the expansion process to facilitate spontaneous mandibular repositioning. This is generally evaluated by having the patient protrude to their lower jaw during tooth contact. Any interferences that could reduce the possibility of stable mandibular repositioning should be eliminated by adjusting the expander or adding composite on the teeth surface. RPE treatment in cross-bite cases can result in a significant improvement to occlusion, including spontaneous mandibular migration (sometimes with asymmetrical migration) (Fig. 9.11).

Generally, RPE is effective in immediately resolving mild TMD cases. By reducing freeway space, the condyle is freed from being forced into a distal position

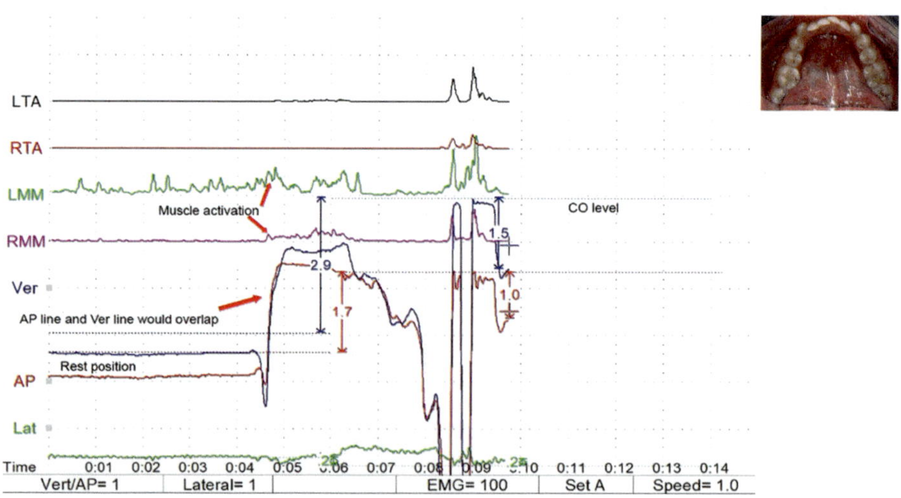

Fig. 9.10 On the left: showing scan 21 (Polygraphic scan) in which very similar results as in Fig. 9.9 are repeated with a testing in sweep mode. Scan 21 (pre-treatment) showing the vertical, anterior-posterior, and lateral movements of the mandible in sweep mode during filtered EMG and swallowing. The patient was instructed to swallow normally and then close to CO, making a “tap-tap” motion in ICP. During swallowing, the patient did not move to CO, indicating that the swallowing occurred with the tongue between the teeth. On the right: occlusal of lower arch showing the amount of incisor compensation due to Class III occlusion compensation (front wall). The masseter activation during swallow confirms that the tongue is between the teeth

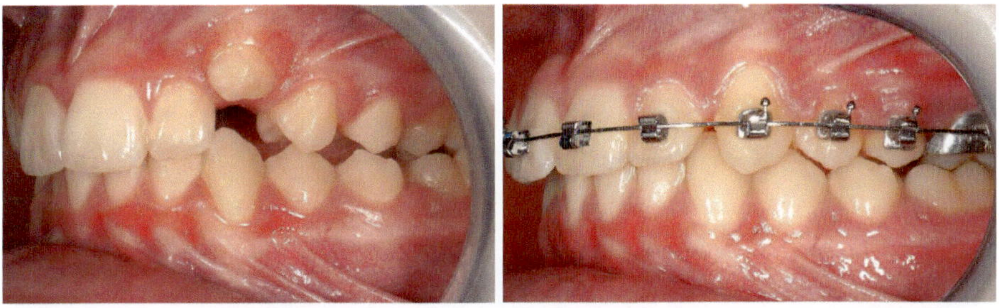

Fig. 9.11 Spontaneous mandibular migration before and after RPE and upper arch alignment. Total time 4 months

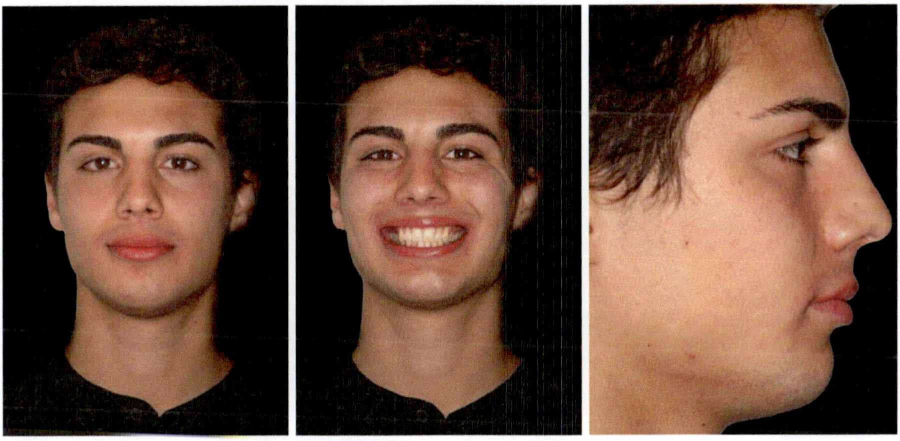

Fig. 9.12 Extraoral photos of adult patient. Note the upper arch shape and buccal corridors

during deglutition. When SMM occurs, the condyle typically changes position in the fossa, moving to a lower and slightly more forward position [22]. Most craniomandibular pain dysfunction syndromes are associated with posterior condylar displacement [23–27], and this is quite frequent in children too [28–31]. Do reverse OJ Class III occlusal malocclusions suffer from TMD?

RPE is a procedure usually reserved for growing patients but can be performed in adults as well with a simple surgical procedure (SARPE, Surgically Assisted Rapid Palatal Expansion). SMM can occur in the adult too. Figures 9.12 and 9.13 show a patient age 19 with a Class II occlusion and some periodontal problems. Figure 9.14 shows the same patient 15 days after SARPE. Immediate Class I is achieved spontaneously, just by eliminating the anterior, transverse, and vertical walls.

Figures 9.15 and 9.16 show the competition of treatment with alignment and Class I intercuspation. During this phase, vertical elastics are placed on premolar region for extrusion.

Figure 9.17 is a digital overlapping of cephalograms taken before treatment and 7 months after SARPE procedure. The changes in mandibular position and consequent profile changes are the bases of Neuromuscular Orthodontics. Consequently,

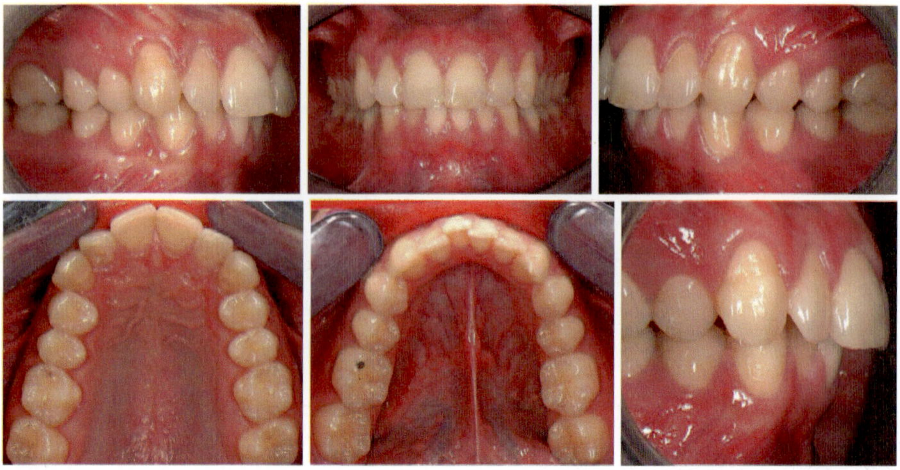

Fig. 9.13 January 2021. Showing adult patient intraoral photos before treatment. Bilateral Class II occlusion

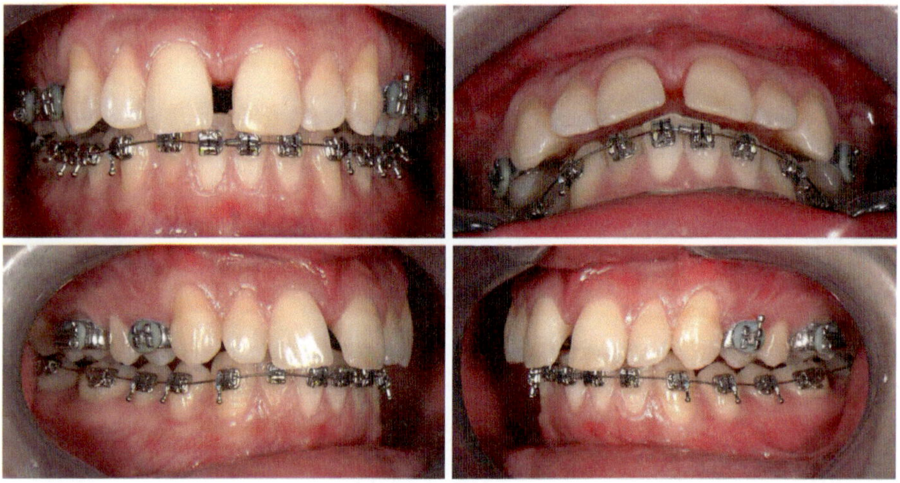

Fig. 9.14 January 2021. Showing 20 days after SARPE procedure. SMM developed immediately at the termination of expansion. Here shown with the application of a lower fixed appliance and 0.014 NiTi wire. Bilateral Class I occlusion

the position of the condyle is lower and more forward during ICP. SMM is proof that the Neuromuscular Theory is a physiological treatment.

Figure 9.18 Shows scan 5 before SARPE procedure. The identification of a sagittal discrepancy by means of CMS is an important diagnostic step before planning any surgical/orthodontic intervention. This scan confirms clinical suspect the mandible is forced in a distal position by occlusion and that the sagittal discrepancy is 2.0 mm on the current horizontal reference plane of occlusion. The frontal shows a physiologic rest position that is circa 1 mm to the right.

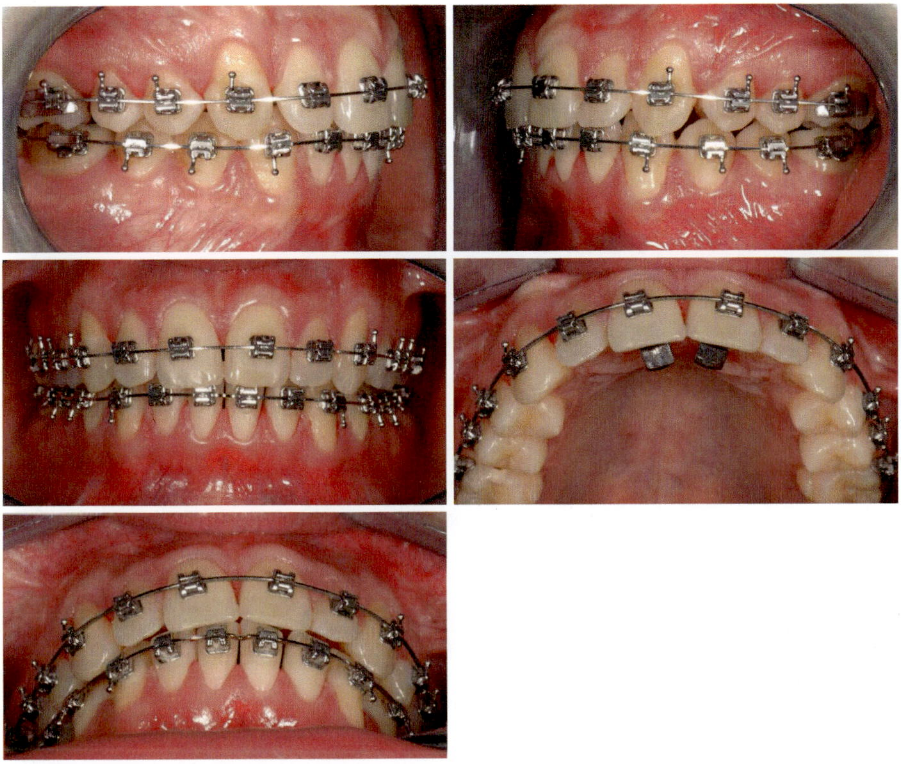

Fig. 9.15 April 2021: intra-oral photos. Application of bite turbo's to correct freeway space

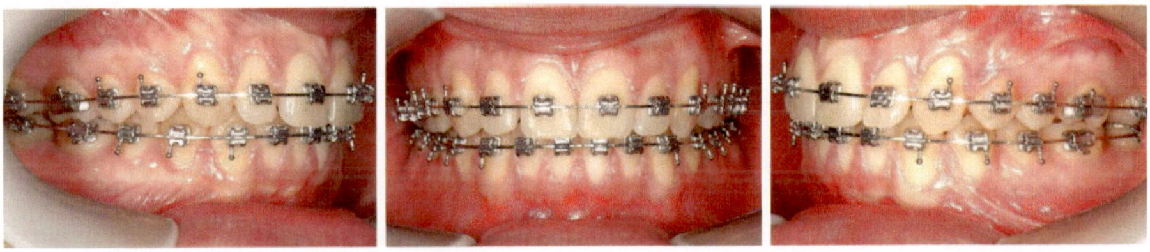

Fig. 9.16 Intra-oral photos, October 2021

Figure 9.19 shows scan 5 after SARPE procedure. Mandibular Freedom (MF) is achieved immediately after SARPE and this facilitates SMM. *The Habitual path of closure* and the *Physiologic path of closure* (Myotrajectory) are now coincident. The HRP and PRP are coincident also. This is an ideal result obtained during treatment procedures. The reduction of the sagittal discrepancy is usually frequently seen, sometimes it is immediate like in this case, in other circumstances it may take up to several weeks. Hidden walls not easily identified must always be explored.

Figure 9.20 shows intra- and extra-oral photos after treatment. In addition to improving the patient's profile, reducing the size of buccal corridors has enhanced the appearance of the smile.

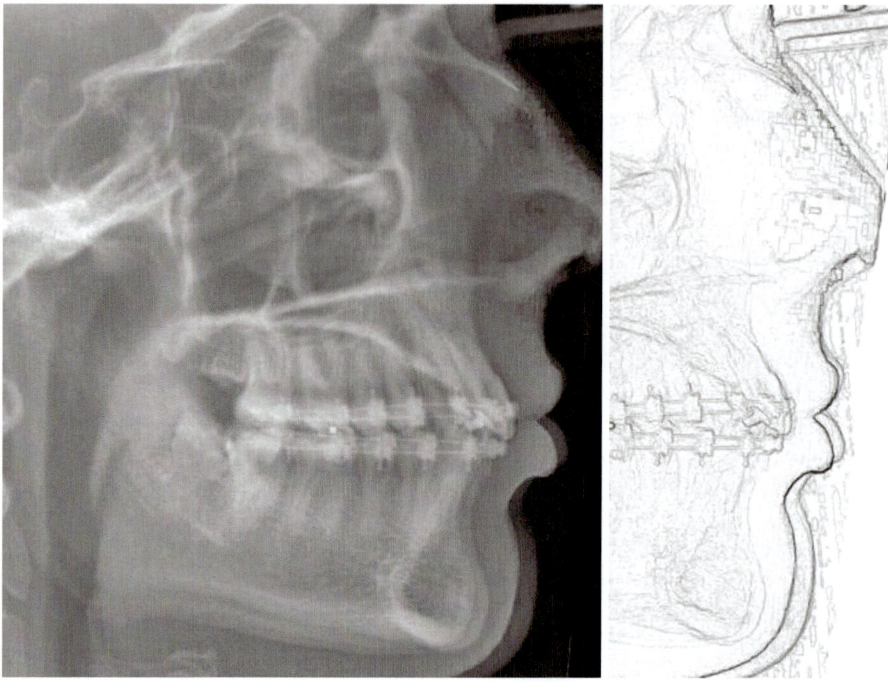

Fig. 9.17 December 2022: Radiologic digital overlapping on S-N, before and after SARPE

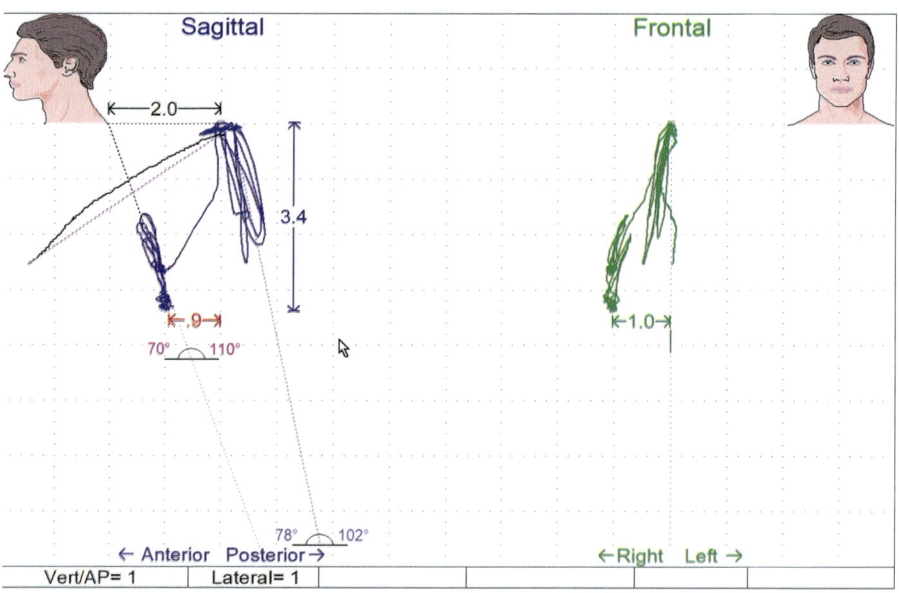

Fig. 9.18 Scan 5 before SARPE. Showing a sagittal discrepancy on the horizontal plane of occlusion of 2.0 mm

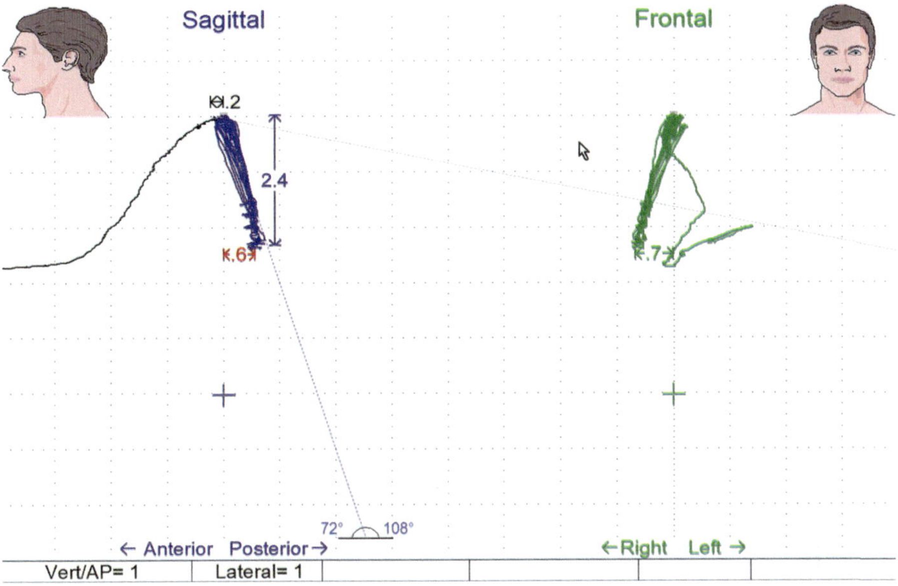

Fig. 9.19 Scan 5 after SARPE. Showing how SMM has reduced sagittal discrepancy. HRP and PRP overlap and habitual path of closure is coincident with the Neuromuscular Trajectory

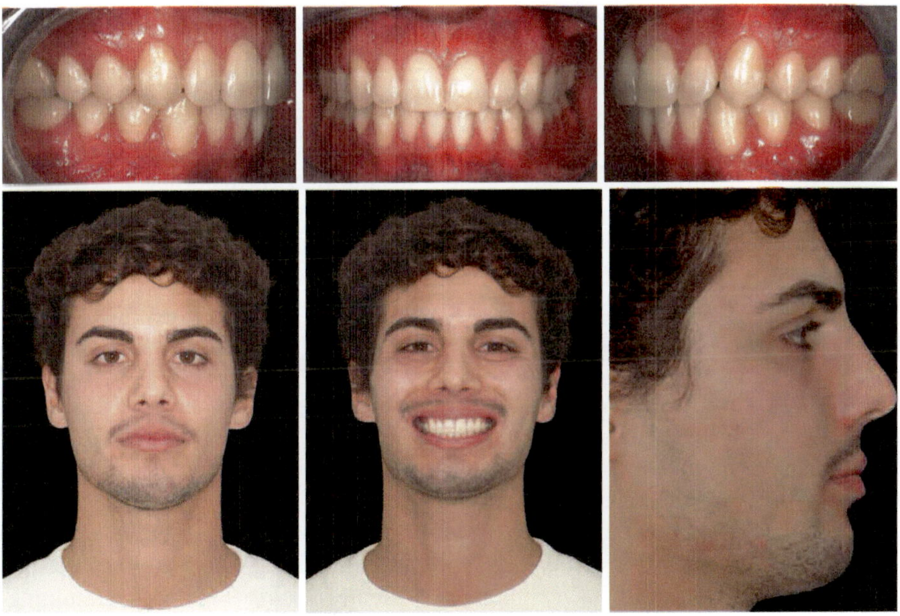

Fig. 9.20 Intra- and extraoral photos after treatment

In some cases, after RPE, the upper incisors may still be so under-torqued and/or extruded to need correction. To avoid these problems, a + 17° minimum torque for upper central incisors is suggested. While some extrusion of the upper incisors may be present at initail diagnosis, a correction by intrusion should only be considered necessary after determining the extrusion required on the posterior/mid sectors of the dental arches due to kinesiographic calculation. In fact, reducing the freeway space and increasing posterior support can minimize the need for anterior intrusion, which may result in bone loss. However, a slight and gradual intrusion may be necessary for aesthetic and prosthetic purposes.

Achieving mandibular freedom can be done through various methods, but it is essential to ensure that the selected procedure does not use up all available freeway space. Rapid palatal expansion (RPE), for example, utilizes freeway space, resulting in an increase in vertical contacts and extrusion. This factor must be taken into consideration before proceeding with orthodontic and prosthetic treatments. Physiological vertical freeway space can be measured through mandibular tracking after TENS application. Ideally, if there is a slight excess in freeway before RPE, spontaneous mandibular migration may occur.

However, when posterior support is necessary after RPE, and freeway space is abundant, spontaneous mandibular migration is unlikely to happen because the posterior gap remains excessive, regardless of the positive effects of RPE. Therefore, it is crucial to understand the dynamics of mandibular stabilization from a neuromuscular perspective. Typically, cases like these are characterized by an altered tongue posture, between the teeth, that prevents spontaneous eruption of the lower premolar-molar district.

If there is a resulting generalized residual excess of freeway space after RPE, the occlusal plane should be corrected by selectively extruding the upper mid/ posterior segments while avoiding lower posterior interferences by the second molars. The excess curve of Spee should also be corrected by extruding the premolar sectors without incisal flaring, and this can be done easily during growth but special attention is required for adult treatments in which total lower arch distalization becomes necessary. Careful attention to these factors can lead to successful treatment outcomes while minimizing adverse effects. Thanks to the use of TADs (Temporary Anchorage Devices), this has become easier in orthodontic treatment. In these cases, the occlusal plane inclination after posterior vertical correction (extrusion) should be the result of upper and lower toque/extrusion procedures that promote a counterclockwise rotation of the occlusal plane. Positional Class II occlusions, most of all Class II malocclusions, *are, for these considerations,* ***essentially a vertical problem***, not a sagittal one as many orthodontists believe. The vertical correction must focus on the change of the occlusal plane inclination and lower correction of the excess curve of Spee.

The best way to obtain a SMM is by MF in which *periodontal occlusal afferent inputs to the CNS are not completely interrupted.* Functional treatments must focus on periodontal feedback for the mandibular position/re-positioning. Deprogramming and reducing accommodation are not functional orthodontic treatment modalities and remain essentially diagnostic procedures. Using a bite plane or similar appliances can determine MF, but at the cost of eliminating tooth contact and consequent neurological feedback of the mandibular position. For these reasons, the author suggests to always search for SMM without interruprting occlusal proprioception. Bite turbos do give some feedback to the neurological system, a sort of incisor-to-incisor contact. For this reason, it can be a dis-occluding and distraction technique of choice when using fixed appliances.

SMM has several advantages. One of which is avoiding Class II mechanics and distalization, that as previously discussed, can cause condylar retrusion. Furthermore, classical Class II mechanics determines a clockwise rotation of the occlusal plane and extrusion of the lower molars.

Figures 9.21, 9.22, and 9.23 show a young girl affected by positional Class II occlusion complicated by lower canine misposition. Obviously, the primary concern is canine recovery.

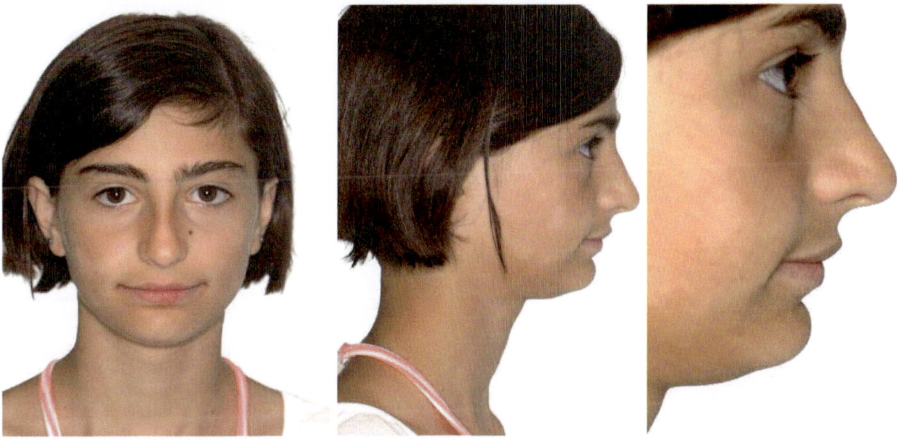

Fig. 9.21 Extra-oral photos showing a concave profile and a retruded mandible

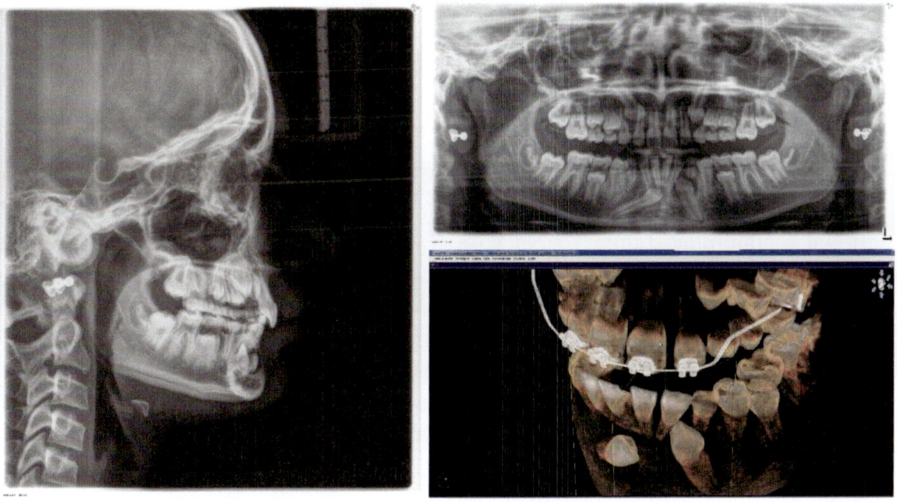

Fig. 9.22 Initial X-Rays and a CBCT photogram. Cephalogram, panoramic, and CBCT are all useful for canine position diagnostics. Lateral cephalogram shows a skeletal deepbite

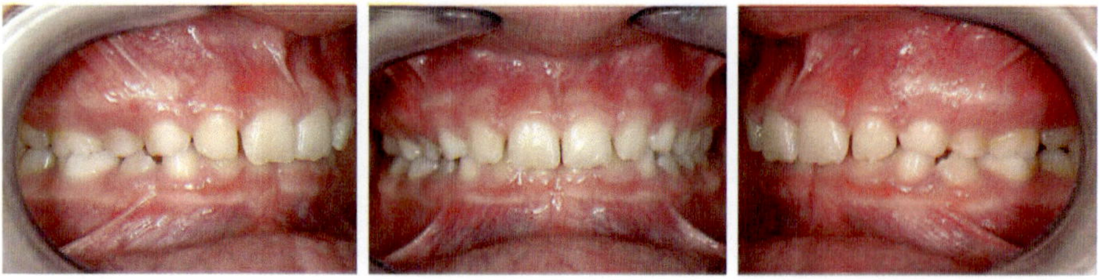

Fig. 9.23 Intraoral photographs showing dental deep-bite and molar Class II occlusion

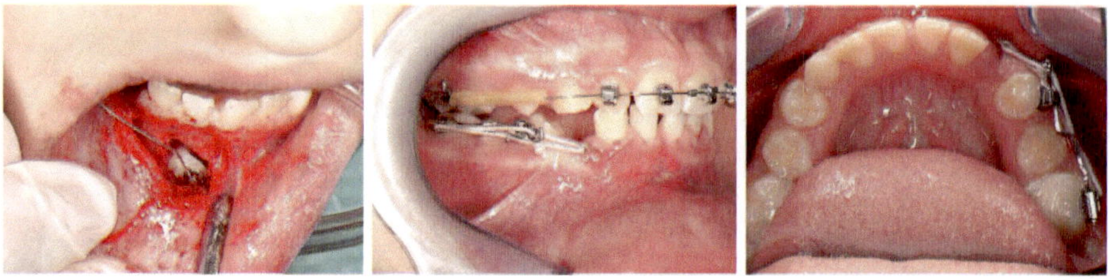

Fig. 9.24 (Cont. intraoral photos) showing from left to right: surgical procedure, after 1 week traction with a very light force applied, occlusal photo

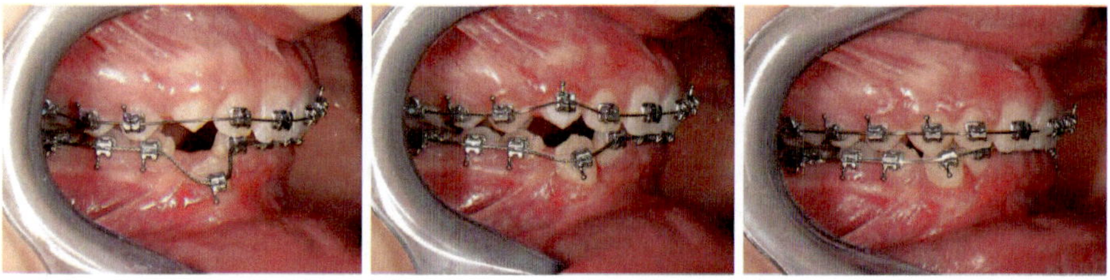

Fig. 9.25 (Cont. Intraoral photos) shows a sequence during an 8-month period in which the lower right canine was extruded and positioned in the lower arch. SMM occurred while correcting the upper arch

Surgical treatment was necessary to save and reposition the lower right canine. A sectional rectangular stainless steel wire was passively placed on lower arch and very light forces were applied to lower right canine. (Fig. 9.24).

As the lower right canine was repositioned, SMM was the result of lower curve of Spee correction coupled with upper alignment and torque adjustment of the front incisors. Applying bite turbos for lateral premolar extrusion finally favored a complete Class I occlusal relationship (Figs. 9.25 and 9.26).

Figures 9.27 and 9.28 show intra- and extra-oral photos taken 2 years after treatment. Radiologic superimposition in Fig. 9.29 shows how SMM has improved its

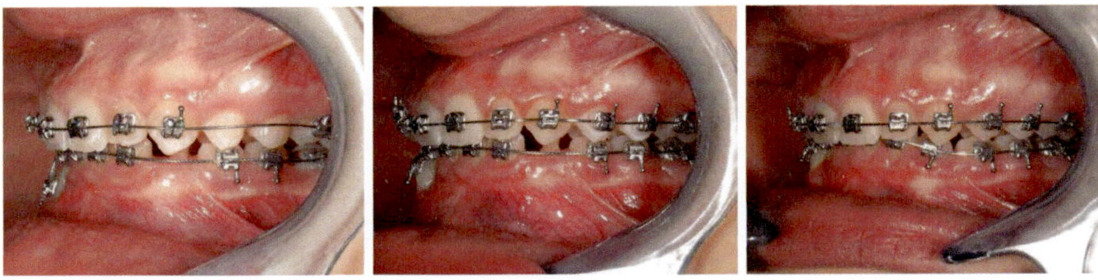

Fig. 9.26 (Cont. intraoral photos) showing SMM on the left side as patient prepares for bite turbo's and extrusion of lower premolar/molar segments

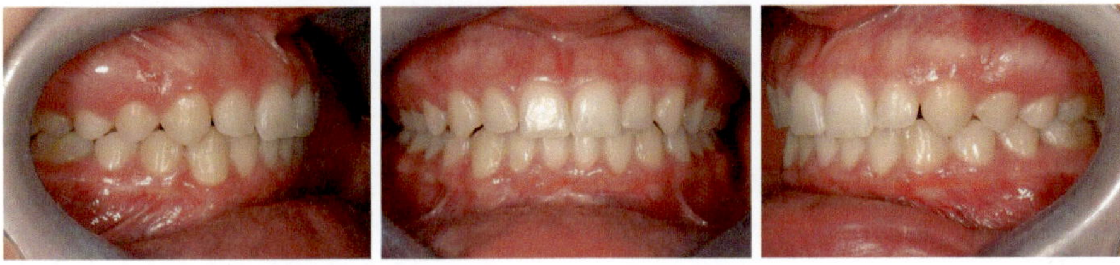

Fig. 9.27 (Cont. intraoral photos) showing stable occlusion 2 years after treatment

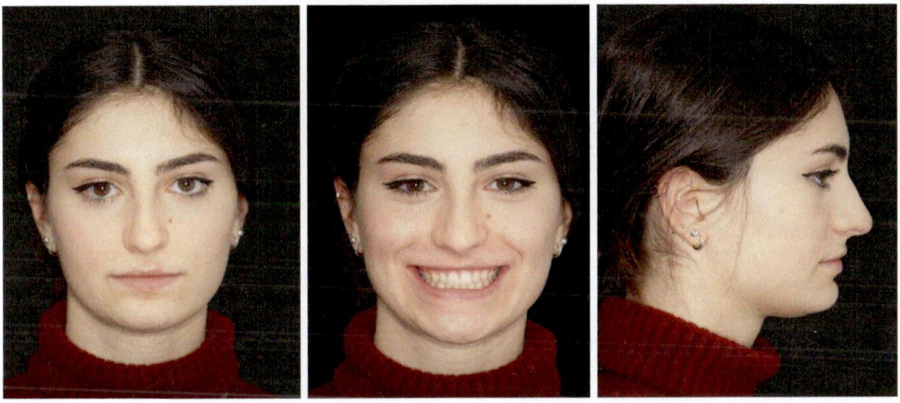

Fig. 9.28 Extraoral photos 2 years after treatment

profile. It must be noted that this new position of the mandible is a new position of the condyle in the fossa.

While it may not be mandatory to perform a comprehensive functional analysis on every orthodontic patient, using bioelectric instrumentation in neuromuscular treatment procedures can greatly benefit the practitioner. The continuous use of bioelectric instrumentation allows for the acquisition of knowledge and expertise, leading to improved *clinical* evaluation skills.

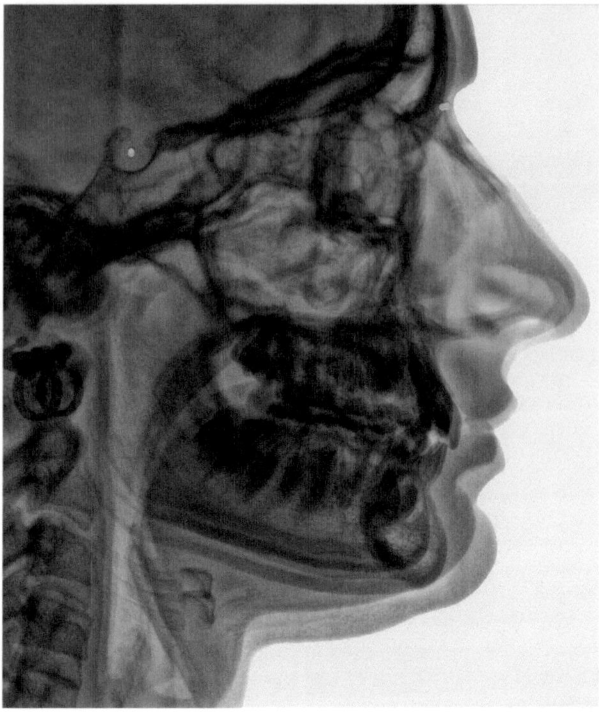

Fig. 9.29 Superimposition of initial and final cephalograms on S-N. Note the increase in the vertical dimension and forward mandibular positioning. Profile changes are significant also

References

1. Silveira S. e.a., The increased prevalence of malocclusion in modern humans: an integrative review. EC Dent Sci. 2018;17:2097–107.
2. Mew M. Craniofacial dystrophy. A possible syndrome? Br Dent J. 2014;216(10):555–8.
3. Doraczynska-Kowalik A, et al. Genetic factors involved in mandibular prognathism. J Craniofac Surg. 2017;28:5.
4. Hartsfield Jr JK, Morford LA, Otero LM. *Genetic factors affecting facial growth.* Orthodontics-Basic Aspects and Clinical Considerations; Bourzgui, F., Ed, 2012: 125–152.
5. Kærn M, et al. Stochasticity in gene expression: from theories to phenotypes. Nat Rev Genet. 2005;6(6):451–64.
6. Jaenisch R, Bird A. Epigenetic regulation of gene expression: how the genome integrates intrinsic and environmental signals. Nat Genet. 2003;33(3):245–54.
7. Lerman MD. A revised view of the dynamics, physiology, and treatment of occlusion: a new paradigm. Cranio. 2004;22(1):50–63.
8. Tanaka EM, Sato S. Longitudinal alteration of the occlusal plane and development of different dentoskeletal frames during growth. Am J Orthod Dentofac Orthop. 2008;134(5):602e1-11. discussion 602-3
9. Fushima K, et al. Significance of the cant of the posterior occlusal plane in class II division 1 malocclusions. Eur J Orthod. 1996;18(1):27–40.
10. Nakasima A, et al. Hereditary factors in the craniofacial morphology of Angle's Class II and Class III malocclusions. Am J Orthod. 1982;82(2):150–6.

11. Balkhande PB, Lakkakula BVKS, Chitharanjan AB. Relationship between matrilin-1 gene polymorphisms and mandibular retrognathism. Am J Orthod Dentofac Orthop. 2018;153(2):255–61.e1
12. Lima Filho RM, Lima AC, de Oliveira Ruellas AC. Spontaneous correction of class II malocclusion after rapid palatal expansion. Angle Orthod. 2003;73(6):745–52.
13. Volk T, et al. Rapid palatal expansion for spontaneous Class II correction. Am J Orthod Dentofac Orthop. 2010;137(3):310–5.
14. Planas P. The Planas law for minimum vertical dimension. Rev Esp Parad. 1968;6(4):215–47.
15. Schiavoni R, Grenga V. Management of the Herbst splint appliance in Class II malocclusion with different growth pattern. Prog Orthod. 2009;10(1):48–57.
16. Kai S, et al. The significance of posterior open bite after anterior repositioning splint therapy for anteriorly displaced disk of the temporomandibular joint. Cranio. 1993;11(2):146–52.
17. Perez CV, et al. The incidence and prevalence of temporomandibular disorders and posterior open bite in patients receiving mandibular advancement device therapy for obstructive sleep apnea. Sleep Breath. 2013;17(1):323–32.
18. Tallents RH, et al. Occlusal restoration after orthopedic jaw repositioning. Cranio. 1986;4(4):369–72.
19. Clark W. Design and management of twin blocks: reflections after 30 years of clinical use. J Orthod. 2010;37(3):209–16.
20. Li P, et al. Severe Class II division 1 malocclusion in an adolescent patient, treated with a novel sagittal-guidance twin-block appliance. Am J Orthod Dentofac Orthop. 2016;150(1):153–66.
21. Hiyama S, et al. Neuromuscular and skeletal adaptations following mandibular forward positioning induced by the Herbst appliance. Angle Orthod. 2000;70(6):442–53.
22. Melgaco CA, et al. Immediate changes in condylar position after rapid maxillary expansion. Am J Orthod Dentofac Orthop. 2014;145(6):771–9.
23. Weinberg LA. Role of condylar position in TMJ dysfunction-pain syndrome. J Prosthet Dent. 1979;41(6):636–43.
24. Weinberg LA. An evaluation of occlusal factors in TMJ dysfunction-pain syndrome. J Prosthet Dent. 1979;41(2):198–208.
25. Weinberg LA, Lager LA. Clinical report on the etiology and diagnosis of TMJ dysfunction-pain syndrome. J Prosthet Dent. 1980;44(6):642–53.
26. Weinberg LA. The role of stress, occlusion, and condyle position in TMJ dysfunction-pain. J Prosthet Dent. 1983;49(4):532–45.
27. Shokri A, et al. Comparative assessment of condylar position in patients with temporomandibular disorder (TMD) and asymptomatic patients using cone-beam computed tomography. Dent Med Probl. 2019;56(1):81–7.
28. Owen AH 3rd. Orthodontic/orthopedic treatment of craniomandibular pain dysfunction. Part 3: anterior condylar displacement. Cranio. 1984;3(1):31–45.
29. Egermark-Eriksson I, Carlsson GE, Magnusson T. A long-term epidemiologic study of the relationship between occlusal factors and mandibular dysfunction in children and adolescents. J Dent Res. 1987;66(1):67–71.
30. da Silva CG, et al. Prevalence of clinical signs of intra-articular temporomandibular disorders in children and adolescents: a systematic review and meta-analysis. J Am Dent Assoc. 2016;147(1):10–18 e8.
31. Al-Khotani A, et al. Prevalence of diagnosed temporomandibular disorders among Saudi Arabian children and adolescents. J Headache Pain. 2016;17:41.

Treatment Procedures

10

The application of the various orthodontic treatment techniques to establish a new centric, the Myocentric, is not a simple task. This is because orthodontics is, per se, a slow procedure. Orthodontics has several methods to change occlusion and mandibular position in the adult and the growing patient. Which fixed, functional or removable appliance is chosen by the practitioner is based on his personal experience and knowledge.

Growth simplifies orthodontic treatment and must be taken into consideration during therapy. Unfortunately, most orthodontic treatments are considered finished well before the end of mandibular growth. This is especially true for boys, where mandibular growth and remodeling can still occur over 18 years of age [1]. Orthodontists know very well that several attempts have been made to accurately predict mandibular growth and that these methods have failed what promised. There seems to be a correlation between statural and mandibular growth, but it is difficult to understand the potential of these factors for orthodontic treatment even if it helps us by identifying mandibular peak growth.

When employing bioelectric instrumentation for function assessment, the measurements are sensitive to a precision of one-tenth of a millimeter. This introduces an unprecedented dimension to functional analysis in orthodontics. The key therapeutic insight derived from this instrumentation lies in our ability to align treatment objectives with a distinct developmental growth ***direction***. It is not important to speculate on how much the mandible will grow in millimeters, but rather assess *where the muscles are posturing the mandible.* The neuromuscular theory puts the muscles at the center of the development of the face and its structures. A Class III individual with a longer-than-normal mandible will always have an altered tongue posture and often a past or persistent history of respiratory dysfunction. Besides rare genetic family-based Class III skeletal subjects [2–4], sporadic Class III develops for respiratory/postural problems and is accompanied by alteration of tongue function. We cannot dismiss the importance of some sort of genetic predisposition for Class II and Class III skeletal malocclusions, but it remains difficult to interpret phenotype variability, penetrance, and expressivity for the morphological influence on

F. Savastano, *Neuromuscular Orthodontics*,
https://doi.org/10.1007/978-3-031-41295-0_10

malocclusion. In these cases, mandibular tracking pinpoints a new mandibular posture, a mandibular advancement, and an increase in freeway space. Needless to say, all the information we get from our instrumentation must be correctly interpreted and all conclusions and therapeutic decisions set according to our clinical experience.

There are several limitations to the diagnostic neuromuscular protocol. There is no possibility to accurately measure mandibular rest position when there is a lack of freeway space. Skeletal open bites are always characterized by head extension as a physiologic response to scarcity of freeway space. This postural compensation is usually sufficient in creating a minimal freeway space, but the price to pay is linked to muscle tenderness and neck pain. Other limitations for a complete functional analysis include lack of collaboration, intolerance to TENS, pacemaker.

Extrusion

Tooth extrusion is necessary to alter the vertical dimension. Excess freeway space is one of the main reasons for which extrusion is necessary. In general, when extruding you consume freeway space.

The dental arches are characterized by two main curves: the curve of Spee and the Curve of Wilson. Together they shape the upper and lower arch as a part of a helicoid (and this reminds me of the DNA filaments). It seems that evolution has granted this anatomy to facilitate mastication and swallow [5, 6]. Studies on lower arch, mandibular, and condylar movements and how function determines form can be understood according to George Monson's "spherical Theory of Mandibular Movement" [7]. Extrusions performed on the lower arch have two direct consequences:

1. They increase the ray of the Monson's sphere.
2. They tend to create protrusion of the lower incisors.

Increasing the ray of the sphere implies a need for it. It is not uncommon that positional Class II with increased overjet has an excess curve of Spee. This excess curve of Spee represents a smaller than normal sphere for the individual that occludes in a more distal position (Monson describes three main sizes of the sphere according to age and sex). When repositioning the mandible forward and correcting the Class II relationship according to neuromuscular needs, the correction of the curve of Spee allows a wider ray of Monson sphere. Fortunately, if the orthodontic correction takes place during growth, lower incisor protrusion can be controlled and avoided by correct intra-arch mechanics. When occlusal recording re-positions the mandible forward and down because of muscular needs, an increase of posterior vertical dimension is inevitable. This increase in freeway space on the posterior section of the dental arches must be occupied by dental extrusion to create stability and avoid relapse. It is only when extrusion is applied mainly to the upper arch that there is a change in the plane of occlusion. The application of the Monson Theory has been tested and applied to the Artex® articulator by Dr. Piero Silvestrini [8]. He developed the Kalot System that resembles the part of the Monson Sphere that

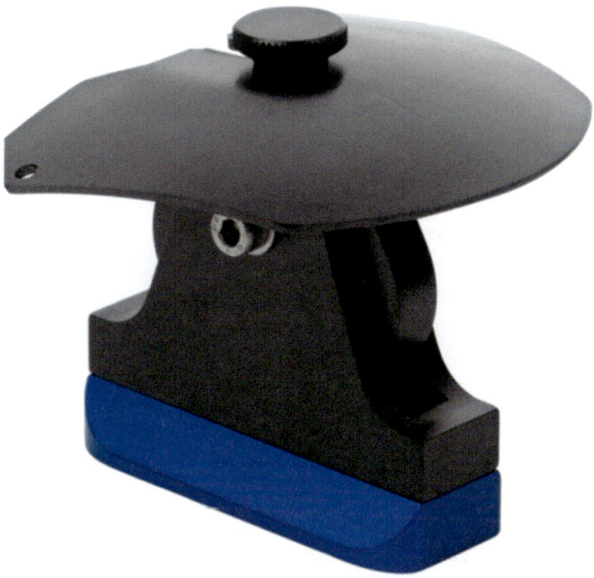

Fig. 10.1 Partial of the Kalot add-on for Artex® Articulators. *Source*: Amann Girrbach AG, Herrschaftswiesen 1, AT-6842 Koblach, AUSTRIA

creates the plane of occlusion for complex prosthodontic rehabilitation cases (Fig. 10.1).

Probably any change in the condylar position due to neuromuscular and/or functional repositioning, produces changes in condylar shape [9]. The question arises on how to extrude and most of all what sectors to extrude, because this can determine a change in the inclination of the plane of occlusion. There has been some debate on the rotation of the plane of occlusion and how it should be carried out during the correction of Class II occlusion. Orthodontic mechanics can modify the inclination of the occlusal plane. For example, Class II elastics or forced protrusion/bite jumping devices, change the occlusal plane through a forced extrusion (and mesialization) of the posterior segments of the lower arch, while the upper arch is slightly distalized. Class II elastics extrude the upper anterior segments for the vertical force component on the canines. These effects produce a clockwise rotation of the occlusal plane [10] (Fig. 10.3). It is important to remember that the natural development of the occlusal plane is *counterclockwise* for the untreated healthy population [11]. There is some evidence that Positional Class II's have a relatively more clockwise rotation of the occlusal plane (OP) in respect of Class I and III subjects, that on the contrary, have flatter and more counterclockwise OP inclination [12]. This suggests that the correction of Class II should be carried out with *a major extrusion of the upper mid/posterior maxillary sectors* and *not the lower posterior mandibular teeth*. The change in the inclination of the occlusal plane must have a maxillary component of intrusion or extrusion of the posterior sectors because, for example, an extrusion alone of the molars of the lower arch, without any intrusion of the maxillary, will not produce a clockwise rotation of the OP, but only a change in the mandibular plane inclination (Go-Mn). Sadao Sato corrects Class II occlusions with a counterclockwise rotation of the OP and suggests a possible relationship between OP and mandibular position relative to the cranium [13]. This is a remarkably interesting matter because it is recognized that Class II occlusions, defined generally *skeletal,* are, de facto ***positional.***

So, coming back to extrusion, it seems logical that extrusion can be achieved if there is enough freeway space to do so, but we still must question how to quantitatively distribute it for each dental arch. The author suggests approaching Class II correction extruding the upper mid/posterior maxillary teeth for the previously so-called "posterior support." My clinical observation is that when the OP is clockwise rotated, it forms a sort of a "sliding ramp" that prevents anterior mandibular stabilization thus the correction of the mandibular position in centric occlusion. Furthermore, if the spherical occlusion hypothesis seems logical, then the correction of the excess curve of Spee must accompany an anterior repositioning of the mandible because the ray of the sphere increases in size. The correction of the occlusal plane by counterclockwise rotation reduces the chances of creating a posterior occlusal plane with an inclination similar to that of the condylar pathway [14]. Furthermore, it is important to understand that the occlusal plane can be effectively divided into two components, the anterior occlusal plane (AOP) and the posterior occlusal plane (POC). The steepness of these planes is in relation to several types of malocclusions, but skeletal Class II which are characterized by mild open-bite morphology benefit the most by reducing the steepness of the POC; this may seem a contradiction in cases with open bite morphology, but the correction proposed by Sato et al. is described as an increase in posterior freeway space by intrusion of the posterior mandibular sectors and then applying a final correction by reducing the POC steepness by extrusion/intrusion of the upper second and first molar. The posterior lower sectors remain tipped back and flattened. The final result is a counterclockwise correction of the occlusal plane [15]. This permits an increase in freeway space and forward anterior mandibular closure that reduces OJ.

Mounting casts on the articulator is important for all complicated orthodontic cases. Most of all, the use of the face bow allows us to visually measure maxillary vertical asymmetries with occlusal plane canting. The majority of asymmetric maxilla is linked to an underdeveloped condyle that can occur for several reasons, from trauma, malocclusion, to inflammatory diseases of the Tmj [16–23]. Except for hyperplasia of a condyle, which is an uncommon finding in asymmetries, all other vertical loss of one side of the maxilla should be treated with extrusion of the dental segments on the same side enough to pair and regain a correct, maxillary occlusal plane perpendicular to the maxillary mid-sagittal plane (Na-ANS-Ba). This forced orthodontic extrusion tends to create a condylar *distraction* that facilitates condylar remodeling [23]. This is much easier in children than in the adult patient, but it does not change the choice for extrusion or intrusion. It can be hypothesized that intrusion of the maxillary dentition where the vertical *seems* increased will stimulate degenerative reactions to the condyle (Fig. 10.2).

There are several ways to extrude teeth. I would say that there are two main methods that can be accomplished differently. Active extrusion (AE) is when force

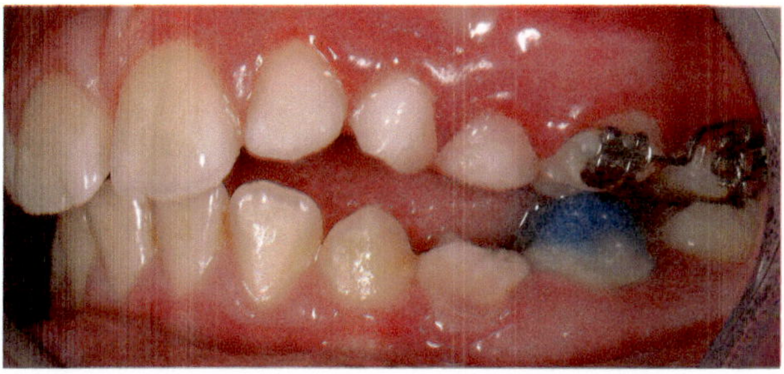

Fig. 10.2 Forced eruption with vertical distraction in a case with condylar asymmetry

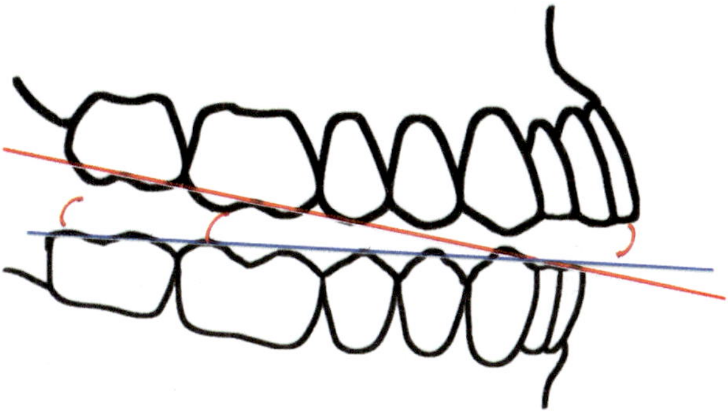

Fig. 10.3 Blue line = starting Class II MP (mandibular Plane), Red Line = OP after Class II elastics due to superior anterior extrusion. *OP* occlusal plane

is applied mechanically to vertically move the tooth along its main axis or in a vertical fashion. It is important to say, that high forces should not be applied in the extrusion process, since there is a possibility of consequent anchylosis of the tooth. Passive extrusion (PE) is generally obtained with functional appliances like a Bionator or an activator where you have carved out resin for selected teeth. It is generally said among functionalists that passive extrusion is more stable, and that active extrusion may relapse a bit with occlusal forces and for intrinsic behavior of the structural fibers in the periodontium.

Active Extrusion (AE)

Fixed or removable appliances can be used to actively force eruption of the dentition. Elastics are frequently used for this task. Every time Class II elastics are used, there is an application of an extruding force to the lower molars and the upper canines. There is no way of controlling extrusion of these segments nor limiting lower incisor flairing. These forced extrusions on both arches are part of the requested mechanics for the classical treatment with Class II elastics. The OP rotates clockwise and the changes are mostly dento-alveolar [24] (Fig. 10.3).

When you apply an elastic between teeth of the upper and lower arch, you are always extruding teeth on both arches. You can limit forced eruption on one arch by applying a robust stainless steel arch wire, but there will always be some degree of extrusion. The only exception is if you apply a fixed anchorage with TADs.

During fixed appliance therapy, vertical elastics are often used to create the "posterior support" in Class II correction. Once bite opening has been established with a posterior block on the upper incisors (bite turbos), box elastics are applied vertically on the premolar region of both sides. Since the desired extrusion is selectively orientated to the upper arch, the lower arch should carry stainless steel wires with a minimum of 0.017 × 0.022 in., while the upper a 0.016 Copper NiTi (Fig. 10.4). Wire bending is also effective to favor selected tooth extrusion.

For example, let us consider a Class II/1 occlusion (Fig. 10.5). A bite registration for a functional appliance may look like in Fig. 10.6. Besides specific cases in which the bite is very deep and the mandibular plane Go-Me is almost parallel to the maxillary plane ANS-PNS, correction of the posterior gap should be achieved with extrusion *mainly* on the upper arch (Fig. 10.7). In more severe skeletal deep-bite cases that exhibit excess freeway space, the curve of Spee must be improved without complete flattening. These cases benefit the most when upper and lower extrusion is obtained aggressively. Usually, the occlusal plane angulation does not change as expected and seems not to play a major role in stability. Unfortunately severe skeletal deep-bite tends to relapse due to the specific morphology associated with this type of malocclusion. Therefore, occlusal plane inclination should not change while extrusion is equally achieved on upper and lower mid-posterior sectors. Correcting excess curve of Spee is an extrusion procedure and consumes freeway space.

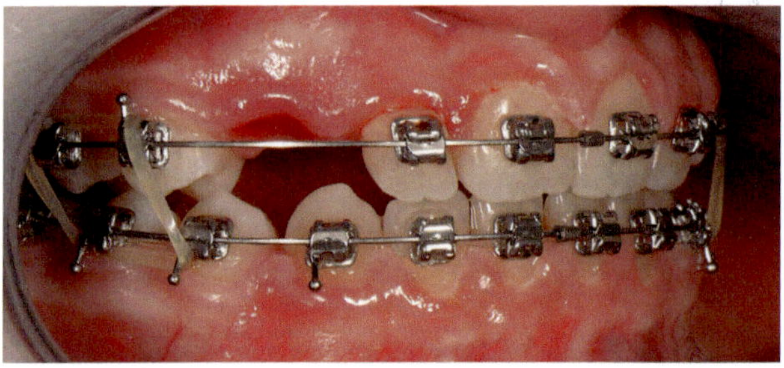

Fig. 10.4 Intra oral photo showing vertical elastics on premolars and bite turbos

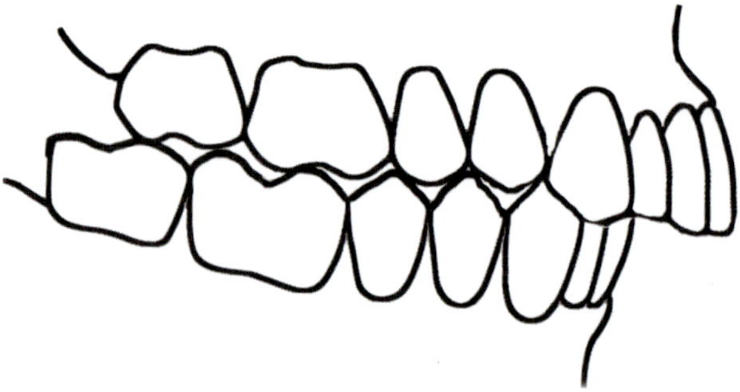

Fig. 10.5 Class II occlusion

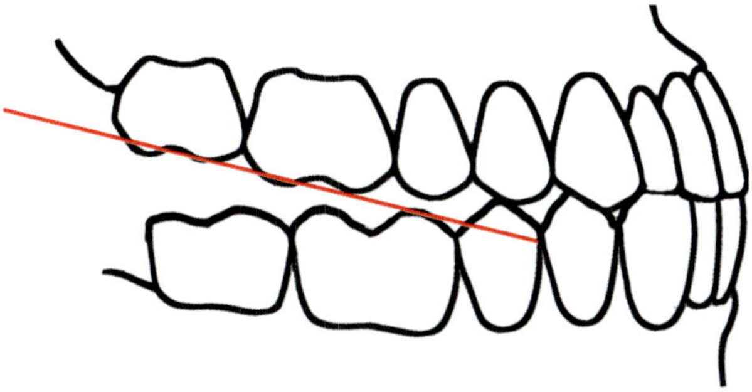

Fig. 10.6 Posterior occlusal plane shown during bite registration (edge to edge) for functional appliance. Note the inter-occlusal space in the distal section of the bite registration

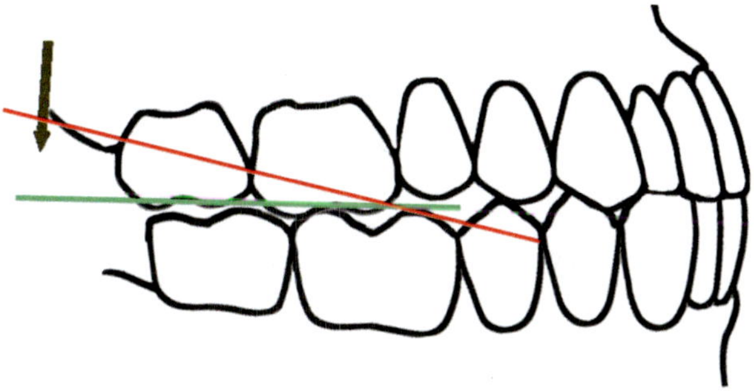

Fig. 10.7 Correction of occlusal plane inclination with a counterclockwise rotation. Main extrusion in mid/posterior sections

Removable appliances can be used for extrusion also. In general, any removable appliance can be used to force tooth eruption. It will be necessary to add a bracket to the selected tooth and wiring from the removable appliance. The limitation and efficacy are limited by collaboration. Unfortunately, to obtain an effective extrusion, cooperation must be continuous without any exception: a 12-h a day cooperation/extrusion will be without doubt useless, as the other 12 h remaining a day are left for relapse. Constant gentle forces are necessary to stimulate bone formation and to reduce the risk of reduced blood supply to the periodontium. When the process of appositional bone has consolidated, there is little room for massive relapse. We cannot change the skeletal characteristics of the individual, but we can satisfy muscle requests by positioning teeth accordingly.

The Class II/1 occlusion as described in Fig. 10.5 is corrected with a neuromuscular orthodontic procedure. As an example, a bite registration after TENS reveals a PRP as seen in Fig. 10.8. The fabrication of a Bionator or a Sava 1 Extruder is accomplished by sending to the technician a bite recording in PRP. If utilizing a resin-like Bosworth® Sapphire®, recording can be performed with the TENS-Only technique as previously described. My personal experience is with both techniques, kinesiographic and TENS-only. For obvious reasons, it is much easier to record a mandibular position in the child with the TENS-only technique. Figures 10.9, 10.10, and 10.11 show the correct procedure on how the extrusions should be carried out. Usually it is advisable to extrude the upper premolar sector at first, in order to obtain a Class I occlusion with only premolar contacts. Figure 10.11 shows the results

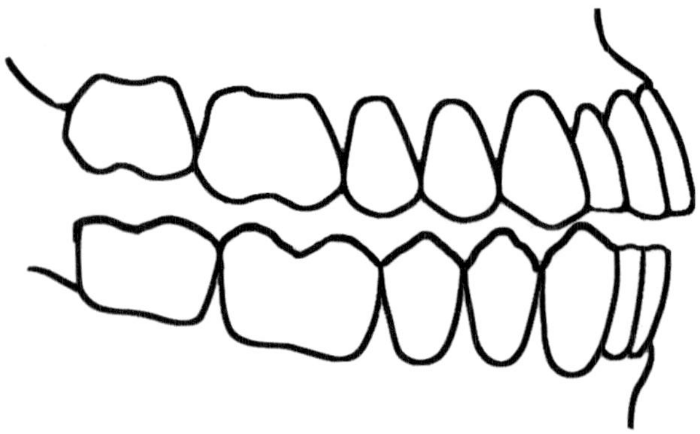

Fig. 10.8 Schematic representation of occlusal Class II after TENS application, rest position. There is a freeway space within 5 mm circa. The interocclusal space is recorded and this recording is used to create an appliance that permits extrusion while maintaining the PRP

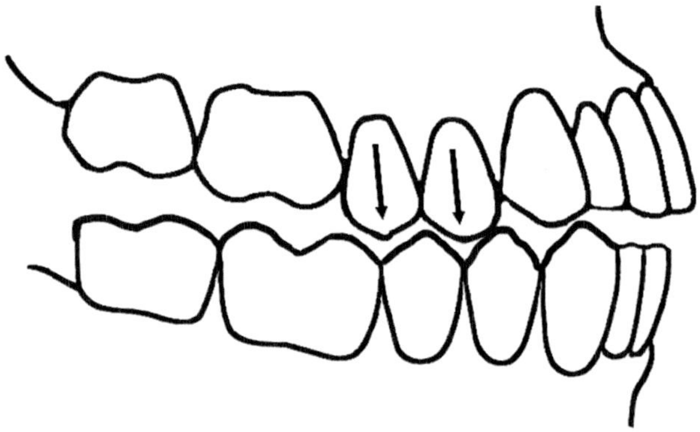

Fig. 10.9 First step of Neuromuscular correction is extrusion of the premolar area

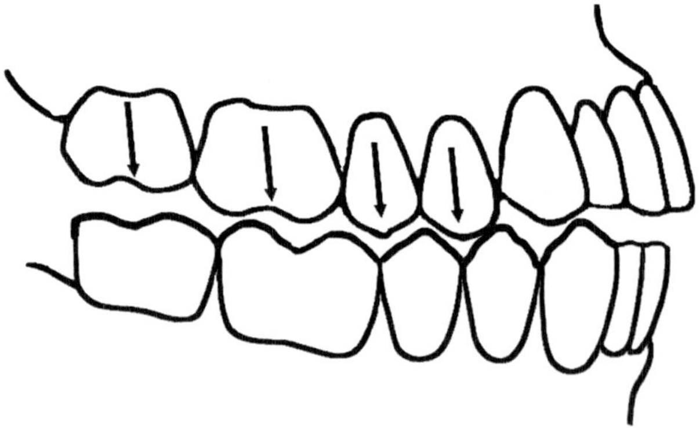

Fig. 10.10 Second step for Neuromuscular correction is extrusion of upper molars

obtained at the end of this procedure: it can take several weeks to complete this vertical correction. It is very important to keep in mind that the vertical correction in positional Class II can be done only after RPE. It is imperative to correct transverse discrepancies before any sagittal/vertical correction. When extrusions and alignments are completed, a natural spontaneous freeway space, usually 1–3 mm, is present.

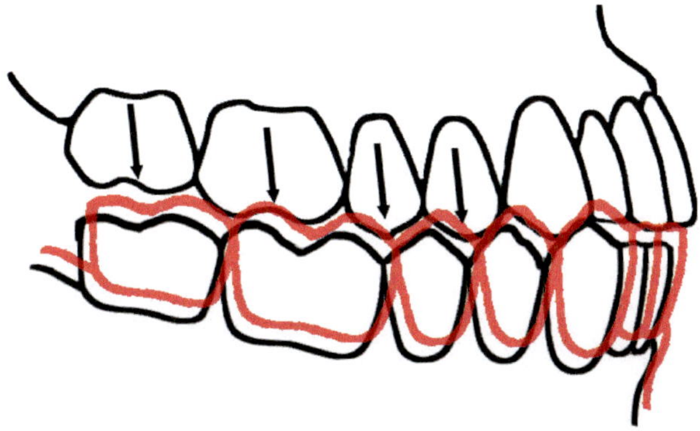

Fig. 10.11 From RP to CO. Natural freeway space is present at the end of the extrusion phase

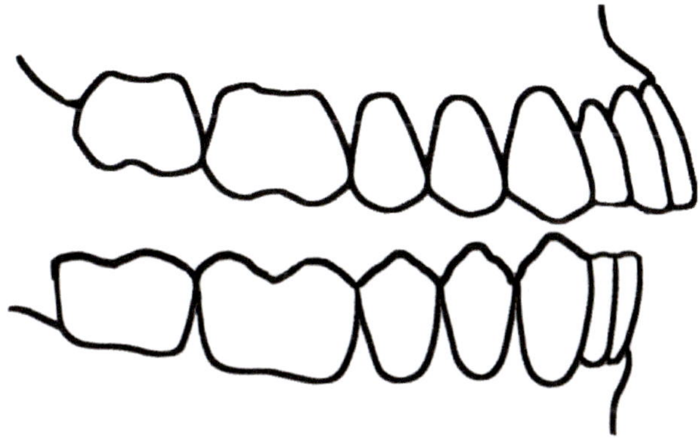

Fig. 10.12 Result of TENS on occlusal Class II with excess freeway space and RP on or behind vertical from CO. Closure toward the upper plane of occlusion on the neuromuscular trajectory would place mandible correctly for a class I occlusion. A pure extrusion would retain a Class II occlusal relationship

One of the advantages of extruding mainly on the upper arch, is that you do not need to worry about lower incisal flaring. Even though there is no consensus on the position of the lower incisors, the author suggests controlling lower flaring, not much for bone/periodontal issues, but more for the fact that excessive flaring will reduce the possibility of Class I occlusion [25, 26]. Class I occlusion is not the main objective of NO, but when correcting positional Class II occlusion with this technique, there is a good opportunity to do it with fashion.

Another neuromuscular orthodontic treatment procedure is that referred to as the "phase II" treatment of patients that have undergone orthotic treatment for a TMD problem. The general idea that a second-phase treatment is possible by simply using the orthotic as an extrusion guide is misleading. This is especially true for patients that have a TMD problem in a severe Class II occlusion. As described in Chap. 7, there are various possibilities for the correction of the mandibular position by orthodontic means. Chapter 7, Fig. 7.13 illustrates schematically these various possibilities. When RP is on or behind the vertical of CO, the vertical occlusal relationship is Class II (Fig. 10.12). This means that you cannot simply extrude teeth and leave 1.5 mm of freeway space: this could be functionally valid (if you reduce the overjet properly) but the result would be a class II occlusion with OJ. Instead it is necessary to set the Myocentric closer to the HP, thus leaving a greater freeway space than the usual 1.5–2 mm. Doing so would solve orthodontically the malocclusion and finish the case in a Class I occlusion. The objective of this correction is not an ideal freeway space, but rather setting a new centric occlusion on the Myotrajectory with an increased freeway space. This is a practical demonstration of why, in certain cases, it is more important to identify a "new centric" on the Myotrajectory than an ideal MyoCentric with 2 mm of freeway space. It is not infrequent to see posterior open bites on patients who have undergone excessive orthotic wear. These cases require a new Kinesiographic assessment to identify proper orthodontic objectives.

The following is a clinical example of this treatment procedure with the use of the TENS only technique. This approach takes a little more experience from a clinical point of view in respect of a full MKG assessment: there is no possibility to *measure* the PRP recording.

Case 10.1

Class II Occlusion with Increased OJ and Increased Freeway Space

Summary A 13-year-old female was visited in my office and was complaining for misalignment of her upper front teeth. Medical/dental anamnesis revealed common headaches and inadequate forward head posture, with tendency of head rotation to the right. Physical examination showed a slight reduction in total mouth opening.

Pre-treatment		
Extraoral analysis (Fig. 10.13a)		
Facial Profile	Convex	
Facial Height	Upper: Normal, Lower: Reduced	
Occlusal Plane	Normal	
Facial Symmetry	Normal	
Lips	Normal	
Mandibular posture	Retrognathic	
Head posture	Rotated to right	
Intraoral Analysis (Fig. 10.13)		
Teeth	123456/123456	7 s and 5 s erupting, 8 s present
	123456/123456	7 s erupting, 8 s present
Molar Class	Class II bilaterally	
Canine Class	Class II bilaterally	
Overjet	7 mm	
Overbite	6 mm	
Oral Hygiene	Fair	
Rotations	Upper central incisors	
Crossbite	Box-bite upper left 4	
Diastemas	Lower arch, distal to canines	
Crowding	Moderate upper	
Agenesis	No	
Missing teeth	No	

Pre-treatment	
Functional Analysis	
Swallow	Swallows with tongue between teeth
Tongue Tie	No
Tongue posture	Good
Tongue thrust	Yes
Slurred speech	No
Cephalometrics (Fig. 10.14)	

Neuromuscular Diagnosis	
Freeway Space (clinical evaluation)	Increased ≥4 mm
Skeletal Class	I
Anterior Wall	Yes
TMJ Left	Occasional click during opening
TMJ Right	Normal
Problem list	
Dental	No important dental problems
Skeletal	Class II positional: Mandible is distally positioned during ICP
	Maxillary width is restricted.
Functional	TMJ Clicking

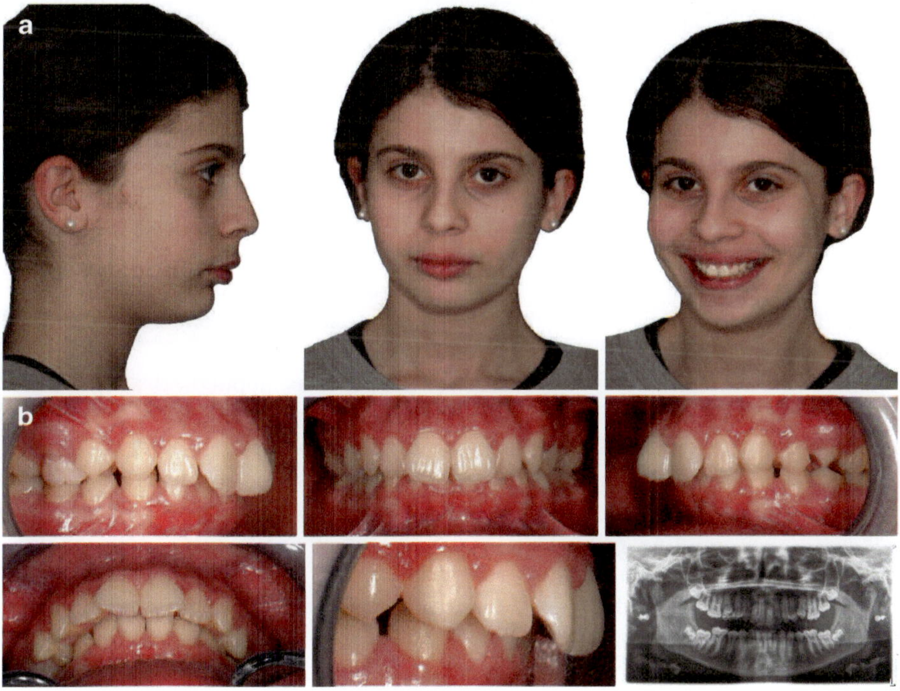

Fig. 10.13 (**a**, **b**) Extra- and Intraoral photos. March 2018

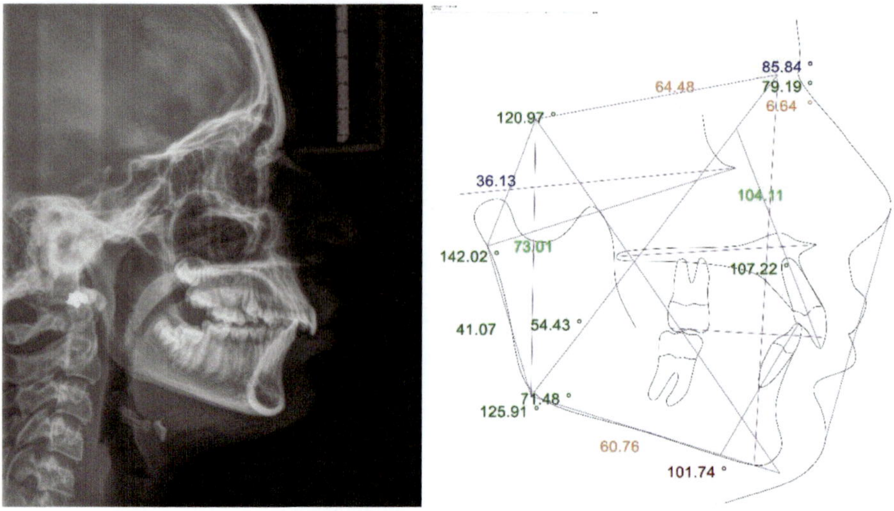

Fig. 10.14 Lateral cephalogram and cephalometric analysis, pretreatment. Jarabak analysis

Neuromuscular Treatment Objectives and Therapeutic Steps

- Reduction of freeway space by RME and lower immediate alignment for torque correction.
- Mandibular Repositioning with a modified Functional Appliance after bite registration via "TENS only technique."
- No change of occlusal plane inclination is necessary.

Treatment Sequence

Rapid palatal expansion was completed in **April 2018** (Fig. 10.15). Note that the expansion may seem excessive because it must be taken into consideration a need for lower torque correction and expansion. Furthermore, mandibular anterior repositioning will reduce the transverse gap visible at this stage.

Lower arch expansion and levelling started in **June 2018** with lower fixed appliances. In September 2018, a bite registration was taken in PRP and sent to the lab for a modified Bionator (Fig. 10.16).

By **October 10th, 2018,** a modified Bionator was applied. Brackets were attached to upper 6 s, 5 s, and 4 s, bilaterally. The modified Bionator was carefully carved to allow extrusion of the premolar areas of both arches (Fig. 10.17). Vertical elastics, bilaterally, between upper and lower premolars were applied. The patient was instructed to wear them on a 24/24 h basis with the only exception when eating. One elastic was worn for each side (1/4 4.5 oz.), creating a "square" between premolars (not shown).

On **November 21st, 2018**, a video recording and intraoral photos (Fig. 10.18) were taken. Intraoral photos show that in ICP occlusal Class I is achieved in the premolar relationship. Arrows show premolar relationship/contact and highlight the second step for occlusal extrusion of the posterior sectors, that is, torque correction

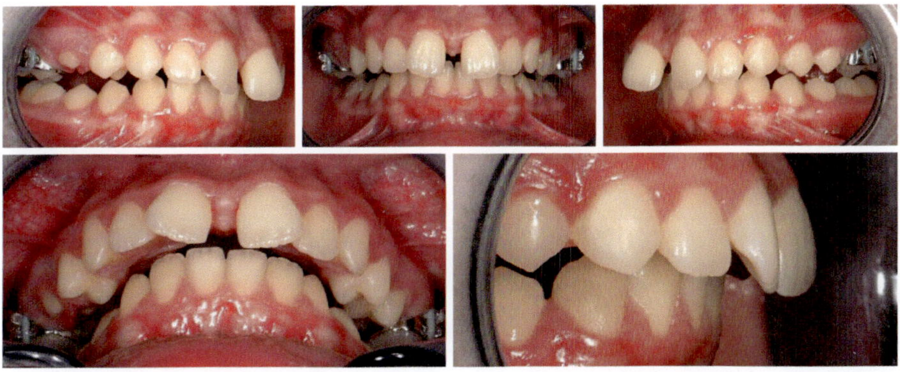

Fig. 10.15 April 2018. End of RPE active phase

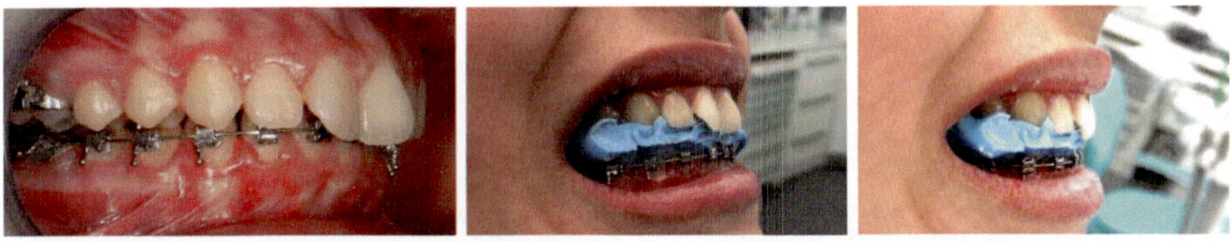

Fig. 10.16 September 2018. Bite recording of new mandibular position in PRP for the construction of a modified Bionator

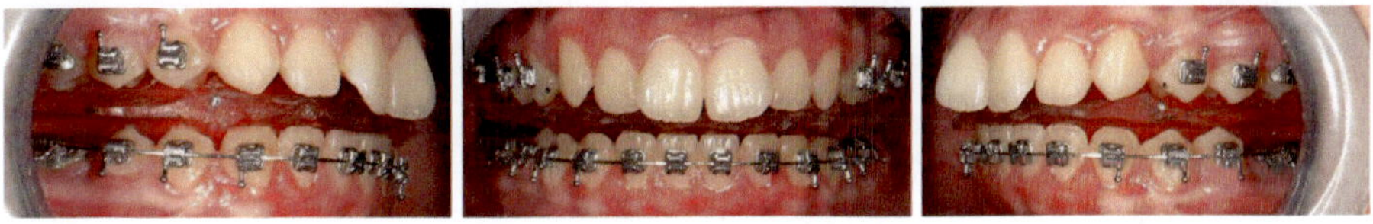

Fig. 10.17 Modified Bionator is manufactured on occlusal registration taken during TENS session. Brackets are applied to upper arch selectively to premolar and first molar. Carving of resin to selectively extrude premolar/molar area. Note lingual torque of lower molars. October 2018

and extrusion of first upper and lower molars. Note that at this stage lower incisors become visible in CO as overbite is reduced due to reduction of freeway space due to premolar extrusion and reduction of OJ is achieved by the new mandibular position (Fig. 10.18).

RPE has been useful in creating space for crowded teeth in this case, although extra space for alignment may not always be ready for crowding solutions. Alignment of the upper arch is now necessary. Brackets were applied to the remaining teeth of the upper arch from canine to canine; we are now ready for extrusion of the first molars and alignment of the upper arch (Fig. 10.19).

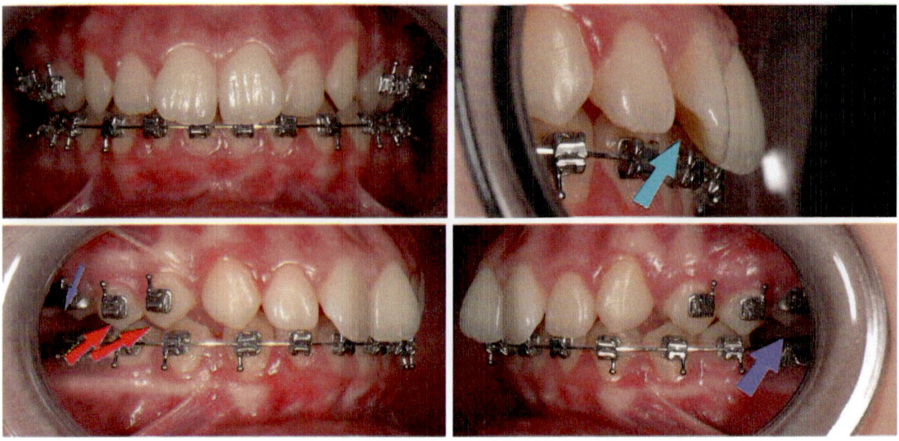

Fig. 10.18 Centric occlusion after 40 days of treatment. From top: Overjet is completely reduced (blue arrow). Class I occlusion at premolar region (red arrows). There is about 5 mm vertical gap to extrude in the molar region to have tooth contact (purple arrows). Note diastemas between upper canines and first premolar, bilaterally

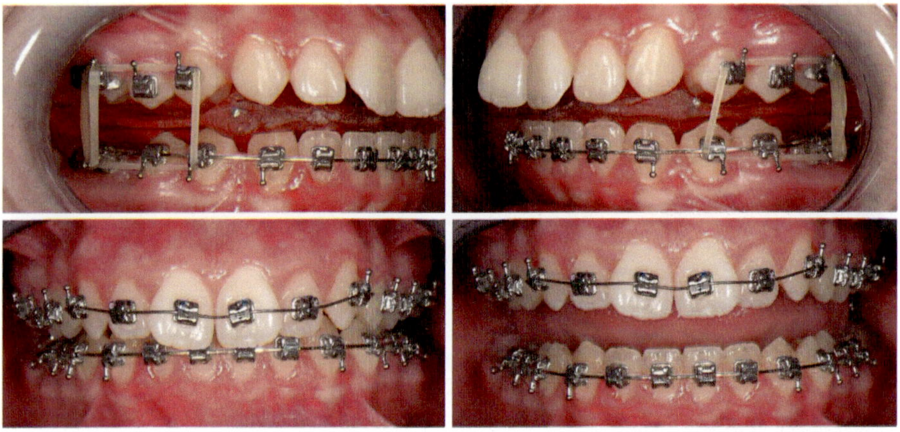

Fig. 10.19 November 21, 2018: alignment of the upper arch. Elastics now include lower and upper molars

The alignment of the upper anteriors is characterized by a segmental arch limited from 3–3. This is done to avoid intrusion forces on the just extruded premolars. Now the ¼ 4.5 oz. includes the lower and upper molars. An extra elastic 1/8 6 oz. is added during the day between upper and lower molars when the modified Bionator is worn (full day except for schooltime). By May 2019, final alignment regimen has started. The modified Bionator has been suspended. Molar contact between the arches is present at this stage. Upper canines have been distalized by class II elastics to close posterior diastemas (Fig. 10.19) only during the Bionator phase. Upper 0.018 × 0.025 NiTi insures control over the upper arch. Lower 0.016 × 0.022 NiTi is sufficient for arch control. It is not necessary to flatten the lower arch. It is always necessary to verify anterior incisal contacts that could prevent mandibular neuromuscular repositioning (Fig. 10.20).

June 2019. Bite turbos are added lingually to the upper incisors. This is a standard procedure to control freeway space with vertical elastics (not shown). November 2019: now the arches are aligned and there is no more active treatment with elastics, Fig. 10.21. Patient is now at a stabilization phase for 2–3 months with the bite turbos in place for vertical control. I prefer avoiding possible interferences from second molars during this stabilization phase; temporary posterior build-ups could open the bite a millimeter or so, which naturally is reduced over time with a slight intrusion of the lower second molars.

Fixed appliance therapy ended in June 2020. A Hawley-type upper removable retention appliance applied for 18 h/day was prescribed and a lower fixed 3–3 composite retention was built.

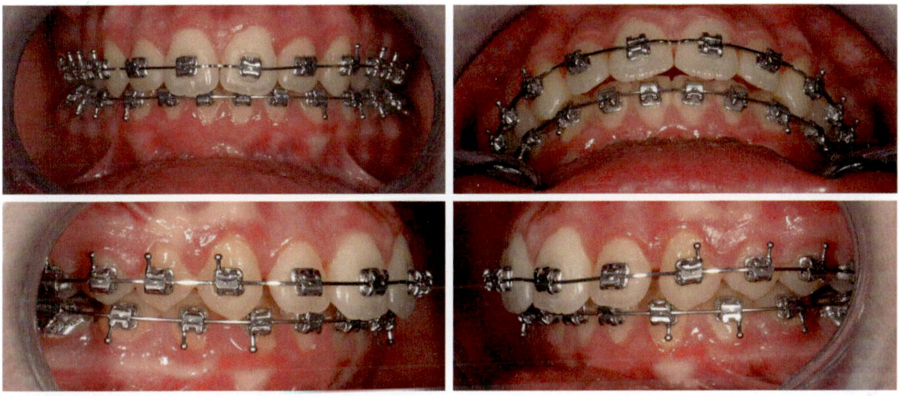

Fig. 10.20 May 2019. Final alignment phase

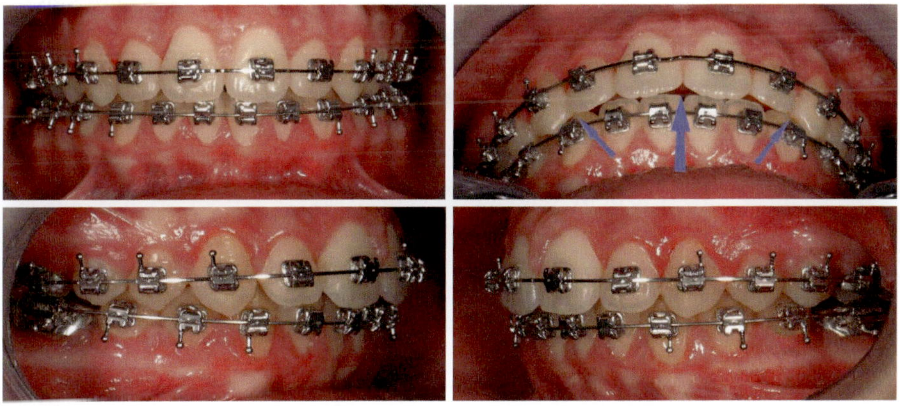

Fig. 10.21 Alignment is good. Always checking for the involuntary creation of an anterior wall (purple arrows)

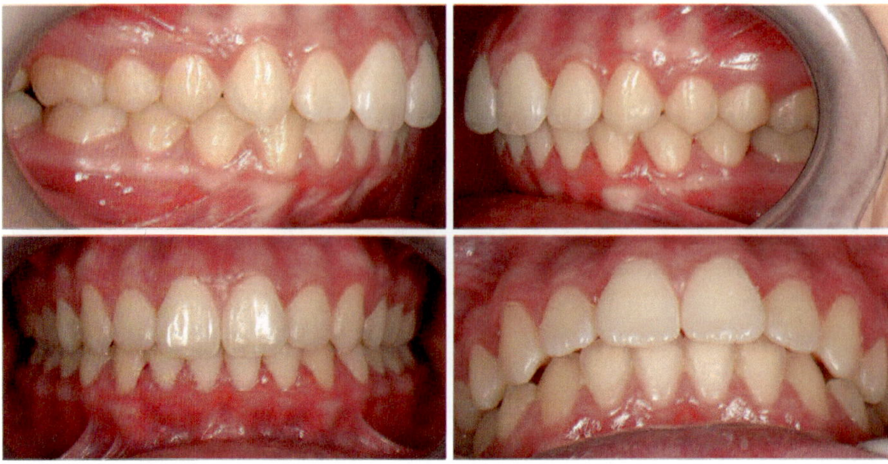

Fig. 10.22 Intraoral photos, 10 months after treatment

Lateral Cephalogram X-ray and panoramic were done in April 2021. Intra- and extraoral photos were also taken at this time and are shown in Figs. 10.22 and 10.23.

Treatment Results—Discussion

The increase in VD is visible in both frontal and lateral aspects (Figs. 10.24, 10.25, 10.26 and 10.27). Since photos are taken in a natural head posture, it could be that the cranio-cervical posture has changed due to mandibular repositioning and reduction of freeway space. Patient seems more upright. A loss on torque control of the lower incisors is a common finding when aligning and reducing the curve of Spee. It is not possible to reduce the curve of Spee without sacrificing incisor protrusion. To avoid this, a lower arch preparation in young growing children with lip bumper or lower arch distalization in adults with TAD is advisable.

From a dental point of view, Class I occlusion was obtained bilaterally with a normal OJ. This TENS-only technique is a fast, effective, and inexpensive method. It represents the first step in acknowledging neuromuscular diagnosis with a bite registration. It is necessary to execute with meticulous precision every step without modifying the suggested protocol:

- Depending on the type of Myomonitor® (J4 or J5) apply Myotodes® accordingly.
- Have patient relax with an Aqualizer® between teeth.
- Adjust balance and pulsing of ULF-TENS to a minimum for a perceivable spike of 1 mm circa. This is done by gently applying a finger to the lower incisors.
- Have patient pulse for a minimum of 40 min. Check that patient is in a relaxed state and let mandible “drop.”
- Ask patient to not consider operators presence.
- Turn off TENS device.
- Gently register with fast-setting putty the front incisor relationship.

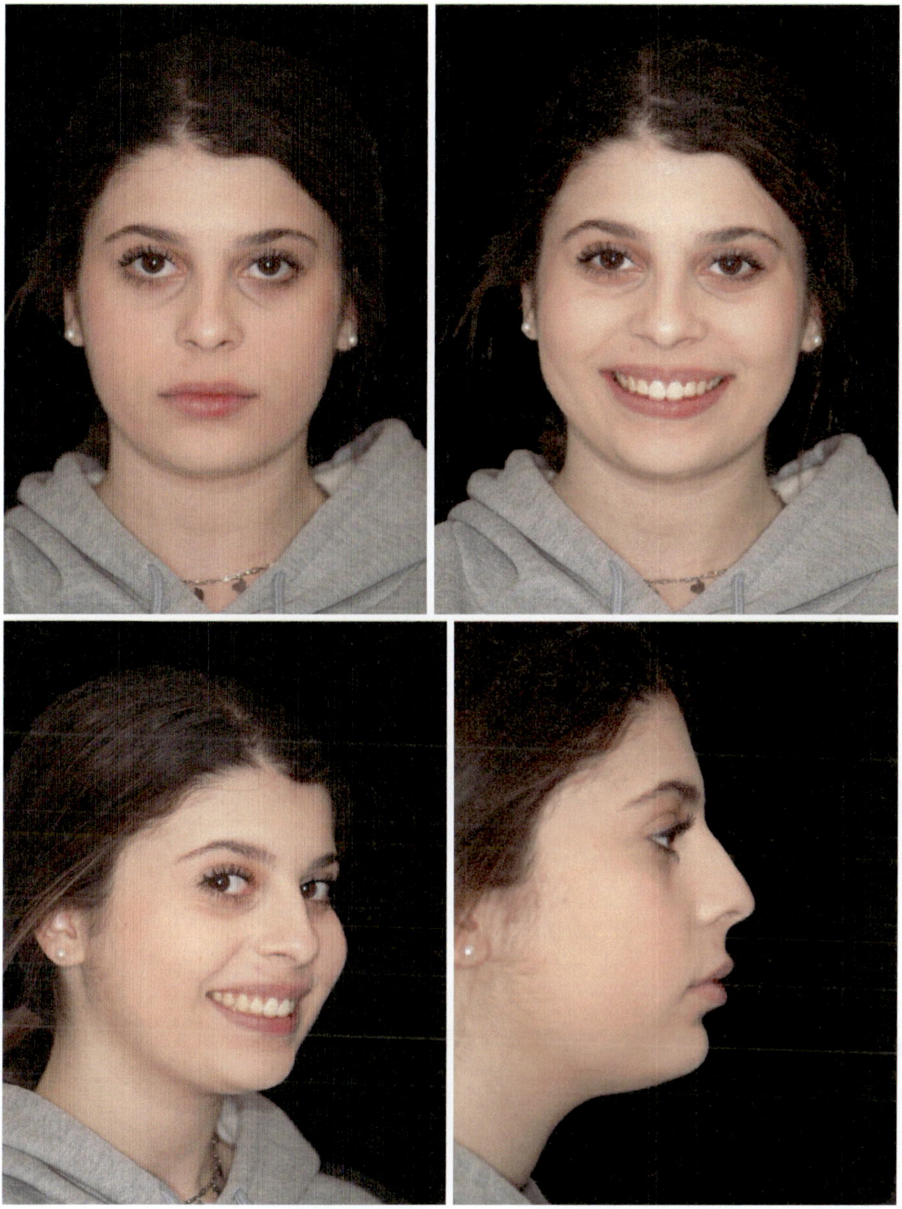

Fig. 10.23 Extraoral photos, 10 months after treatment

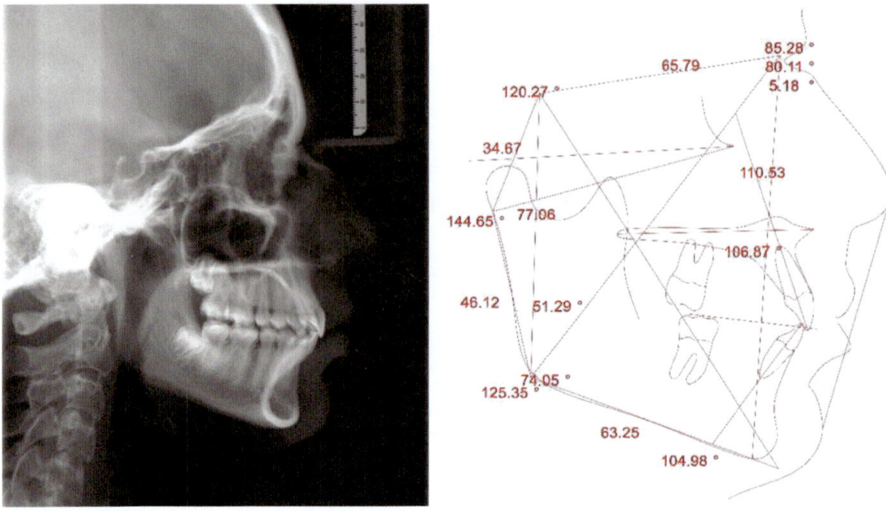

Fig. 10.24 Lateral Cephalogram and cephalometric tracing. Jarabak analysis

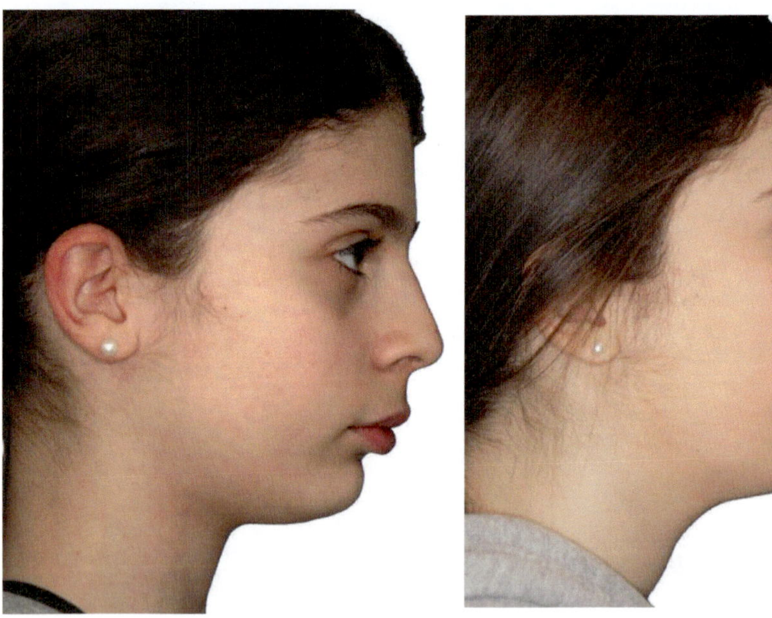

Fig. 10.25 Pre- and Post-treatment lateral profile photos. Natural head posture

Fig. 10.26 Superimposition of initial cephalometric tracing (black) with final cephalometric tracing (red). Note the increase of 3° angle of lower incisor to mandibular plane

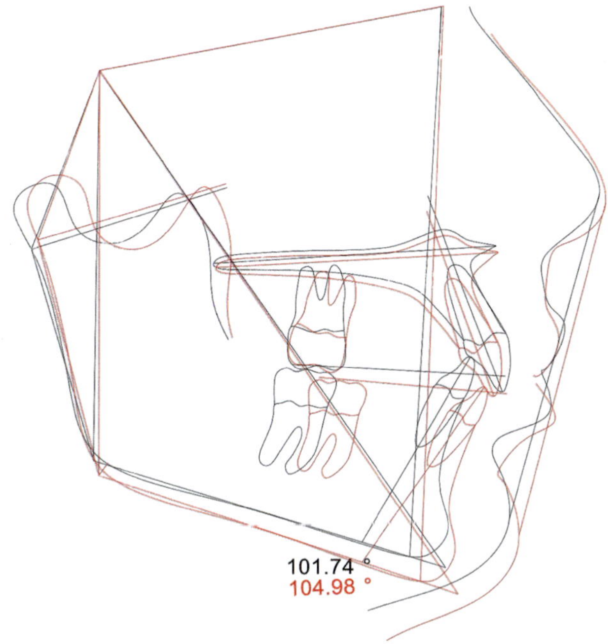

MEASUREMENT		NORMAL VALUE	VALUE	DIFFERENCE	BIAS
Dental Analysis					
OcP/MeGo	°	14.0	14.9	0.9	
Interincisal angle	°	135.0	129.3	-5.7	
+1/SN	°	102.0±2.0	100.1	-1.9	
+1/NL	°	110.0±6.0	107.2	-2.8	
-1/MeGo (anatomic)	°	90.0±3.0	101.7	11.7	•••
+1i/NPg	mm	5.0±2.0	10.5	5.5	••
-1i/NPg	mm	0.0±2.0	4.7	4.7	••
Ls/E-line	mm	-1.5±2.5	0.0	1.5	
Li'/E-line	mm	1.0±1.0	-1.8	-2.8	••
Skeletal Analysis					
N-S-Ar	°	123.0±5.0	121.0	-2.0	
S-Ar-Go	°	143.0±6.0	142.0	-1.0	
Gonial angle (anatomic)	°	130.0±7.0	125.9	-4.1	
Bjork (anatomic)	°	396.0±5.0	388.9	-7.1	•
S-N	mm	71.0±3.0	64.5	-6.5	••
S-Ar	mm	32.0±3.0	36.1	4.1	•
Ar-Go-N	°	53.5±1.5	54.4	0.9	
ML/NGo	°	72.5±2.5	71.5	1.0	
Go-Ar	mm	44.0±5.0	41.1	-2.9	
S-Ar/Ar-Go	%	67.5±7.5	88.0	20.5	••
Go-Me	mm	71.0±5.0	60.8	-10.2	••
Go-Me/N-S	%	100.0±5.0	94.2	-5.8	•
Angle SNA	°	82.0±2.0	85.8	3.8	•
Angle SNB	°	80.0±2.0	79.2	-0.8	
ANB	°	2.0±2.0	6.6	4.6	••
SN/ML (anatomic)	°	36.0	28.9	-7.1	
N-Go	mm		106.0		
S-Me II FH	mm		48.3		
Y/SN	°	66.0±3.0	66.3	0.3	
S-Go/N-Me	%	63.5±1.5	70.1	6.6	•••
SNPg	°	81.0±3.0	80.1	-0.9	
NAPg	°	175.0±3.0	168.7	-6.3	••

MEASUREMENT		NORMAL VALUE	VALUE	DIFFERENCE	BIAS
Dental Analysis					
OcP/MeGo	°	14.0	14.5	0.5	
Interincisal angle	°	135.0	125.6	-9.4	
+1/SN	°	102.0±2.0	99.2	-2.8	•
+1/NL	°	110.0±6.0	106.9	-3.1	
-1/MeGo (anatomic)	°	90.0±3.0	105.0	15.0	•••
+1i/NPg	mm	5.0±2.0	8.0	3.0	•
-1i/NPg	mm	0.0±2.0	6.3	6.3	•••
Ls/E-line	mm	-1.5±2.5	2.3	3.8	•
Li'/E-line	mm	1.0±1.0	-0.7	-1.7	•
Skeletal Analysis					
N-S-Ar	°	123.0±5.0	120.3	-2.7	
S-Ar-Go	°	143.0±6.0	144.7	1.7	
Gonial angle (anatomic)	°	130.0±7.0	125.3	-4.7	
Bjork (anatomic)	°	396.0±5.0	390.3	-5.7	•
S-N	mm	71.0±3.0	65.8	-5.2	•
S-Ar	mm	32.0±3.0	34.7	2.7	
Ar-Go-N	°	53.5±1.5	51.3	-2.2	•
ML/NGo	°	72.5±2.5	74.1	1.6	
Go-Ar	mm	44.0±5.0	46.1	2.1	
S-Ar/Ar-Go	%	67.5±7.5	75.2	7.7	•
Go-Me	mm	71.0±5.0	63.2	-7.8	•
Go-Me/N-S	%	100.0±5.0	96.1	3.9	
Angle SNA	°	82.0±2.0	85.3	3.3	•
Angle SNB	°	80.0±2.0	80.1	0.1	
ANB	°	2.0±2.0	5.2	3.2	•
SN/ML (anatomic)	°	36.0	30.3	-5.7	
N-Go	mm		109.7		
S-Me II FH	mm		51.9		
Y/SN	°	66.0±3.0	66.8	0.8	
S-Go/N-Me	%	63.5±1.5	69.7	6.2	•••
SNPg	°	81.0±3.0	80.6	-0.4	
NAPg	°	175.0±3.0	170.6	-4.4	•

Fig. 10.27 Cephalometric results

- When putty has hardened, have patient finally open mouth: remove Aqualizer®, add fast-setting putty to all lower arch and have patient reposition with previously created anterior bite registration.
- When putty has hardened, trim and check bite registration.

It is important that after Aqualizer® removal, the patient does not have any tooth contact between the dental arches.

Passive Extrusion (PE)

Teeth erupt spontaneously. Functional appliances keep away anything that can reduce this eruption: tongue, cheeks, and occlusal forces. This is the preferred method for gaining an increased eruption. The limitations are not only represented by collaboration, but also by speed. Forced orthodontic eruption is faster and more aesthetic.

Passive spontaneous extrusion of selected sectors of the dental arch are accompanied by fixed appliance therapy for finishing. In growing patients, passive extrusion should always be attempted as the correction of choice whereas, in the adult it is more likely that first choice would be fixed appliance therapy. The main advantage of PE is that with the use of functional appliances such as the Bionator, mandibular reposturing can be added as part of the treatment procedure. This treatment option is ideal for children that have a good compliance.

Correcting freeway space by extrusion does have some limitations. You cannot correct an excess curve of Spee only by passive extrusion; if using a functional appliance like the Bionator, control over the entire arch is necessary to take advantage of potential growth of the mandible and thus avoid lower incisor flaring.

In other words, what erroneously is called *phase two* or orthodontic treatment after orthotic re-functioning (or *phase one*), extrusion and reduction of the curve of Spee is ***impossible*** without lower molar distalization or any other specific orthodontic treatment able to gain enough space to preserve lower incisor torque and avoid flaring. Therefore, extrusion and correction of the curve of Spee are easily achieved during growth, where the correct use of lee-way space and mandibular length increase from mandibular growth gives the orthodontist enough space to reduce or even preserve incisal position of the lower arch. The author is not convinced that the ideal cephalometric angulation of the lower incisor to the mandibular plane should be limited to 90–95°. There is no evidence that moderate incisor flaring is dangerous for the periodontal tissues [25, 26]. Lower proclination may have a more important side effect: *posterior condylar displacement.* The entity of the lower flaring on posterior condylar displacement is dependent on the level of overbite. When overbite is severe, any flaring of the lower incisors will displace distally the condyle. Note that in severe Class II deep-bite cases, lower flaring can already be present. This explains the importance of reducing OB as soon as possible and with dental extrusion. This reduction of freeway space increases tongue space in ICP. The orthodontic mechanics for the correction of excess curve of Spee in the adult are complex when TADs, stripping, and special techniques for posterior tipping are used. The first step in the correction of the curve of Spee should be extrusion of the premolar area. This means that space is needed: lower expansion is a reaction to upper rapid palatal expansion, and it should be carried out on all Class II occlusions. RPE lowers and positions the condyles in a more forward position [27], thus setting the first step toward mandibular freedom and SMM. Tip back of the lower posterior molars is very useful and total arch distalization can be achieved with TADs as well. Furthermore, reducing torque in the lower posterior sectors increases total posterior diameter.

Any extrusion on any of the two arches will produce a reduction of freeway space, and this is especially true for the adult patient. Growing patients may produce freeway space as they develop. A skeletal deep-bite will remain a deep-bite no matter what extrusion you induce with your treatment. It could be that early interceptive orthodontics in severe deep-bite children could produce impressive results, but the author remains skeptical on transforming a skeletal deep-bite into a skeletal normal bite. It is probably not possible to influence the mandibular angle too much during growth. It could hypothetically be possible, but collaboration and intense use of functional appliances to an extreme is not part of my personal experience. So, when extruding on a severe deep-bite case during growth, do not expect to see a miraculous reduction of the freeway space. On many occasions, you will preserve the excess freeway you have recorded with the bioelectric instrumentation during the first diagnostic assessment. Other times collaboration and growth pattern can deliver surprising results.

Functional Appliances and Extrusion

Every orthodontist should have a preferred method of treatment to pursue proper objectives. For functional orthodontists, ***functional appliances*** (FA) are the daily instruments to work with. My personal opinion is somewhat critical in defining what is or is not a functional appliance. There are two types of FA based on how they act on Class II occlusion. They have one common feature: mandibular repositioning.

(a) The Frankel Appliance

By far the most *functional* appliance of all. There is truly little space taken from the oral cavity, thus leaving excellent space for tongue function. Mandibular repositioning is achieved without hard "bite jumping" to a new mandibular position. The appliance has some intrinsic elasticity and stimulates muscular function for the recorded bite position. 97% of acrylic is vestibular and participates in *stretching* oral tissues. This appliance helps stabilize a previous RPE by keeping away soft tissues (muscle) away from the maxilla. There is no other quality functional appliance like the Frankel. The stimuli for the lip competence are fundamental factors for functional rehabilitation of occlusion. Of all the positives that can be said on the Frankel, this device does have some limitations. Extrusion of the dentition with this device is limited and not as good as with functional appliances with inter-occlusal acrylic. This should be the appliance of choice when freeway space does not exceed 7–8 mm at initial diagnosis. The bite recording procedure for the neuromuscular orthodontist is represented by recording the PRP.

(b) The Bionator

This is the device of choice when vertical control (extrusion) is important. Some variations include an expansion screw or acrylic filling of the vestibular wires. I use this appliance without any vestibular wires or pads together with fixed appliance therapy to force extrusion of selected arch sectors. The Bionator permits selected anchorage (you carve acrylic only where you desire to extrude). Although bite recording position of the mandible is achieved via bite jumping, this is the acrylic device of choice for its versatility. Bite recording is done in PRP.

I have used, tested, and modified most of the FA on the market. There are several remarkably effective appliances like the Planas and Bimler. Most neuromuscular orthodontic cases with functional appliances can be carried out with these two appliances. Appliances cannot be considered functional when the only correction is a sagittal repositioning of the mandible ("sagittal first" techniques), nor when they are hard bite jumping devices like the Herbst. I like to consider appliances *functional* when they *stimulate* a new *function* and set a new mandibular "muscular" position. Hard reset of the mandibular position like a Herbst or twin block appliance force to a new hinge that is not acceptable by neuromuscular standards. There are although, a limited number of other bite jumping devices like the Jasper Jumper® or Gentile Jumpers® that do not create a new hinge but can promote mandibular anterior repositioning. These orthodontic devices typically produce lower anterior flaring and posterior intrusion/distalization, and can be used in conjunction with a lower fixed lingual arch and posterior vertical elastics. One advantage of using these devices is that they offer a viable alternative for noncompliance therapy. There will always be a significant percentage of individuals who do not cooperate with treatment, making it necessary to utilize these appliances even if they do not comply with our preferred neuromuscular approach. These devices function similarly to Class II elastics, causing a clockwise rotation of the occlusal plane.

The use of FA in Neuromuscular Orthodontics is regulated by a bite recording that differs from the ones these appliances were intended for. In the growing patient, the PRP/Myocentric is used for bite registration. An easiest alternative to a complete K7 scan is to use an ULF-TENS device to record a new mandibular position. The use of the TENS and functional appliances together with fixed appliance therapy and forced extrusion can correct Class II occlusions remarkably fast. Patient acceptance of the Frankel appliance or the Bionator is generally very good, and the bite recording we use for the appliance construction is based on a mandibular position with reduced or zero accommodation.

From a more specific and technical point of view, the Frankel 2 appliance can be constructed with occlusal stops on the lower molars, so that extrusion will take place mainly on the upper arch, favoring a slight counterclockwise rotation of the occlusal plane. These stops can be useful also for leeway space management of the lower arch too and this permits an easier correction of the curve of Spee during the mixed dentition phase. The Bionator can be used in the same way: the acrylic can be directed to contact the occlusal surfaces of the molars of the lower arch.

Intrusion

Tooth intrusion is needed to gain freeway space. Open-bite patients usually have very little freeway space or none and adjust head posture to create some freeway space. Head extension is the reactive response to loss of FWS and it frequently causes neck pain/discomfort. Open-bite occlusions are accompanied by several other characteristics which make them more vulnerable to articular pathologies such as arthrosis and pain. Any treatment which provides an increase in freeway space will improve symptoms in a short time. It is logical to think that interceptive orthodontics plays a major role in open-bite cases, since the intrusion and the consequent production of freeway space immediately correct head posture. Could this change in head posture together with freeway space stimulate growth of the mandibular ramus?

There are several ways to intrude teeth. Let us look at the most frequently used methods for tooth intrusion.

(a) High Pull Head Gear (HPHG)
(b) Build-ups
(c) Fixed appliance therapy
(d) Functional appliances
(e) Vertical springs

High Pull Head Gear (HPHG)

HPHG is generally applied with functional appliances. The Teuscher [28] appliance is very effective and has a very strong vertical effect. The author uses this appliance to treat skeletal Class II. Class II open bites cannot be treated with mandibular reposturing: the mandible is not expected to grow normally and is smaller than normal for age and sex. The Teuscher appliance may have some effect on condylar growth since the construction bite is somewhat taken at a maximum 5 mm of mandibular advancement. The reduction and limitation of vertical growth of the maxilla are achieved by the appliance's very strong vertical component and with a good control of torque of the maxillary incisors. Changing the upper maxillary plane of occlusion by **anterior rotation/intrusion** mimics what a surgeon does when correcting Class II open-bites: maxillary impaction/rotation. The rotation of the maxillary plane permits overclosure of the mandible thus reducing OJ and correcting dental class. The force needed is at least 500 gr., face bow should be short and external arch activated at circa $-15°$ relative to occlusal plane (personal experience). When the pull is applied on the external bow, it will produce an intrusion of all of the maxillary teeth and reduction/elimination of the excessive steepness of the posterior occlusal plane. The appliance has also an effect on the lower posterior segments due to occlusal forces therefore limiting extrusion and somewhat intruding lower first and second molars. All these characteristics favor an anticlockwise rotation of the occlusal plane which determines an increased mandibular overclosure and reduction of OJ.

Orthodontic diagnosis is complete when adding an occlusal plane appraisal to the skeletal morphological evaluation. Extrusion of the posterior segments in normo-bite individuals will cause only an opening/rotation along the hinge axis. In deep-bite cases, with excess freeway space, posterior interferences due to extrusion (reduction of freeway space) will provide anterior displacement by forward rotation of the mandible. The increase of the occlusal plane inclination relative to the condylar path, determines a pivot effect of posterior contact thus favoring mandibular anterior repositioning. In open-bite cases, the posterior occlusal plane inclination is similar to that of the condylar path and therefore any correction should be directed to the correction of the steepness of the posterior occlusal plane [13, 14]. Obviously, this correction does not mean that the posterior vertical dimension increases, but according to Sato et al., proper biomechanics flatten/reduce excessive inclination of the posterior occlusal plane also by correction of the lower posterior segments that are tipped and intruded. *There is an increase in freeway space and a reduction of posterior interferences*. This allows anterior displacement of the mandible with the possibility of condylar remodeling.

Build-Ups

Build-ups are especially useful for selective intrusion. When build-ups are constructed within freeway space and respect the totality of the dental arch, no intrusion will occur. To be successful, you must be sure to completely deplete all freeway space. This effect stretches the muscles, and the neuromuscular system will react trying to overcome the interference and regain freeway space. This reaction of the neuromuscular system is expressed with an increase in bite force against the build-up. Another consequence of muscle stretching is that there is no freeway space left and that teeth tend to be constantly in contact with the build-ups. This is in contrast with several studies that affirm the contrary [29, 30]. These studies are focused on the measurement of the *Habitual* freeway space and consider any increase in Vertical Dimension (VD) beyond this as muscle stretching. Muscle stretching for the neuromuscular orthodontist occurs only when the increase in the vertical relationship overcomes freeway space as measured after muscular deconditioning. There is obviously a misconception of freeway space between the general practitioner and the neuromuscular dentist. There is a muscular reaction of increased hyperactivity when the increase is close to or beyond Physiological Freeway Space (HRP). Some studies agree on this type of muscular reaction even if they have not been conducted with a neuromuscular setting [31].

There is also a physiologic reaction to this increase of the vertical and depletion of freeway space: head extension.

The occlusal force stimulated as a reaction to muscle stretching is usually sufficient for intrusion. Like build-ups, rapid palatal expanders constructed on acrylic base can achieve the same result. High-angle cases with little or no freeway space in growing patients should always undergo RPE on acrylic base when possible (Fig. 10.28).

Fixed Appliance Therapy

Brackets can selectively be placed more occlusally. Wire bending for intrusion (with torque control) and the use of TADs for anchorage seem effective methods for tooth intrusion. While there are several well-established mechanics for upper and lower incisor intrusion, molar intrusion is at times a more complicated task. Coronal torque loss is frequent when using only vestibular TADs. It is advisable to use both lingual and vestibular TADs, or at least control torque with fixed lingual arches or fixed trans-palatal bars (Fig. 10.29).

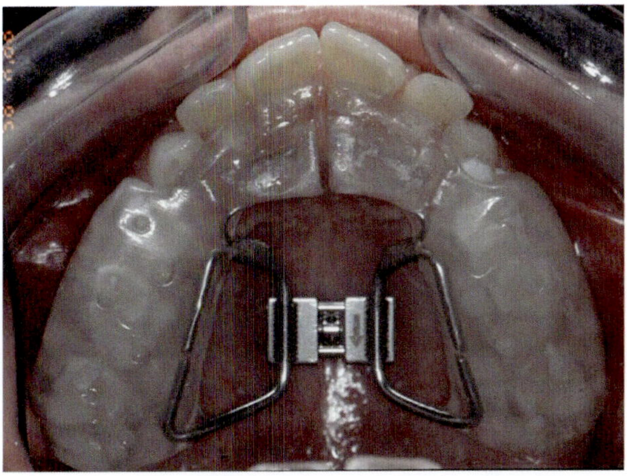

Fig. 10.28 A bonded RPE expander, modified with anterior sliding acrylic

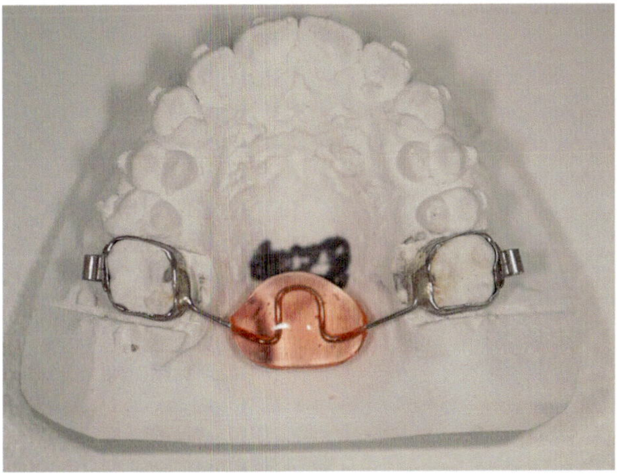

Fig. 10.29 Intrusion bar. The Nance button must be distant at least 4 mm from mucosae

Some techniques can be effective in creating freeway space and correcting open-bites by molar tipping/intrusion [32]. A modified fixed trans-palatal bar with a large Nance button can be easily activated by tongue force during deglutition to intrude the posterior teeth (Fig. 10.29).

Functional Appliances

Functional appliances are not frequently used for molar intrusion but in conjunction with HP. Until some time ago, there were some success stories of vertical growth controlled by remarkably high-bite construction activators. The use of TADs has definitively changed this scenario.

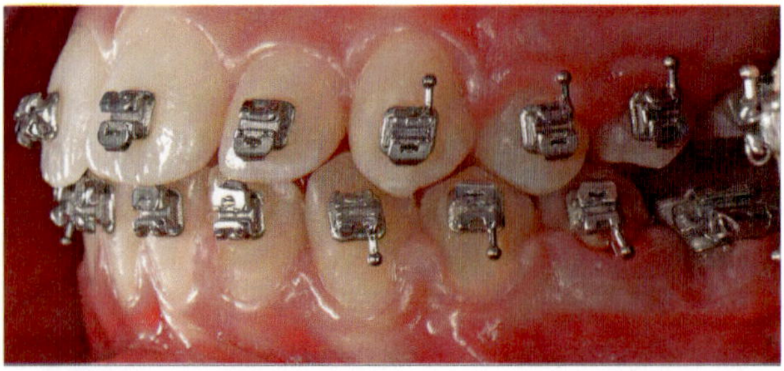

Fig. 10.30 6 mm intrusion on posterior molars with Rapid Molar Intruder®, American Orthodontics, USA

Vertical Springs

The Rapid Molar Intruder® by American Orthodontics is by every means the easiest and most effective way for molar intrusion [33–36]. Since the applied forces act on both arches, you can limit intrusion of molars according to orthodontic needs. This is the author's choice when freeway space is needed in mild cases of open-bite. It also plays an important role as an efficacious method for interceptive orthodontics (Fig. 10.30).

Bite Jumping Devices and Intrusion

The modus operandi of these devices is well documented. The rotation of the occlusal plane is similar to other Class II with extrusion of the lower molars and intrusion/distalization of the upper molars. The slight rotation of the maxillary plane of occlusion is clockwise. By adding a robust lingual arch, lower molar extrusion can be prevented, while upper intrusion/distalization takes place. This new tool gains indication for those Class II borderlines for open-bite, where it is desirable to gain some freeway space. The intrusion effect can be increased if you chose to select elastic metal jumpers by placing them more distally in the lower arch in respect of the canines. The same cannot be done with the telescopic type of jumpers because these are more rigid and adapt differently. Noncompliance therapy comes at a price. Even though there is some effect on mandibular reposturing for Class II correction, the lack of posterior support is tangible. Vertical posterior elastics may reduce the upper intrusion effect while applying a lower lingual arch with some success, but again the results are linked once more to collaboration.

Case 10.2

Class III Occlusion with No OJ and Reduced Freeway Space (Open Bite)

Summary A 12-year-old female was visited in my office and was complaining open-bite and large mandible. Medical/dental anamnesis was negative except for a medical problem that would impede her to total anesthesia.

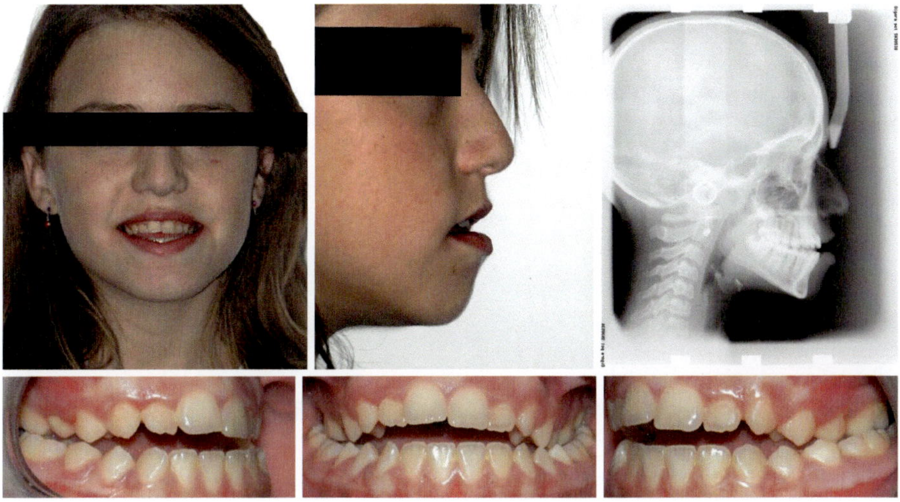

Fig. 10.31 November 2007. Extra- and intraoral photos and lateral cephalogram before treatment

It was explained that the treatment of choice would have been maxillofacial surgery. Any other orthodontic treatment would have not improved facial aesthetics (Fig. 10.31).

Pre-treatment	
Extraoral Analysis (Fig. 10.31)	
Facial Profile	Convex
Facial Height	Upper: Normal, Lower: Increased
Occlusal Plane	Posterior steep
Facial Symmetry	Normal
Lips	Incompetent, lower hypotonic
Mandibular posture	Forward
Head posture	
Intraoral Analysis (Fig. 10.31)	
Teeth	
Molar Class	III
Canine Class	III
Overjet	0
Overbite	−4
Oral Hygiene	Fair
Rotations	
Crossbite	Bilateral, premolar-molar
Diastemas	
Crowding	Slight upper crowding
Agenesis	
Missing teeth	
Intraoral Functional Analysis (Fig. 10.14)	
Swallow	Secondary dysfunction
Tongue Tie	
Tongue posture	Forward
Tongue thrust	Yes

Pre-treatment	
Slurred speech	Yes
Cephalometrics	
Neuromuscular Diagnosis	
Freeway Space	Reduced or absent
Skeletal Class	III
Anterior Wall	
TMJ Left	
TMJ Right	

Problem List
Class III profile and occlusion. Absent lip seal.
Bilateral crossbite

Neuromuscular Treatment Objectives
Create freeway space by intrusion. Expansion of upper arch.

Treatment Sequence

Treatment started in December 2007 with RPE and orthopedic face mask. By November 2008 a lower fixed lingual arch and 0.018 × 0.025 upper and lower stainless steel wires were applied to the upper and lower arch. Alignment was completed and by February 2009 bilateral Bite Fixers® (ORMCO) were applied with a modification to the original prescription. On the lower arch, the bite fixers were placed distal to the first premolars bilaterally (Fig. 10.32). This type of application results in a vector that favors intrusion the upper posterior segments providing a clockwise rotation of the occlusal plane. This encourages bite closure and at the same time provides a reduced anterior-posterior vector that guarantees avoidance of mandibular entrapment during bite closure. The extrusion of the lower posterior sectors is inhibited by the lower lingual arch and is anyways very limited due to a more vertical placement of the spring on the lower arch. Furthermore, Class III elastics, ¼ 6 oz. were added at 18 h/day to cover the distalizing effect of the resulting vectors (not shown). This type of biomechanics resembles the Rapid Molar Intruder® from American Orthodontics, which reduces and almost eliminates Anterior-Posterior (AP) vector forces.

The Bite Fixer was suspended by May 2009, while the patient continued Class III elastics 18 h/day. By December 2009, alignment was completed and by June 2010 the upper wire was segmented distal to the canines to favor intercuspation with

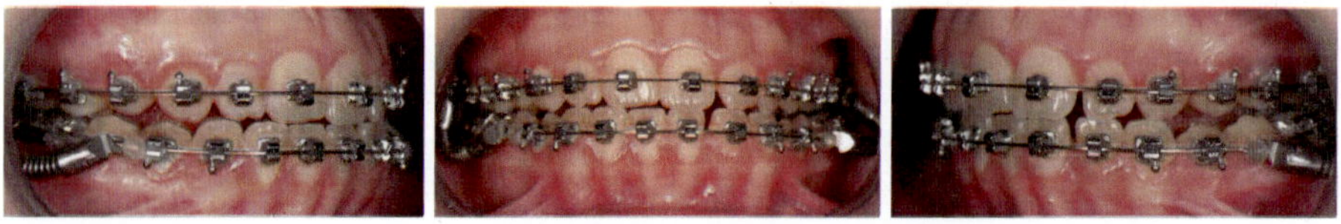

Fig. 10.32 Application of Bite Fixer® after ERP/Facemask and alignment

vertical elastics as shown in Fig. 10.33. The patient was instructed to wear an elastic that would include "box-like" the 4 front incisors during sleep (5/16 4 oz., not shown).

Patient completed the active treatment by August 2010, Fig. 10.34 shows the final occlusion and profile photo.

Figure 10.35. Photos taken at 18 months post treatment.

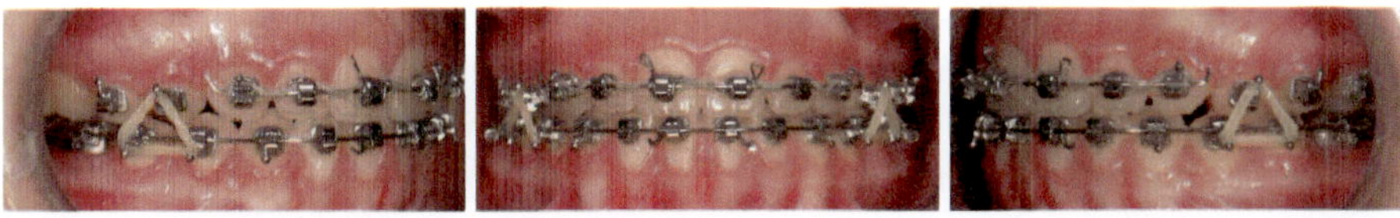

Fig. 10.33 Vertical elastics for intercuspation

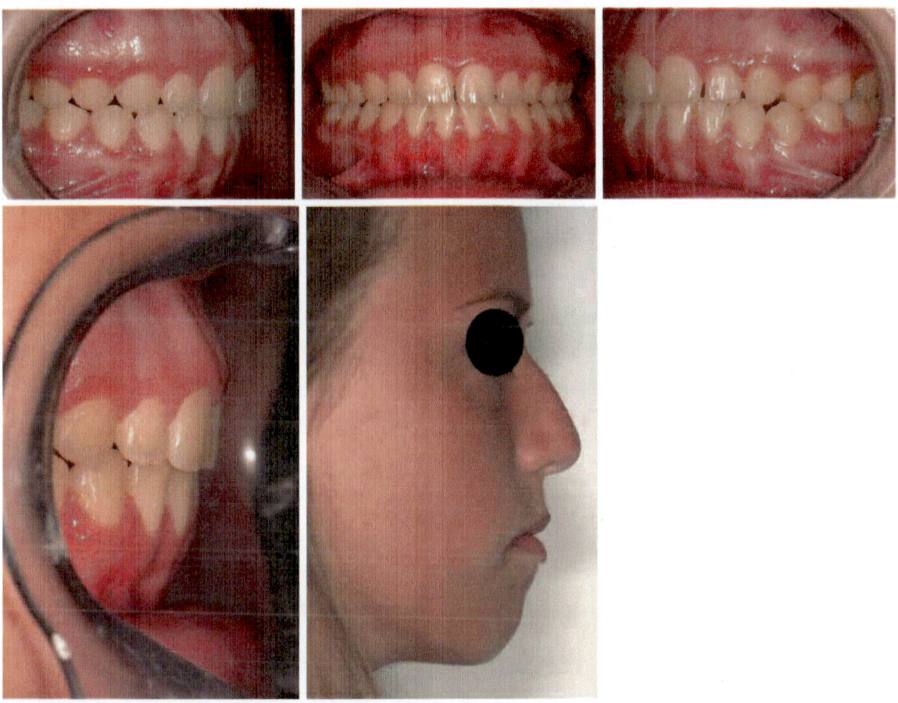

Fig. 10.34 Final occlusion and profile

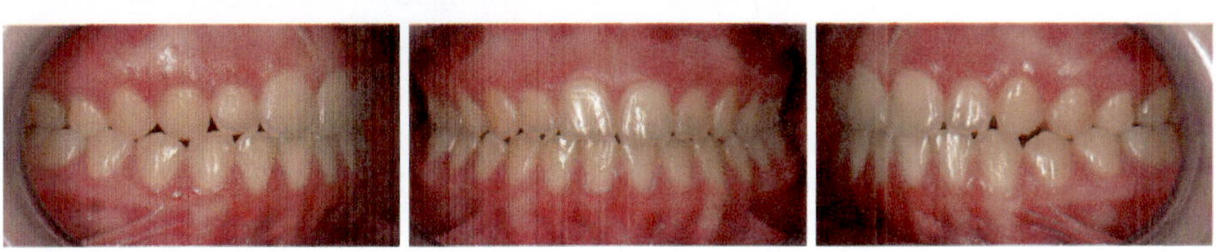

Fig. 10.35 Photos at 18 months post treatment

Treatment Results—Discussion

Unfortunately, this case has several limitations, one most important of which is the impossibility of general anesthesia for surgical treatment. RPE and resolving cross-bite increases bite opening. Therefore, the main objective was intrusion and correction of secondary swallow disorder.

Habit Correction

Habit correction is fundamental to orthodontic therapy success. There cannot be any swallow disorder or malocclusion related phonetic problem at the end of treatment. Tongue function and tongue posture must be corrected, may it depend on OSAS or thumb sucking just to name some causes.

Children who have undergone surgical treatment for adenoids and/or tonsils and have had a story of mouth breathing, will sometime continue to use their mouth to breathe as a habit. The use of tape to keep the mouth closed during day and night may be useful for treating a mouth breathing habit. Today, you can buy specific tape to do this that is indicated for snoring too. Most orthodontic patients should be evaluated by an ENT specialist before undergoing treatment. Swallow disorders may accompany mouth breathing. For this reason, it is important to evaluate deglutition with SCAN 3+ EMG of the sub-mandibular and perioral musculature. Interceptive therapy with Froggymouth® [37], a tongue education device, can be particularly useful. Other myotherapy exercises can help secondary tongue dysfunction when young patients are slow in recovering a correct deglutition spontaneously after orthodontic treatment.

Myofunctional therapy has gained some momentum in the recent years. Undoubtedly, the benefits are well described in literature and progress in the techniques continues. Unfortunately, collaboration is usually scarce and highly specialized centers are far from rural areas. Not all patients who have the need for such therapies benefit from it.

Thumb sucking, nail biting, and other conscious habits must be eliminated during orthodontic treatment, because they can jeopardize results in all aspects, functional and aesthetic. At times it can be requested that instrument playing be suspended when it compromises dental occlusion and or TMJ function. Parafunctional habits are mostly conscious and therefore their correction is linked to will. Unconscious habits are involuntary and may be a residue of a functional adaptation to primary needs. Treatment of these habits should be carried out creating a "one only" path treatment which recreates a *correct* habit. As an example, the use of tape to keep mouth closed during nighttime to restore nasal function after surgery. The use metal spikes to correct erroneous tongue posture for a resolved oral habit. The spikes also act as a daytime feedback mechanism which allows consciousness of erroneous tongue position.

Retention

It is important to note that there is ongoing research and discussion within the orthodontic community regarding the duration and type of retention required after orthodontic treatment. While some orthodontists may use fixed retainers to avoid any potential complaints during the post-treatment phase, it is important to view retention as a recovery period for the function and occlusion of the teeth.

Even though fixed therapy may create a stable occlusion and the patient may swallow in Inter-Cuspal Position (ICP), the majority of tooth contacts will form in the coming months. Therefore, the retention phase should leave the occlusal contacts free to allow for these natural adjustments to occur.

Recent advancements in technology, such as surface electromyography (s-EMG), have increased our understanding of the muscular reaction to occlusal changes. While there may be a general improvement in muscle EMG output after treatment, changes in muscle function can continue for over a year after treatment. When it comes to the use of fixed lower 3–3 retention, it is important to consider the neuromuscular effects. It may be wise to wait for the majority of mandibular growth before applying the fixed 3–3 retention, as it reduces the compensation that lower incisors can do by lingual tipping in case of mandibular post-treatment growth. This can result in an increase in condylar distal positioning. For this reason, it may be advisable to favor this retention method for female patients rather than male patients.

Functional appliances can be an effective form of retention, and the Frankel appliance is a well-accepted option. Depending on the skeletal discrepancy of the orthodontic case, this functional appliance can act as an active retention method, promoting lip competence and tone while also controlling the vertical freeway space.

Positioners, both preformed and with a setup, are commonly used as a retention method. However, due to potential neuromuscular stresses, it is use should not exceed 45 days. This allows for potential benefits of the device while minimizing any negative effects on the patient's neuromuscular system. When used after fixed appliance therapy, positioners can stimulate muscle contraction and activation, promoting improved muscular function after treatment. Typically, the positioner is worn passively during nighttime and for a maximum of 4 h during the day. During this daytime application, the patient is instructed to clench on the positioner.

Removable Hawley appliances and their variations are a suitable retention option because they allow for occlusal contacts, which is important for maintaining proper function and occlusion. These appliances can be an ideal option to use following the positioner phase of retention. Hawley appliances are custom made and designed to fit comfortably in the patient's mouth. They are typically made of acrylic and have a metal wire that holds the appliance in place. The appliance can be easily removed for cleaning and oral hygiene purposes. Hawley appliances can be customized to meet the individual needs of the patient, such as incorporating additional wire components. These variations can further aid in retaining proper occlusion and function after orthodontic treatment.

References

1. Ochoa BK, Nanda RS. Comparison of maxillary and mandibular growth. Am J Orthod Dentofac Orthop. 2004;125(2):148–59.
2. Litton SF, et al. A genetic study of class III malocclusion. Am J Orthod. 1970;58(6):565–77.

3. Cruz CV, et al. Genetic polymorphisms underlying the skeletal class III phenotype. Am J Orthod Dentofac Orthop. 2017;151(4):700–7.
4. Bui CH. Phenotypic characterization of skeletal class III: establishing the basis for genetic analysis. Am J Orthod Dentofac Orthop. 2006;129(5):711.
5. Smith BH. Development and evolution of the helicoidal plane of dental occlusion. Am J Phys Anthropol. 1986;69(1):21–35.
6. Spears IR, Macho GA. The helicoidal occlusal plane—a functional and biomechanical appraisal of molars. In: Proceedings of the 10th International Symposium on Dental Morphology, at Berlin; 1995. p. 391–7.
7. Benson CW. Spherical occlusion: a logical deduction**read before the section on full denture prosthesis at the seventy-sixth annual session of the American Dental Association, St. Paul, Minn., Aug. 8, 1934. J Am Dent Assoc (1922). 1935;22(3):456–67.
8. Silvestrini PB. Definizione di un piano occlusale curvo individuale sulla base di misure scheletriche funzionali. Parodontologia e Stomatologia Nuova. 1991:2.
9. Rabie AB, She TT, Hagg U. Functional appliance therapy accelerates and enhances condylar growth. Am J Orthod Dentofac Orthop. 2003;123(1):40–8.
10. Proffit WR, Fields H, Larson B, Sarver DM. Contemporary orthodontics. 6th ed. Elsevier; 2018. Hardback ISBN: 9780323543873. eBook ISBN: 9780323543880.
11. Riolo ML. An Atlas of craniofacial growth: cephalometric standards from the University school growth study, the University of Michigan. Craniofacial growth series. Monograph no. 2. 1974, Ann Arbor: Center for Human Growth and Development, University of Michigan. 379 p.
12. Li J-L, Kau C, Wang M. Changes of occlusal plane inclination after orthodontic treatment in different dentoskeletal frames. Prog Orthod. 2014;15(1):41.
13. Tanaka EM, Sato S. Longitudinal alteration of the occlusal plane and development of different dentoskeletal frames during growth. Am J Orthod Dentofac Orthop. 2008;134(5):602 e1-11. discussion 602-3
14. Fushima K, et al. Significance of the cant of the posterior occlusal plane in class II division 1 malocclusions. Eur J Orthod. 1996;18(1):27–40.
15. Greven M, Cazacu I, Piehslinger E. Correlation of occlusal-plane-inclination with functional condylar displacement in different skeletal classes. Int J Dent Oral Health. 2020:6.
16. Krisjane Z, et al. The prevalence of TMJ osteoarthritis in asymptomatic patients with dentofacial deformities: a cone-beam CT study. Int J Oral Maxillofac Surg. 2012;41(6):690–5.
17. Owen AH 3rd. Orthodontic/orthopedic treatment of craniomandibular pain dysfunction. Part 4: unilateral and bilateral crossbite. Cranio. 1985;3(2):145–63.
18. Fushima K, Inui M, Sato S. Dental asymmetry in temporomandibular disorders. J Oral Rehabil. 1999;26(9):752–6.
19. Miller VJ, et al. The effect of parafunction on condylar asymmetry in patients with temporomandibular disorders. J Oral Rehabil. 1998;25(9):721–4.
20. Zhang Y, et al. Three-dimensional condylar positions and forms associated with different anteroposterior skeletal patterns and facial asymmetry in Chinese adolescents. Acta Odontol Scand. 2013;71(5):1174–80.
21. Chia MSY, Naini FB, Gill DS. The aetiology, diagnosis and management of mandibular asymmetry. Orthodontic Update. 2008;1(2):44–52.
22. Ringold S, Cron RQ. The temporomandibular joint in juvenile idiopathic arthritis: frequently used and frequently arthritic. Pediatr Rheumatol Online J. 2009;7:11.
23. Stoustrup P, et al. Orthopaedic splint treatment can reduce mandibular asymmetry caused by unilateral temporomandibular involvement in juvenile idiopathic arthritis. Eur J Orthod. 2013;35(2):191–8.
24. Zimmer B, Nischwitz D. Therapeutic changes in the occlusal plane inclination using intermaxillary elastics. J Orofac Orthop. 2012;73(5):377–86.
25. Djeu G, Hayes C, Zawaideh S. Correlation between mandibular central incisor proclination and gingival recession during fixed appliance therapy. Angle Orthod. 2002;72(3):238–45.
26. Allais D, Melsen B. Does labial movement of lower incisors influence the level of the gingival margin? A case-control study of adult orthodontic patients. Eur J Orthod. 2003;25(4):343–52.

27. Melgaco CA, et al. Immediate changes in condylar position after rapid maxillary expansion. Am J Orthod Dentofac Orthop. 2014;145(6):771–9.
28. Teuscher U. A growth-related concept for skeletal class II treatment. Am J Orthod. 1978;74(3):258–75.
29. Carlsson GE, Ingervall B, Kocak G. Effect of increasing vertical dimension on the masticatory system in subjects with natural teeth. J Prosthet Dent. 1979;41(3):284–9.
30. Manns A, Miralles R, Cumsille F. Influence of vertical dimension on masseter muscle electromyographic activity in patients with mandibular dysfunction. J Prosthet Dent. 1985;53(2):243–7.
31. Grünheid T, et al. The adaptive response of jaw muscles to varying functional demands. Eur J Orthod. 2009;31(6):596–612.
32. Endo T, et al. Cephalometric evaluation of anterior open-bite nonextraction treatment, using multiloop edgewise archwire therapy. Odontology. 2006;94(1):51–8.
33. Cinsar A, Alagha AR, Akyalçin S. Skeletal open bite correction with rapid molar intruder appliance in growing individuals. Angle Orthod. 2007;77(4):632–9.
34. Mostafa O, El-Beialy A, Bushnak M. Root resorption associated with rapid molar intruder (RMI). IOSR J Dent Med Sci. 2017;16:95–9.
35. Carano A, Siciliani G, Bowman SJ. Treatment of skeletal open bite with a device for rapid molar intrusion: a preliminary report. Angle Orthod. 2005;75(5):736–46.
36. Elsayed E, Abdel Aziz F, Shafik M. Prediction of root resorption and periodontal tissue changes associated with rapid molar intruder. Egypt Orthod J. 2012;2012(42):33–49.
37. Patrick F. The role of biochemistry and neurophysiology in the re-education of deglutition. Med Clin Arch. 2017;1(1):3–3. https://doi.org/10.15761/MCA.1000106.

Head and Body Posture in Relation to Mandibular Position 11

In discussing Neuromuscular Orthodontics, I believe it is important to include a chapter regarding the relationship of the stomatognathic system to body posture. In 1990, I completed a specialty thesis exploring the connection between body posture, dental occlusion, and Applied Kinesiology. This topic has continued to fascinate me, particularly the potential links between dental occlusion and head and body posture. However, for the purposes of this discussion, I will focus on the most significant findings from my years of research and personal experience, which have helped to inform my current perspective on this complex issue.

In the field of orthodontics, there has been a growing interest in the relationship between dental occlusion and body posture. As a specialist in this field, I have explored these connections in depth, particularly regarding the impact of mandibular position on head and body posture. However, I believe it is crucial to approach this subject with caution, given the amount of pseudo-science that has infiltrated this matter in recent years.

One aspect of this issue that I find concerning is the use of postural analysis as a tool for convincing patients that orthodontic therapy is necessary to treat and prevent postural problems. While there are certainly professionals who genuinely believe that occlusion can affect body posture and have developed treatment protocols accordingly, I do not use body posture as a promotional tool or criticize those who do. Instead, I prefer to focus on the most significant findings from my years of research and experience, which have informed my current perspective on this complex issue.

As with many developing specialties, there are often competing views and a lack of consensus on certain topics. Therefore, I approach the postural problem from a more holistic perspective, one that prioritizes scientific analysis over unsubstantiated claims. While I recognize that this subject is beyond the scope of this book, I would like to briefly share my position. Ultimately, I believe that a cautious and informed approach is necessary when considering the impact of dental occlusion on body posture, and we must remain vigilant in distinguishing legitimate research from pseudo-science.

F. Savastano, *Neuromuscular Orthodontics*,
https://doi.org/10.1007/978-3-031-41295-0_11

Concept 1

In reviewing scientific journal articles on the topic of head posture and the stomatognathic system, it becomes clear that the majority of serious publications focus on the relationship between head posture and facial morphology, rather than dental occlusion. While there is certainly some evidence to suggest that dental occlusion can affect head posture, the research in this area is not yet robust enough to draw definitive conclusions. Therefore, it is important to approach the topic with a critical eye and consider all available evidence [1–7]. It is important to note that the starting point for measuring cranio-cervical posture is *natural head posture*. This means that while the potential impact of dental occlusion on head posture should not be dismissed outright, it is necessary to approach the topic with caution and rely on rigorous scientific research to determine the extent of this relationship [8–10] (Fig. 11.1).

Attempting to link dental occlusion to head and body posture is a significant mistake. It is widely known that head extension is determined by skeletal vertical morphology, rather than Angle dental classification. For example, reduced and insufficient physiological freeway space may be related to head extension, and this has nothing to do with dental occlusion. Head extension is a normal reaction to the lack of freeway space. By extending the head position during habitual posture, a functional freeway space is created that is needed to reduce proprioception from

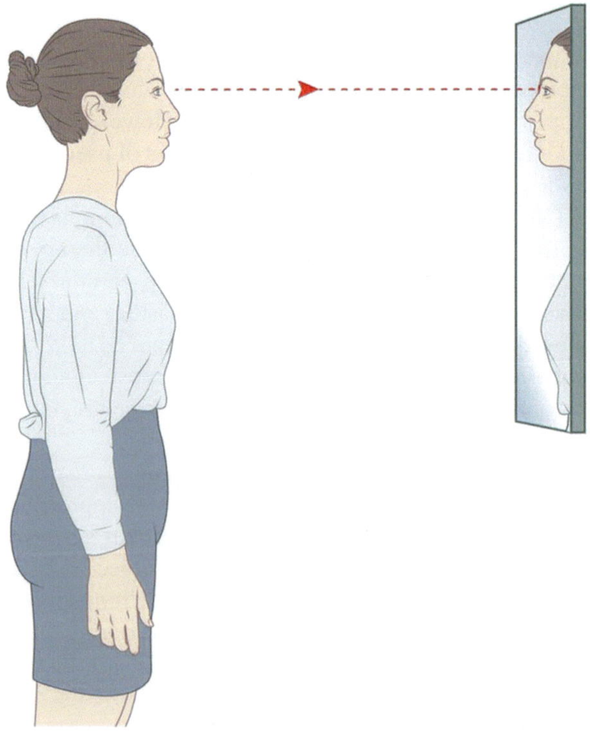

Fig. 11.1 Created-by-Rogier-Trompert-Medical--Art, for Springer Nature

tooth contact. The central nervous system (CNS) does not require continuous proprioceptive information from the oral cavity to function ergonomically. Therefore, this is a natural ergonomic response.

Moreover, it is possible that a deep bite may be linked to forward head posture, which would suggest a direct connection between head posture and excess freeway space. If you have treated deep bite cases through functional orthodontic treatment, which involves extrusion and re-posturing the mandible to reduce excess freeway space, you may have noticed a dramatic correction of forward head posture. This correction is visible in lateral profile photos, as patients become more upright, and there may also be an anatomical increase in posterior airflow [11] (Fig. 11.2). Furthermore, research indicates that airway pathologies can affect cranio-cervical posture and cranio-facial morphology. Therefore, it is important to consider these factors when treating patients with malocclusion [7, 12–15].

Although there is some evidence of how changes in dental occlusion do influence head posture and cervical posture, these remain experimental models that do not refer specifically to any dental class occlusion but rather to mandibular position and consequent occlusal alteration [16, 17].

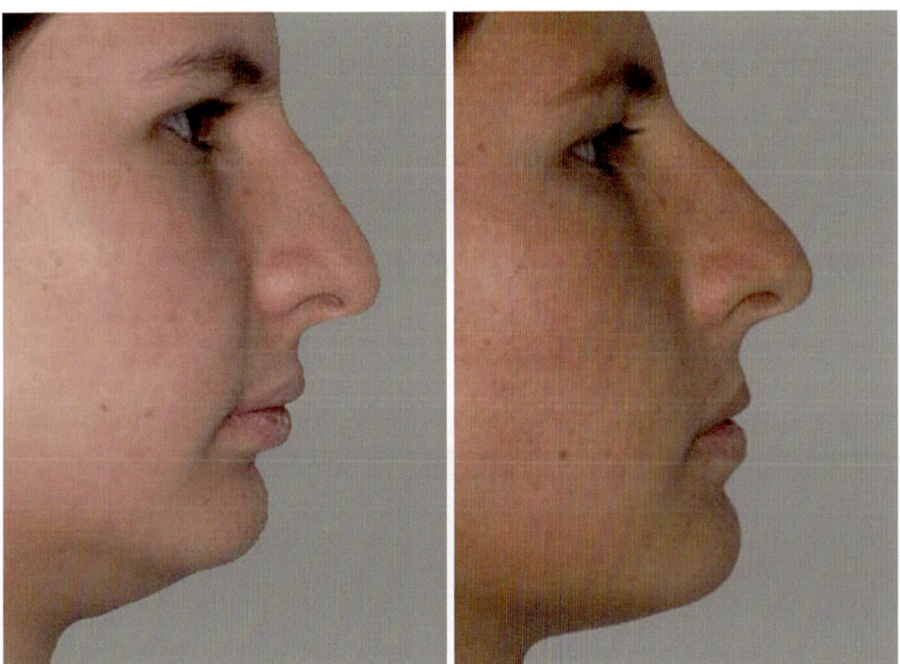

Fig. 11.2 Profile photos before and after neuromuscular treatment of Class II positional occlusion. Natural head posture. From ***Savastano*** *F (2014) Correction of a Class II Occlusion in an Adult. J Dent Oral Disord Ther 2(4): 1-10. DOI:* https://doi.org/10.15226/jdodt.2014.00128

Concept 2

The human body's posture is not a fixed state but a constantly evolving one. Every individual has a unique set of postural habits, which can change with time and external factors. Pain, stress, and mood can significantly impact an individual's posture and result in protective body postures [18]. These changes aim to reduce pain and discomfort and may not always indicate the root cause of the problem. The variability of postural evaluations is vast and diverse, making it challenging to provide a discriminatory comment on what can be considered the norm.

It is important to note that other proprioceptive signals can influence head and body posture by eliciting specific responses from the central nervous system (CNS). For instance, vision and its related pathologies, such as torticollis ocularis, can significantly impact posture. Additionally, several patients who experience chronic incorrect head posture may eventually experience changes in their dental occlusion due to facial asymmetry. There are also variable degrees of congenital muscular torticollis with regard to the SCM. The shortened SCM determines a typical head position tilted toward and rotated away from the affected side. Being able to intercept correctly these problems reduces greatly the probability of severe facial asymmetry [19].

Some specific factors can impact head and body posture and their relationship with dental occlusion. While skeletal vertical morphology plays a significant role in head extension, other variables such as vision-related pathologies and facial asymmetry can be related to body posture. Understanding the complex interplay between these factors is crucial for developing effective treatment plans that address patients' unique needs [20]. When mandibular ***posture*** is altered, compensation mechanisms come into play. It is important to make every effort to screen for *ocular torticollis* since the incidence in the general population is quite high [19, 21, 22]. This condition involves a rotation or tilt of the head, causing the chin to point toward one shoulder and the head to twist to the opposite side. It can lead to asymmetric head and body posture, affecting the temporomandibular joint, and altering the occlusion. By carefully evaluating patients for torticollis, healthcare professionals can take proactive steps to prevent long-term negative consequences. Early ophthalmic correction can help patients avoid developing compensation mechanisms that can lead to significant dental and musculoskeletal problems. Torticollis can be congenital (muscular and sternocleidomastoid) affecting 0.4% of newborn, or acquired to neurological problems or related to dystonia. Since our interest from an occlusal perspective focuses on the chronic forms, ENT and ophthalmic surveillance are necessary. So screening for torticollis regularly should be included in all initial orthodontic evaluations to prevent compensation mechanisms from arising [19, 23].

Facial asymmetry occurs when the shorter condyle is accompanied by a tilting of the head on the same side and lifting of the shoulder. Interestingly, dental crossbites appear to be more commonly observed in individuals with postural and idiopathic scoliosis [24, 25]. Dental crossbites could be related to respiratory problems as well and develop asymmetric condyles [26]. While we could provide several additional examples, it is important to recognize that changes in facial morphology and freeway space are not the sole indicators of an individual's body posture. The relationship between these various factors can often be complex and multifaceted, which can make it challenging to fully understand and accurately diagnose postural issues [27].

Concept 3

Do I believe that body posture should be characterized by symmetry and that achieving it should be a primary goal in our treatment? Absolutely not. While symmetry may improve a patient's comfort and aspect, it should not be our primary objective unless we are dealing with a *severe* postural problem. In fact, I do not view symmetry as an absolute characteristic of the human body. For instance, consider the positioning of internal organs or the fact that even functions like respiration are not perfectly symmetrical.

In my opinion, looking for symmetry in growing children is nonsense as growth occurs with hidden schemes that are not visible to the naked eye and are almost impossible to interpret with postural analysis systems. There is no true symmetry during growth just as there is no symmetry during the eruption of permanent teeth. Furthermore, our movements are naturally right or left-handed, which means that they cannot be the result or the cause of anatomic symmetry. The continuous search for symmetry in our patients has become a new disease among many practitioners. While symmetry may be desirable in certain cases, it should not be viewed as the sole indicator of proper posture or a primary goal of treatment. Treatments with the sole objective of searching for symmetry *may interfere with the physiological compensation mechanisms created by body function.*

Concept 4

There is a clear link between occlusion, dental contacts, and body posture, although the precise nature of this relationship is still uncertain. Although computerized postural analysis platforms can provide a wealth of data, testing posture before and after modifying tooth contact or adjusting the dental arch relationship through orthotics or build-ups can produce inconsistent results. Despite the high sensitivity of these computerized systems, their lack of specificity is why experts in this field tend to disagree on many aspects of this relationship.

Postural computerized platforms are often utilized for rehabilitation purposes and for diagnosing severe neurological issues. However, when these platforms are used to study body posture in relation to occlusion, the results are often contradictory. This has led the scientific community to be divided between those who envision a future where postural treatment can be achieved through dental procedures and those who have become more skeptical after an initial period of passionate interest [3, 16, 28–41]. There are, however, many serious practitioners who understand and utilize scientific data on head and body posture to enhance treatment outcomes and quality. Modern neuromuscular gnathology, which focuses on temporomandibular disorders (TMD) from a holistic perspective, is a prime example of this approach. This field employs precise diagnostic criteria *based on strong scientific foundations*, and treatments are administered by highly qualified specialists who understand the importance of a multidisciplinary approach to treating the individual as a whole. In this approach, treatment is not limited to the symptoms of TMD but extends to its underlying causes, which can include a variety of factors related to head and body posture. By taking a holistic approach, specialists can ensure that they address all contributing factors to TMD, which results in a more effective treatment outcome. The success of this approach is dependent on teamwork and collaboration between different specialists, including dentists, orthopedists, physiotherapists, psychologists, and sleep specialists. By working together, they can develop a comprehensive treatment plan that addresses all aspects of the patient's health and well-being.

Concept 5

Muscle testing is a technique used by some practitioners to evaluate the suitability of a new mandibular position and occlusion. While it is an intriguing method, its effectiveness is currently supported by limited scientific evidence. However, muscle testing may still have value in determining the physiological limits of mandibular re-posturing and could be a useful tool for assessing the range of occlusal tolerance by the neuromuscular system. One advantage of muscle testing is its ability to quickly identify an acceptable new mandibular position. *This methodology is limited by the individual's physiological tolerance, which can be significantly wider than specific occlusal dental and orthodontic requests.* Therefore, it is important to approach muscle testing with caution and consider its limitations [42].

Finally, there are several points that should be outlined that according to the author should be implemented in a clinical diagnostic protocol.

1. Forward or extended head posture. The evaluation should be done with cephalometrics on lateral and PA cephalograms X-rays in *natural head posture*, in centric occlusion or habitual RP [8, 43–48]. Further studies can be done while lateral head cephalograms are taken with occlusal recordings in PRP.
2. Detecting clinically relevant head tipping and rotation to one side. Photography is useful only when it is *standardized and repeatable*. This should include a wider focus on position of head-jaw-shoulder for diagnosing "side-bending" in centric occlusion or in HRP [49–52].
3. Detecting or suspecting vision problems is of utmost importance in our profession. Several issues related to the coordination of eye movements with head posture are relevant because continuously altered head posture can modify occlusion and condylar development. Therefore, it is essential to identify any visual problems that may contribute to or exacerbate these issues. It is worth noting that torticollis can have causes beyond vision problems. Neurological or

hypertonic peripheral issues affecting the trapezius or sternocleidomastoid muscles can also lead to this condition. It is very important to conduct a thorough evaluation of the patient's overall health and well-being to identify any underlying issues that may be contributing to the problem. By taking a comprehensive approach, we can ensure that we provide the best possible treatment outcomes for our patients [19, 20, 49, 53–56].

4. It is crucial to always scan for general health problems that may affect orthodontic and gnathology diagnosis. Many health issues can have an impact on the development and alignment of the teeth and jaw, as well as overall body posture. Therefore, it is important to take a holistic approach when evaluating patients and consider any underlying health conditions that may be contributing to their orthodontic or gnathological issues. For example, patients with respiratory problems may have altered breathing patterns that can affect their overall posture and jaw development. Additionally, patients with chronic pain or autoimmune disorders may experience symptoms that affect their oral health and require a unique treatment approach. By thoroughly evaluating the patient's overall health and taking into account any underlying conditions or concerns, we can provide a more comprehensive diagnosis and treatment plan. This approach can lead to improved treatment outcomes and overall patient satisfaction.
5. Tooth loss can significantly impact masticatory function and contribute to facial asymmetry, as it plays a key role in maintaining a stable occlusion [57–59]. In ICP, the condyle should be viewed as an active anatomical feature that adapts to occlusion.

An important takeaway from this chapter is that there are various factors that can complicate our daily work. As our diagnostic capabilities continue to expand with experience and advanced technology, it becomes clear that a multidisciplinary approach is necessary for our patients. This means that we need to learn how to work as a team and collaborate with other professionals. Incorporating posture, neurology, and vision into our occlusal analysis only adds to the complexity of the stomatognathic system. However, it is important to note that any complication that can arise from excessive computerized data increases the likelihood of bias and errors. It is very important to conduct diagnosis and treatment protocols only when there is a strong scientific base support. As the future of our profession continues to evolve, it is imperative that we keep up with the latest developments and adapt to ensure the best possible outcomes for our patients.

References

1. Leitao P, Nanda RS. Relationship of natural head position to craniofacial morphology. Am J Orthod Dentofac Orthop. 2000;117(4):406–17.
2. Solow B, Tallgren A. Head posture and craniofacial morphology. Am J Phys Anthropol. 1976;44(3):417–35.
3. Sakaguchi K, et al. Examination of the relationship between mandibular position and body posture. Cranio. 2007;25(4):237–49.

4. Lin X, Edwards SP. Changes in natural head position in response to mandibular advancement. Br J Oral Maxillofac Surg. 2017;55(5):471–5.
5. Sandikçioğlu M, Skov S, Solow B. Atlas morphology in relation to craniofacial morphology and head posture. Eur J Orthod. 1994;16(2):96–103.
6. Hellsing E, et al. The relationship between craniofacial morphology, head posture and spinal curvature in 8, 11 and 15-year-old children. Eur J Orthod. 1987;9(1):254–64.
7. Solow B, Siersbæk-Nielsen S, Greve E. Airway adequacy, head posture, and craniofacial morphology. Am J Orthod. 1984;86(3):214–23.
8. Showfety KJ, Vig PS, Matteson S. A simple method for taking natural-head-position cephalograms. Am J Orthod. 1983;83(6):495–500.
9. Vig PS, Rink JF, Showfety KJ. Adaptation of head posture in response to relocating the center of mass: a pilot study. Am J Orthod. 1983;83(2):138–42.
10. Vig PS, Showfety KJ, Phillips C. Experimental manipulation of head posture. 1980;77(3):258–68.
11. Savastano F. Correction of a Class II occlusion in an adult. J Dent Oral Disord Ther. 2014;4:2.
12. Wong ML, et al. Craniofacial morphology, head posture, and nasal respiratory resistance in obstructive sleep apnoea: an inter-ethnic comparison. Eur J Orthod. 2005;27(1):91–7.
13. Muto T, et al. Relationship between the pharyngeal airway space and craniofacial morphology, taking into account head posture. Int J Oral Maxillofac Surg. 2006;35(2):132–6.
14. Wenzel A, Höjensgaard E, Henriksen JM. Craniofacial morphology and head posture in children with asthma and perennial rhinitis. Eur J Orthod. 1985;7(2):83–92.
15. Zepa I, et al. Associations between thoracic kyphosis, head posture, and craniofacial morphology in young adults. Acta Odontol Scand. 2000;58(6):237–42.
16. Motoyoshi M, et al. Biomechanical influences of head posture on occlusion: an experimental study using finite element analysis. Eur J Orthod. 2002;24(4):319–26.
17. Shimazaki T, et al. The effect of occlusal alteration and masticatory imbalance on the cervical spine. Eur J Orthod. 2003;25(5):457–63.
18. Lund JP, et al. The pain-adaptation model: a discussion of the relationship between chronic musculoskeletal pain and motor activity. Can J Physiol Pharmacol. 1991;69(5):683–94.
19. Akbari MR, et al. Ocular abnormal head posture: a literature review. J Curr Ophthalmol. 2021;33(4):379–87.
20. Akbari MR, et al. Facial asymmetry in ocular torticollis. J Curr Ophthalmol. 2015;27(1-2):4–11.
21. Erkan Turan K, et al. The frequency and causes of abnormal head position based on an ophthalmology clinic's findings: is it overlooked? Eur J Ophthalmol. 2017;27(4):491–4.
22. Nucci P, et al. A multi-disciplinary study of the ocular, orthopedic, and neurologic causes of abnormal head postures in children. Am J Ophthalmol. 2005;140(1):65–8.
23. Yoon JA, et al. Development of a questionnaire to identify ocular torticollis. Eur J Pediatr. 2021;180(2):561–7.
24. Saccucci M, et al. Scoliosis and dental occlusion: a review of the literature. Scoliosis. 2011;6(1):15.
25. Ben-Bassat Y, et al. Occlusal patterns in patients with idiopathic scoliosis. Am J Orthod Dentofac Orthop. 2006;130(5):629–33.
26. Kilic N, Kiki A, Oktay H. Condylar asymmetry in unilateral posterior crossbite patients. Am J Orthod Dentofac Orthop. 2008;133(3):382–7.
27. Korbmacher H, et al. Correlations between dentition anomalies and diseases of the of the postural and movement apparatus—a literature review. J Orofac Orthop. 2004;65(3):190–203.
28. Fernández Molina A, Burgueño-Torres L, Diéguez-Pérez M. Influence of the mandibular position on various postural anatomical segments. Cranio. 2021:1–9.
29. Michelotti A, et al. Dental occlusion and posture: an overview. Prog Orthod. 2011;12(1):53–8.
30. Tardieu C, et al. Dental occlusion and postural control in adults. Neurosci Lett. 2009;450(2):221–4.
31. Michelotti A, et al. Postural stability and unilateral posterior crossbite: is there a relationship? Neurosci Lett. 2006;392(1):140–4.

32. Marchena-Rodríguez A, et al. Relationship between foot posture and dental malocclusions in children aged 6 to 9 years: a cross-sectional study. Medicine. 2018;97(19):e0701.
33. Baldini A, et al. Evaluation of the correlation between dental occlusion and posture using a force platform. Clinics (Sao Paulo, Brazil). 2013;68(1):45–9.
34. Iacob SM, et al. Plantar pressure variations induced by experimental malocclusion—a pilot case series study. Healthcare. 2021;9(5):599.
35. Baldini A, et al. Influence of vision and dental occlusion on body posture in pilots. Aviat Space Environ Med. 2013;84(8):823–7.
36. El Zoghbi A, et al. Effect of occlusal splints on posture balance in patients with temporomandibular joint disorder: a prospective study. J Contemp Dent Pract. 2021;22(6):615–9.
37. Amaricai E, et al. Do different dental conditions influence the static plantar pressure and stabilometry in young adults? PLoS One. 2020;15(2):e0228816.
38. Julià-Sánchez S, et al. The influence of dental occlusion on dynamic balance and muscular tone. Front Physiol. 2020;10:1626.
39. Cabrera-Domínguez ME, et al. Dental malocclusion and its relation to the podal system. Front Pediatr. 2021;9:563.
40. Ohlendorf D, et al. The impact of a total hip replacement on jaw position, upper body posture and body sway. Cranio. 2015;33(2):107–14.
41. Munhoz WC, Hsing WT. The inconclusiveness of research on functional pathologies of the temporomandibular system and body posture: paths followed, paths ahead: a critical review. Cranio. 2019:1–12.
42. Melis M, Di Giosia M. Applied kinesiology and dentistry—a narrative review. Cranio. 2022;40(6):509–16.
43. Peng L, Cooke MS. Fifteen-year reproducibility of natural head posture: a longitudinal study. Am J Orthod Dentofacial Orthop. 1999;116(1):82–5.
44. Cooke MS, Wei SH. A summary five-factor cephalometric analysis based on natural head posture and the true horizontal. Am J Orthod Dentofac Orthop. 1988;93(3):213–23.
45. Moorrees CFA, Kean MR. Natural head position, a basic consideration in the interpretation of cephalometric radiographs. Am J Phys Anthropol. 1958;16:213–34.
46. *Neuromuscular dental diagnosis and treatment: Robert R. Jankelson Ishiyaku EuroAmerica, St. Louis: 1990. 687 pages, 1132 illustrations.* American journal of orthodontics and dentofacial orthopedics : official publication of the American Association of Orthodontists, its constituent societies, and the American Board of Orthodontics, 1991. **99**(3): p. 283–284.
47. Mahmoud NF, et al. The relationship between forward head posture and neck pain: a systematic review and meta-analysis. Curr Rev Musculoskelet Med. 2019;12(4):562–77.
48. Hooda S, Souza MD. Evaluation of facial asymmetry using digital photographs with computer aided analysis. J Indian Prosthodont Soc. 2012;12:8–15.
49. Silvestrini Biavati P. Trattamento semplificato in gnatologia: il metodo Global Occlusion. Milano: Edra; 2019.
50. Rahlin M, Sarmiento B. Reliability of still photography measuring habitual head deviation from midline in infants with congenital muscular torticollis. Pediatr Phys Ther. 2010;22:4.
51. Choi KY. Analysis of facial asymmetry. Arch Craniofac Surg. 2015;16(1):1–10.
52. Alhammadi MS, et al. Accuracy and reproducibility of facial measurements of digital photographs and wrapped cone beam computed tomography (CBCT) photographs. Diagnostics (Basel). 2021;11:5.
53. Rao R, Morton GV, Kushner BJ. Ocular torticollis and facial asymmetry. Binocul Vis Strabismus Q. 1999;14(1):27–32.
54. Stellwagen L, et al. Torticollis, facial asymmetry and plagiocephaly in normal newborns. Arch Dis Child. 2008;93(10):827–31.
55. Baratta VM, et al. A quantitative analysis of facial asymmetry in torticollis using 3-dimensional photogrammetry. Cleft Palate Craniofac J. 2022;59(1):40–6.
56. Kim HT, Kang JH, Yoo CI. Head tilt and facial asymmetry in congenital muscular torticollis. J Korean Orthop Assoc. 2003;38(3):217–22.

57. Çağlaroğlu M, Kilic N, Erdem A. Effects of early unilateral first molar extraction on skeletal asymmetry. Am J Orthod Dentofac Orthop. 2008;134(2):270–5.
58. Staudt CB, Kiliaridis S. Association between mandibular asymmetry and occlusal asymmetry in young adult males with class III malocclusion. Acta Odontol Scand. 2010;68(3):131–40.
59. Rodrigues VP, et al. Tooth loss and craniofacial factors associated with changes in mandibular condylar morphology. Cranio. 2019;37(5):310–6.

Clinical Cases 12

Case 12.1

Class I Occlusion with Reduced OJ and Increased Freeway Space [1]

(Please refer to DOI:10.5937/SEJODR4-15529 Corpus ID: 80123300 for 4 in-depth explanation)

Summary An 11-year-old Caucasian boy sought orthodontic treatment at the office for recurrent pain of the right TMJ, misaligned teeth, and irregular clicking noises (associated with the right TMJ) during mouth opening (Figures 12.1, 12.2 and 12.3) Intraoral, extraoral photos, and panoramic and lateral cephalograms. Figs. 12.4, 12.5, 12.6, 12.7, 12.8, 12.9, 12.10, 12.11, 12.12 and 12.13 Pre-treatment scans.

Pre-treatment	
Extraoral analysis (fig. 12.1)	
Facial profile	Concave
Facial height	Reduced
Occlusal plane	Slight right tipping
Facial symmetry	Symmetric
Lips	Thin, competent
Mandibular posture	Forward
Head posture	Forward
Intraoral analysis (fig. 12.1)	
Teeth	
Molar class	1
Canine class	1
Overjet	0
Overbite	3

F. Savastano, *Neuromuscular Orthodontics*,
https://doi.org/10.1007/978-3-031-41295-0_12

Oral hygiene	Good/fair
Rotations	
Crossbite	
Diastemas	
Crowding upper arch	
Agenesis	
Missing teeth	
Intraoral functional analysis	
Swallow	Tongue thrust
Tongue tie	No
Tongue posture	
Tongue thrust	Yes
Slurred speech	No
Neuromuscular diagnosis	
Freeway space	Increased
Skeletal class	III
Anterior wall	Yes
TMJ left	
TMJ right	Clicking during aperturew pain
Problem list • Resolve TMJ pain • Align teeth, possibly in Class I • Nickel allergy • Onychophagy	
Neuromuscular treatment objectives • Elimination of front wall • Mandibular freedom and SMM • Reduction of freeway space	

Introduction

The following case is a prime example of how to conduct orthodontic treatment and diagnosis in a neuromuscular manner. Due to space constraints, some scans are not included in this report. However, it is crucial for the reader to note that a strict scan protocol should be followed. This scan cascade should be viewed as a train track, which will develop a neuromuscular mindset. While the capabilities of bioelectric instrumentation can fulfill practitioners' highest demands, we will stick to the basics for now. The previous chapters have described the basic protocol, which must be followed without exception. One of the significant advantages of the software is the ability to repeat scans for each patient indefinitely, except for scan 4/5. This scan requires deconditioning prior to recording, which entails another 40-min TENS application. The one-shot-only scan 4/5 may require some experience, but it is usually easily accomplished after a few weeks of practice.

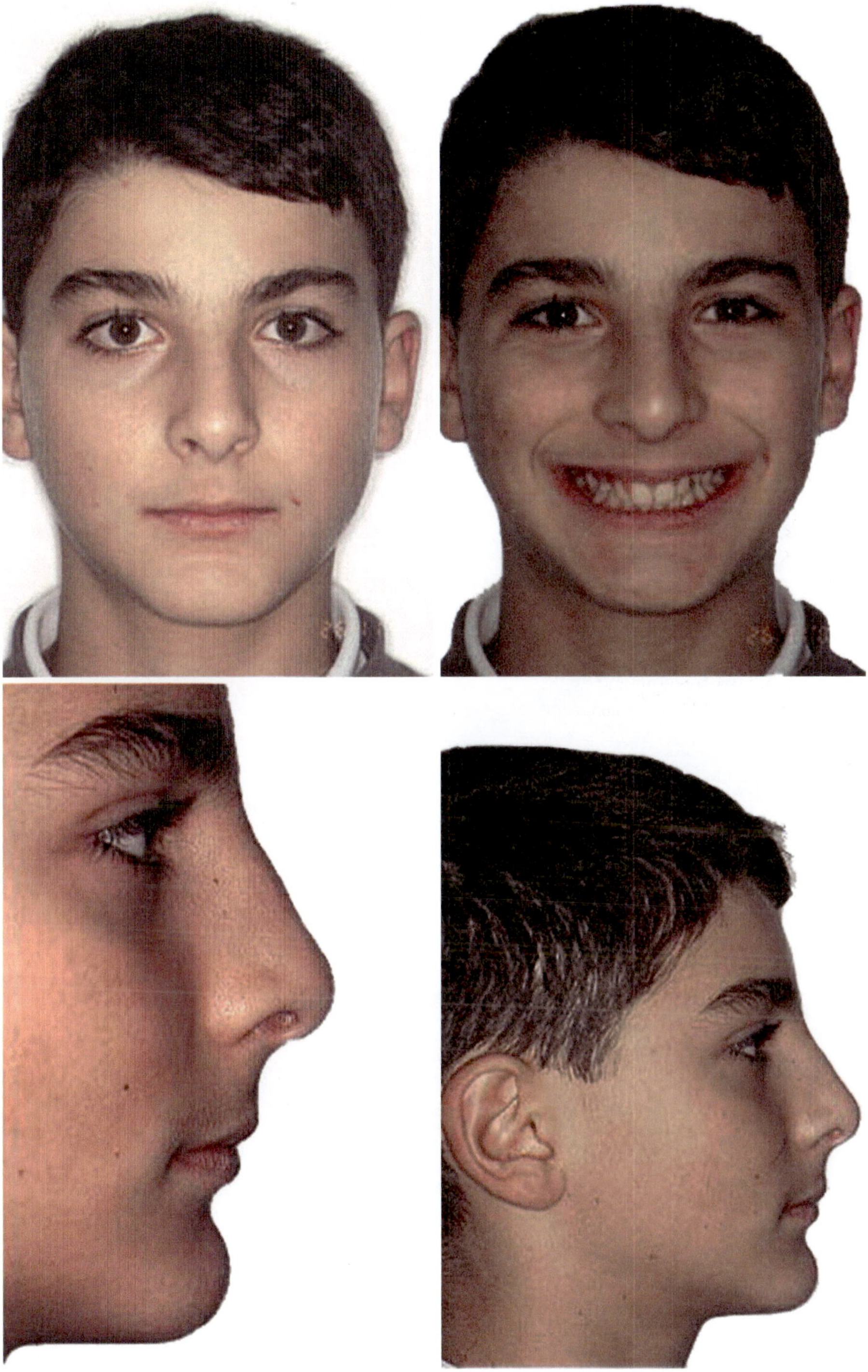

Fig. 12.1 Extraoral photographs showing the patient's concave profile and thin lips, intraoral showing class I relationship bilaterally

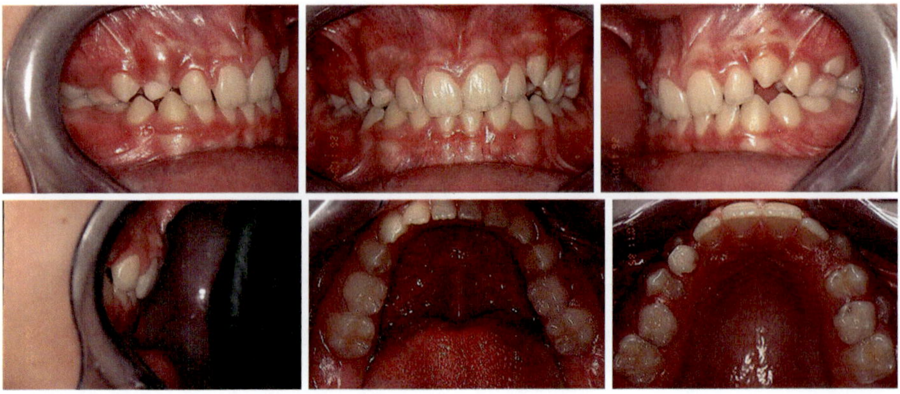

Fig. 12.1 (continued)

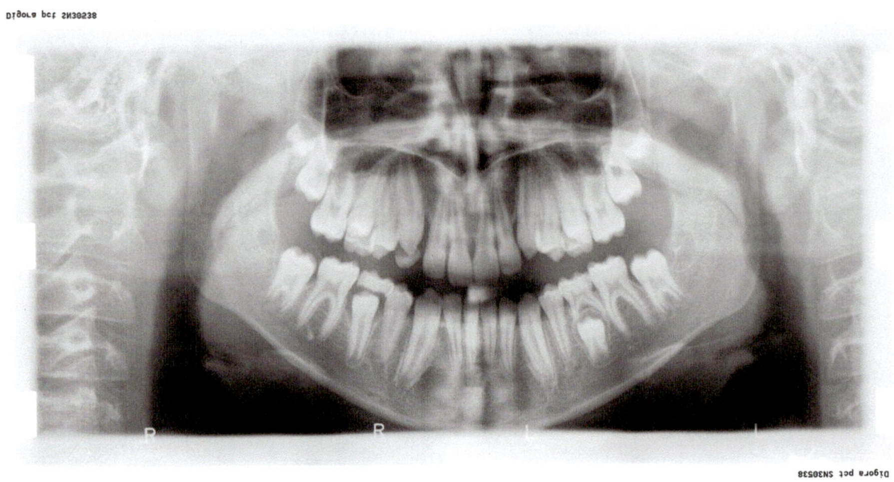

Fig. 12.2 Lateral Panoramic X-ray before treatment

Fig. 12.3 Lateral cephalogram before treatment

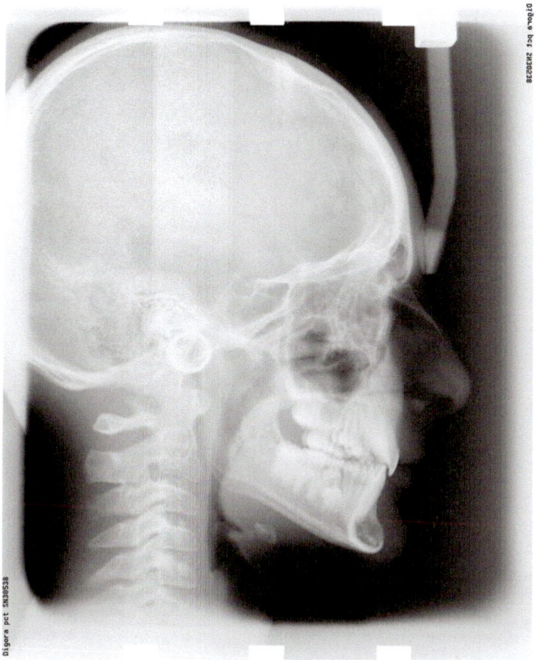

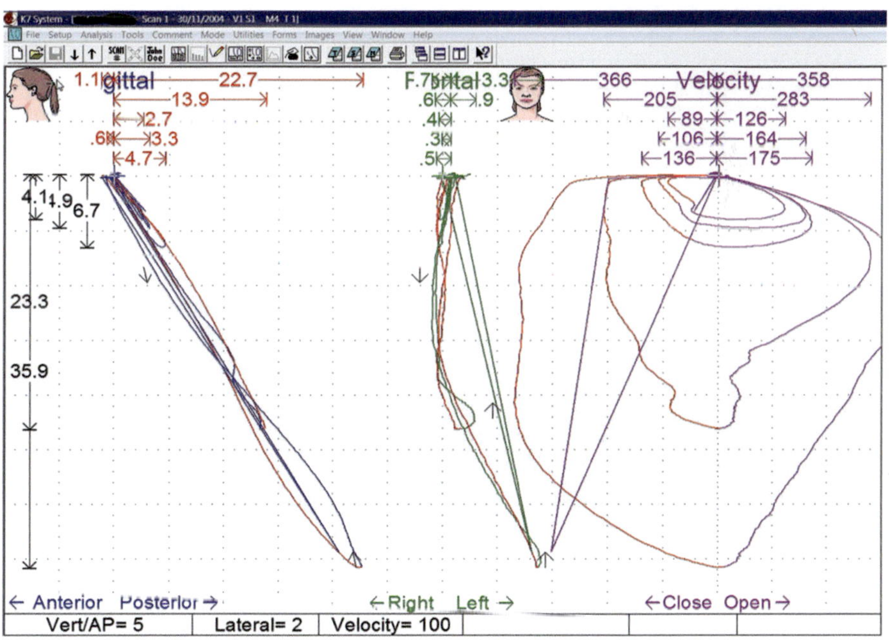

Fig. 12.4 Scan 1 (pre-treatment) shows that the degree of mouth opening was satisfactory (the total mouth aperture was approximately 40 mm), there was a slight lateral deviation to the left upon opening (1.8 mm), and the velocity at tooth contact was also satisfactory. AP: anterior-posterior; Vert: vertical

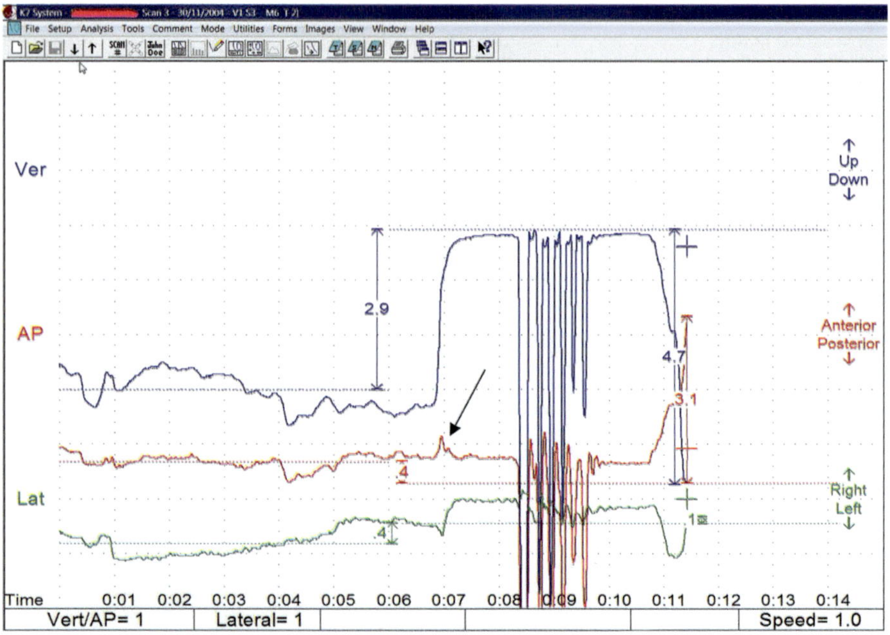

Fig. 12.5 Scan 3 (pre-treatment) shows the vertical, anterior-posterior, and lateral movements of the mandible in sweep mode. The patient was instructed to maintain the mandible in the rest position and then to close it to CO. There was a slight excess in freeway space (2.9 mm). When closing, there was no apparent anterior-posterior movement, a slight movement forward upon closure (which was immediately converted to a backward movement [black arrow]. AP: anterior-posterior; Lat: lateral; Ver: vertical

When neuromuscular practitioners describe and discuss clinical cases, they often have a tendency to dive straight into the analysis of scan 4/5, followed by a consideration of two other crucial factors: skeletal morphology and sEMG. Together, these elements create the foundation of a diagnostic neuromuscular framework. However, this "common way of doing" is only acquired through experience. The resulting conclusions often relate to functional orthodontic treatment considerations. When this is not immediately feasible, a starting phase with a neuromuscular orthotic is typically recommended.

Case Discussion

From a neuromuscular perspective, this case is a classical "mandibular entrapment" case. A simple analysis of the intra-oral photos reveals all the expected signs of mandibular entrapment in a functional Class III, such as lower lingualized incisors, increased overbite with reduced incisor torque, and wear facets where expected. As soon as rapid palatal expansion (RPE) is achieved, all temporomandibular joint (TMJ) symptoms disappear. This suggests that either the upper arch expansion somewhat frees the mandible, allowing for a more anterior and downward position

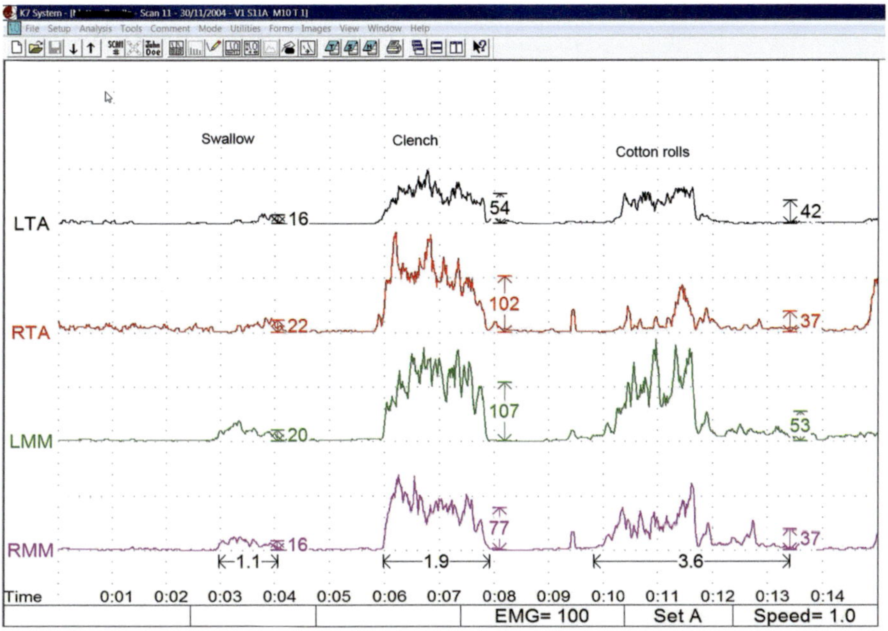

Fig. 12.6 Scan 11 (pretreatment) showing the surface EMG results in sweep mode. The patient was instructed to swallow (first burst), clench in CO (second burst), and then clench with cotton rolls between the teeth, which temporarily prevented occlusion (third burst). Note that during swallowing, the temporalis muscles were slightly unbalanced. During clenching in CO, there was cross-pattern firing. The use of cotton rolls reduced the muscle balance discrepancy. CO: centric occlusion; EMG: electromyography; LMM: left masseter muscle; LTA: left anterior temporalis; RMM: right masseter muscle; RTA: right anterior temporalis

of the condyle with consequent repositioning of the articular disk [2], or RPE has a psychological pain-reducing effect that is currently unknown to me and not described in litterature. The scans and their explanation are presented in Figs. 12.4, 12.5, 12.6, 12.7, 12.8, 12.9, 12.10, 12.11, 12.12 and 12.13. Essentially, two important pieces of data catch our attention. The first is scan 11, which reveals a cross-pattern firing between the masseter and temporalis muscles during clenching in ICP. The second is scan 4/5, which clearly shows how muscle deconditioning leads to a more forward and downward mandibular position. It is important to note that any forward and downward positioning of the mandible necessarily implies a consequent repositioning of the condyle.

There are clear signs of mandibular entrapment that can be observed well before scan 4/5. For instance, scan 3 demonstrates that there is virtually no anterior movement when closing from habitual rest position (HRP) (see Fig. 12.5). Additionally, another important indication of mandibular entrapment and maxillary deficiency is visible in scan 21 (Fig. 12.7). In this scan, the neuromuscular system appears to compensate for the need for more space required for a posterior tongue position by

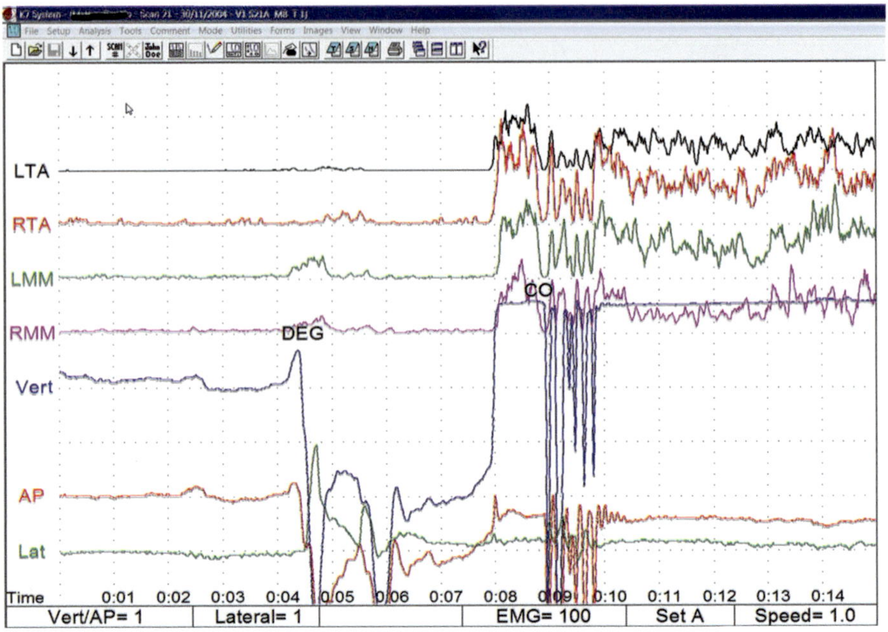

Fig. 12.7 Scan 21 (pre-treatment) showing the vertical, anterior-posterior, and lateral movements of the mandible in sweep mode during filtered EMG and swallowing. The patient was instructed to swallow normally and then close to CO, making a "tap-tap" motion in ICP. During swallowing, the patient did not move to CO, indicating that the swallowing occurred with the tongue between the teeth. The RTA was associated with higher output than the LTA during swallowing. AP: anterior-posterior; DEG: deglutition; CO: centric occlusion; EMG: electromyography; Lat: lateral; LMM: left masseter muscle; LTA: left anterior temporalis; RMM: right masseter muscle; RTA: right anterior temporalis; Vert: vertical

swallowing with the tongue between the teeth. It looks like as if the tongue is indicating where it wants to posture, with a mandible in a more forward position.

The primary reason for the patient's visit to my clinic was TMJ pain, which was easily resolved during RPE. However, our main treatment objectives are more ambitious than simply straightening teeth; we were determined to minimize the likelihood of TMJ pain relapse in the future. It is well-known that individuals who have experienced TMJ pain are at a higher risk for developing TMD compared to the general population. What are the factors that contribute to mandibular entrapment? Undoubtedly, there is a morphological trait that predisposes such individuals to an excessive amount of freeway space during growth. This deep-bite characteristic is often accompanied by a robust lip structure that affects upper incisor torque, ultimately leading to an increased overbite. This increased resting lip pressure has been well described [3]. Current orthodontic therapy tends to overlook the correction of freeway space and instead focuses on actively intruding upper incisors to mitigate the strong effect of the lower lip on them. In contrast, the neuromuscular approach emphasizes the management of freeway space. The overbite is corrected without

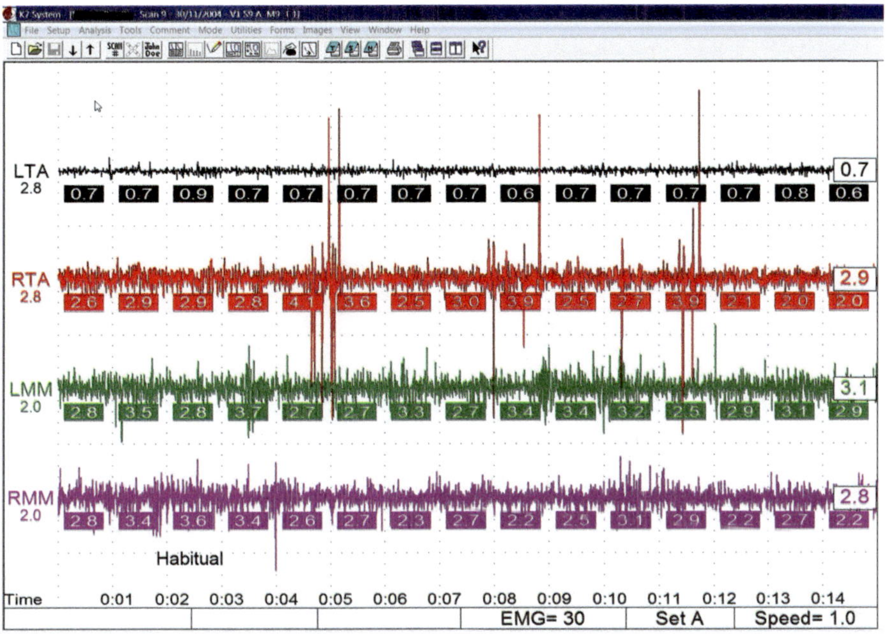

Fig. 12.8 Scan 9 (pre-treatment) showing the surface EMG results for the LTA, RTA, LMM, and RMM. The muscle output at rest was within the normal limits. CO: centric occlusion; EMG: electromyography; LMM: left masseter muscle; LTA: left anterior temporalis; RMM: right masseter muscle; RTA: right anterior temporalis

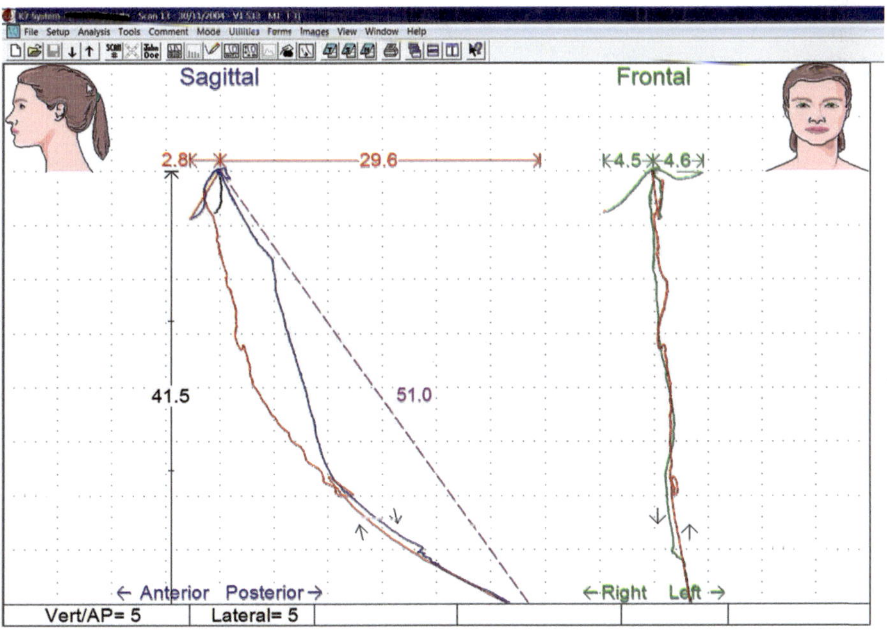

Fig. 12.9 Scan 13 (pre-treatment) showing the range of motion, opening posteriorly and closing anteriorly. AP: anterior-posterior; Vert: vertical

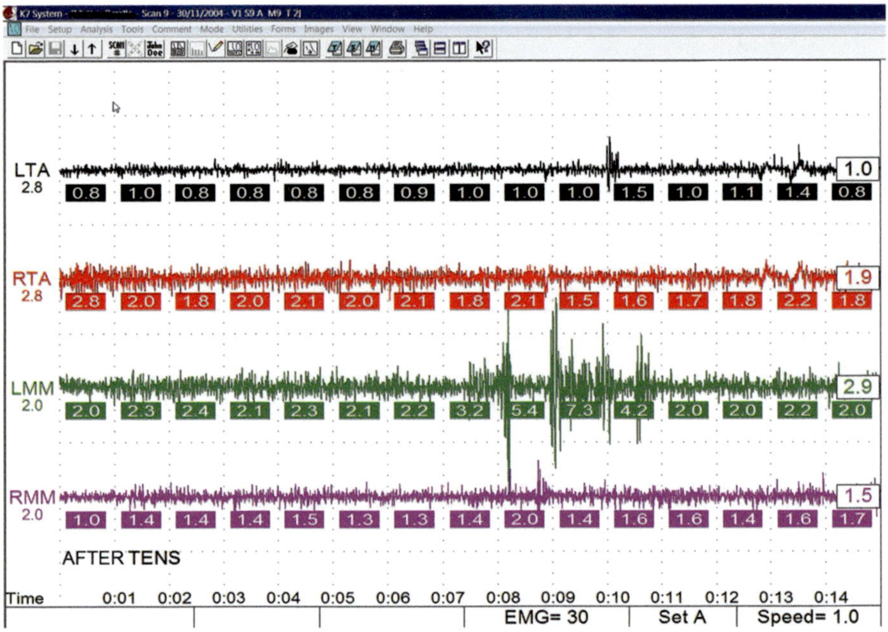

Fig. 12.10 Scan 10 (pre-treatment) showing that the muscles were relaxed(after TENS). An Aqualizer was used to avoid tooth contact for CNS deconditioning. CNS: central nervous system; LMM: left masseter muscle; LTA: left anterior temporalis; RMM: right masseter muscle; RTA: rightanterior temporalis; TENS: transcutaneous electrical nerve stimulation

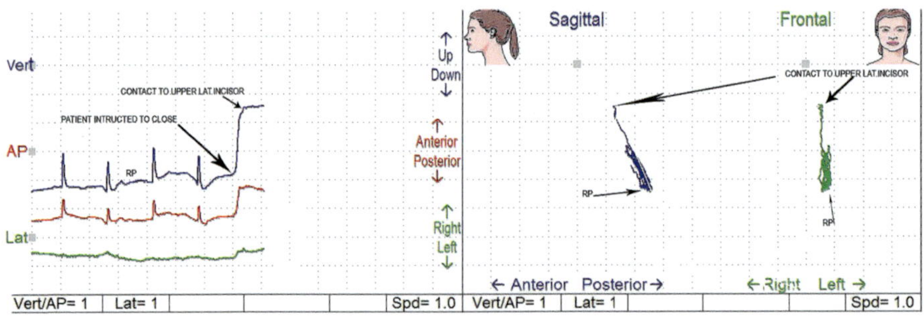

Fig. 12.11 Scan 4/5 (pre-treatment) showing a partial view of scan 5 in split screen mode. On the left-hand side, the patient was instructed to close from resting position to CO. The AP movement was forward (up) because of muscle deconditioning. On the right, the same tracing is shown from the sagittal and frontal views and shows a premature contact with upper lateral left incisor. AP: anterior-posterior; CO: centric occlusion; Lat: lateral; Spd: speed; Vert: vertical

relying heavily on upper intrusion as the main corrective method, but rather through extrusion of the mid and posterior teeth. This increase in lower facial height reduces the lower lip's coverage of the upper incisors, which are only adjusted based on their torquing needs. Moreover, in this particular orthodontic/TMD case, treating the

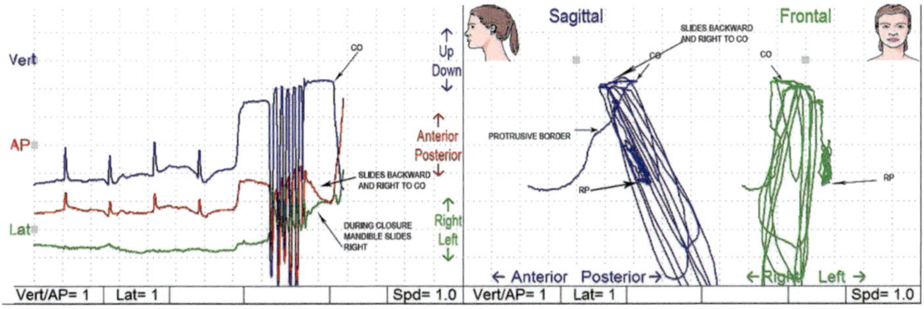

Fig. 12.12 Scan 5 (pre-treatment) showing that, after initial tooth contact, the mandible slid backward and right to CO. AP: anterior-posterior; CO: centric occlusion; Lat: lateral; Spd: speed; Vert: vertical

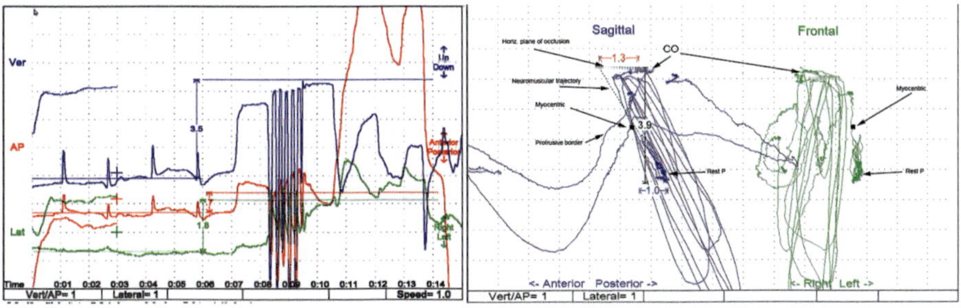

Fig. 12.13 Scan 4 and 5 (pre-treatment) showing a sweeping view of scan 5 and providing a complementary analysis (left). After relaxation/deconditioning, the mandible came forward from the rest position and did not avoid tooth contact. As the patient was instructed to "tap" to CO, the mandible closed upward to CO while sliding back. From the rest position to CO, the mandible closed approximately 2 mm to the right, on the right, Scan 5 showing that, as the mandible moved from the rest position to CO, the computer calculated that 1.3 mm of overjet was needed on the horizontal plane in order to resolve the mandibular retrusion. The black dot on the sagittal view represents the ideal occlusion, with 1.8 mm of freeway space (the myocentric position). AP: anterior-posterior; CO: centric occlusion; Lat: lateral; Vert: vertical

excessive freeway space with extrusion has the added benefit of countering the tendency toward a Class III occlusion when projecting the physiological, ideal path of occlusion onto the horizontal plane of occlusion (Myotrajactory). An extrusion therapy approach is necessary for achieving a Class I dental occlusion without risking posterior condylar displacement. Traditional orthodontic treatments that focus on upper incisor intrusion will not effectively address the issues related to skeletal morphology that result in excess freeway space. Therefore, our neuromuscular treatment objectives should focus on *reducing* freeway space, re-posturing the mandible according to muscular requests, and correcting tooth alignment, with particular emphasis on upper incisal torquing. Since skeletal discrepancy cannot be significantly changed, retention must be considered to prevent/reduce dental intrusion of the posterior/mid-sectors. Extrusion therapy for the pre-molar and molar teeth is effective in reducing freeway space while also improving overall muscle output by increasing muscle fiber recruitment. However, this increase in bite force can lead to relapse in deep-bite patients, especially if they clench during the day as a means of coping with stress.

This figure (Fig. 12.14) illustrates the application of neuromuscular principles following RPE. It is an ideal approach *to create an overjet and a Class II occlusion* when the necessary amount of space for orthodontic treatment is known [4]. It is likely that posterior condylar displacement is present and responsible for TMJ symptoms. Although this anterior advancement of the maxilla may not be sufficient, it remains the only option for preserving TMJ function in adulthood.

Figures 12.15, 12.16, and 12.17 display the intraoral, extraoral, and radiographic results post-treatment. However, satisfaction with the treatment outcome can only

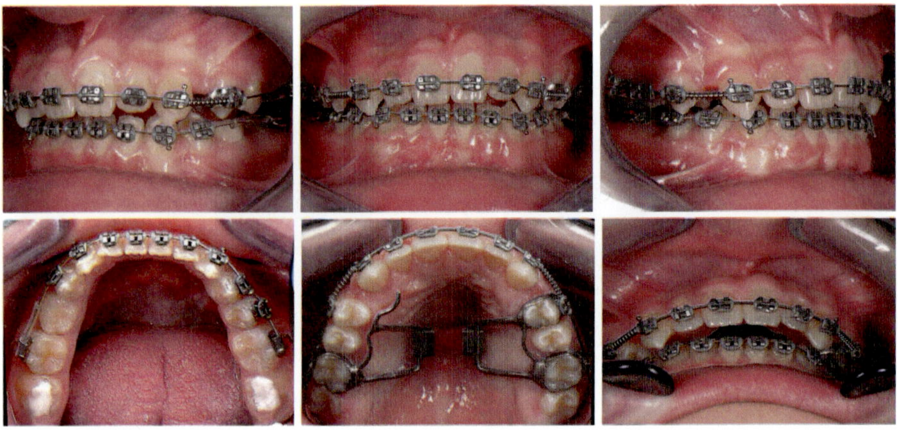

Fig. 12.14 Intraoral photographs showing a canine Class II relationship

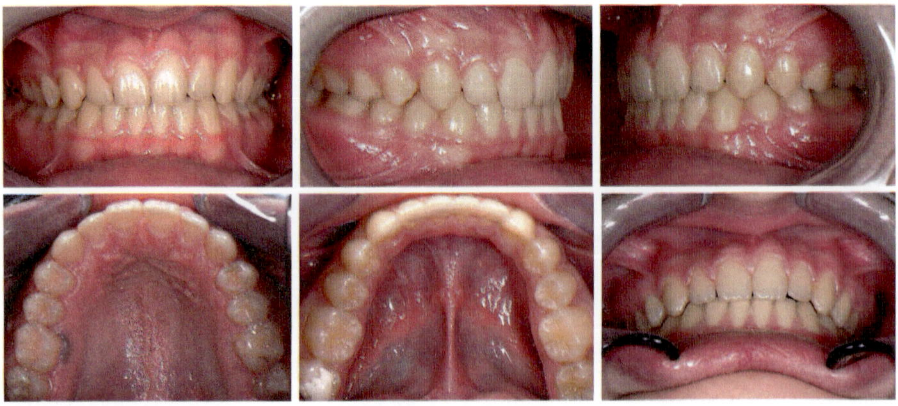

Fig. 12.15 Intraoral photographs at the end of treatment

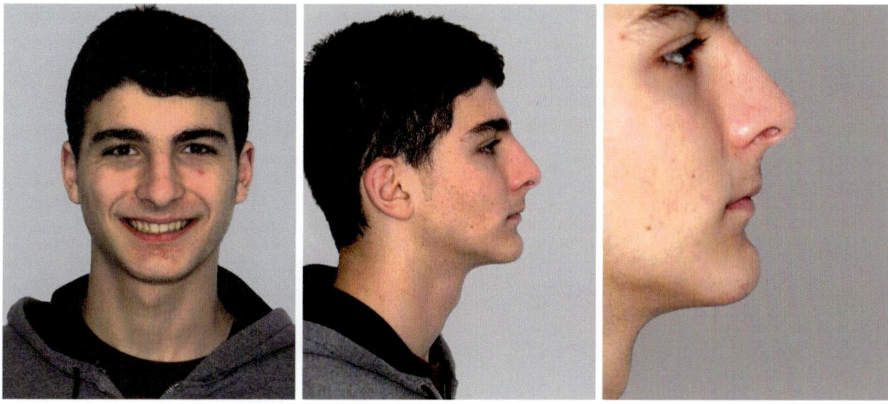

Fig. 12.16 Extraoral photographs at the end of treatment

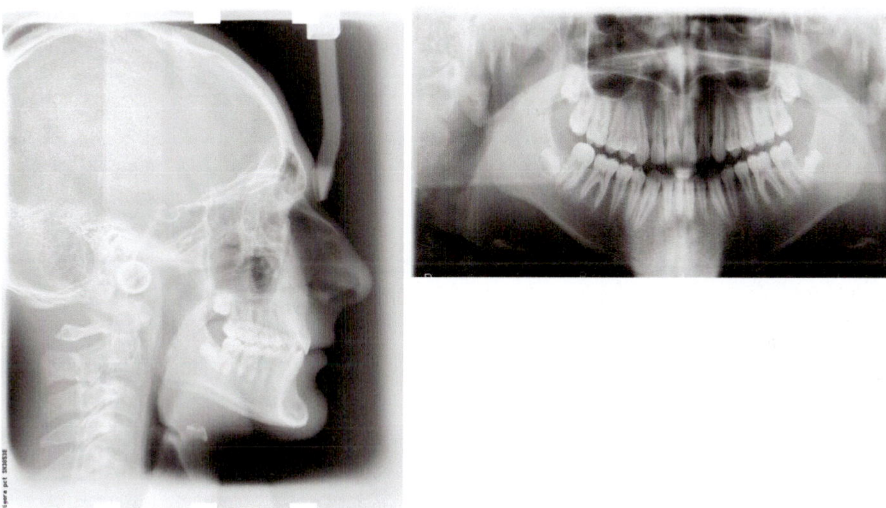

Fig. 12.17 Lateral cephalogram and panoramic X-ray after treatment

be justified from an aesthetic standpoint. Shortly after active orthodontic treatment, a comprehensive functional analysis was conducted, and the results are demonstrated in Figs. 12.18, 12.19, 12.20, 12.21, 12.22 and 12.23. In scan 4/5, the Sagittal relationship was incompletely corrected by 0.8 mm, which can sometimes be remedied by coronoplasty. Additionally, the protrusive border was steep, and the patient maintained the bad habit of nail biting. Despite this, excellent EMG results were obtained, particularly in scan 11, which now shows increased general output and more balanced function. Nevertheless, it should be noted that the temporalis output is superior to the masseter during clenching, indicating that the mandible still

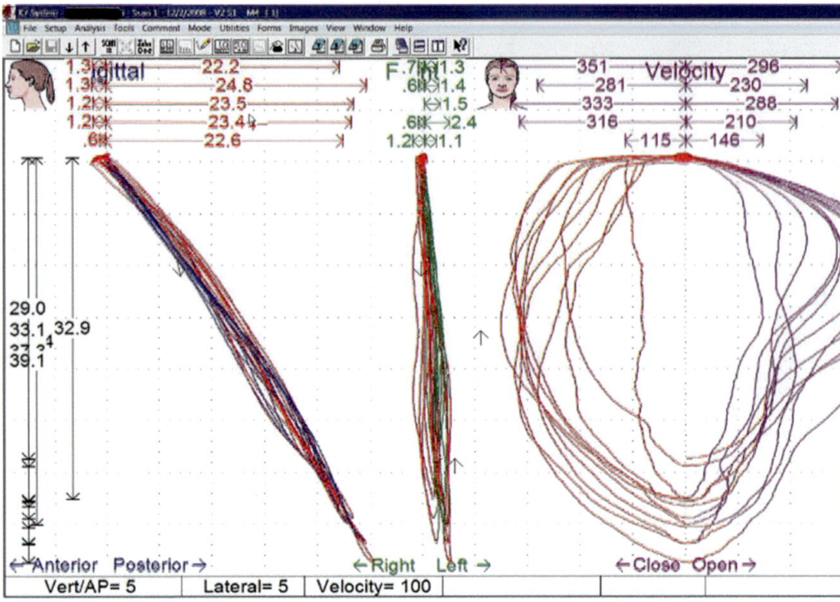

Fig. 12.18 Scan 1 (posttreatment) showing that the sagittal, frontal, and velocity tracings were within the normal limits. The speed at tooth contact to CO was very good. AP: anterior-posterior; CO: centric occlusion; Vert: vertical

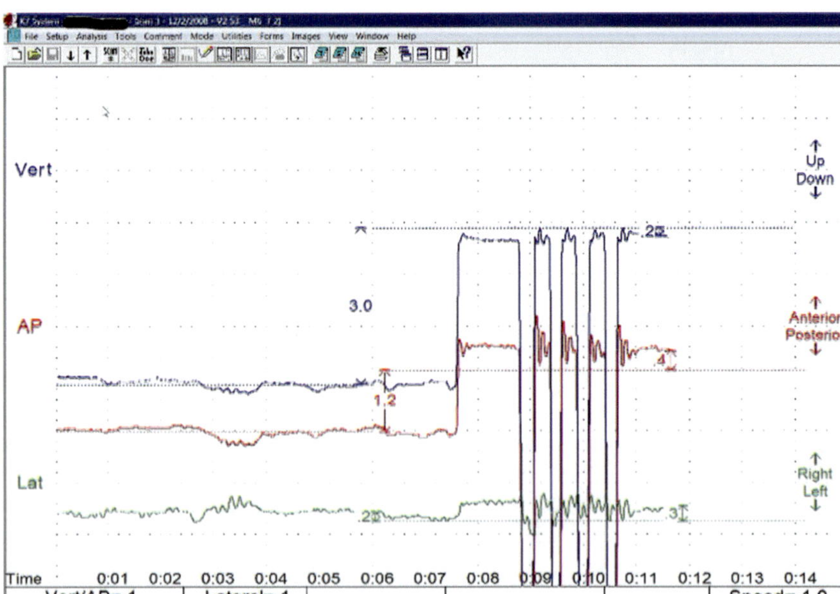

Fig. 12.19 Scan 3 (posttreatment) showing that the freeway space was 3 mm, the mandible moved forward during closure (A/V ratio: 0.4), and the lateral movement was 0.1 mm to the right. AP: anterior-posterior, A/V: anterior/vertical ratio; Lat: lateral; Vert: vertical

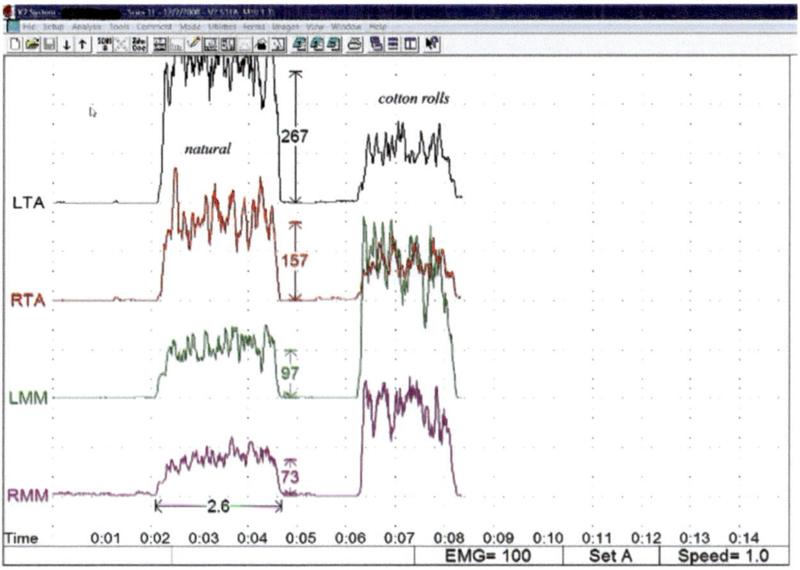

Fig. 12.20 Scan 11 (posttreatment) showing that muscle function was improved (with balanced masseters and unbalanced temporalis muscles) and the overall output was improved. EMG: electromyography; LMM: left masseter muscle; LTA: left anterior temporalis; RMM: right masseter muscle; RTA: right anterior temporalis

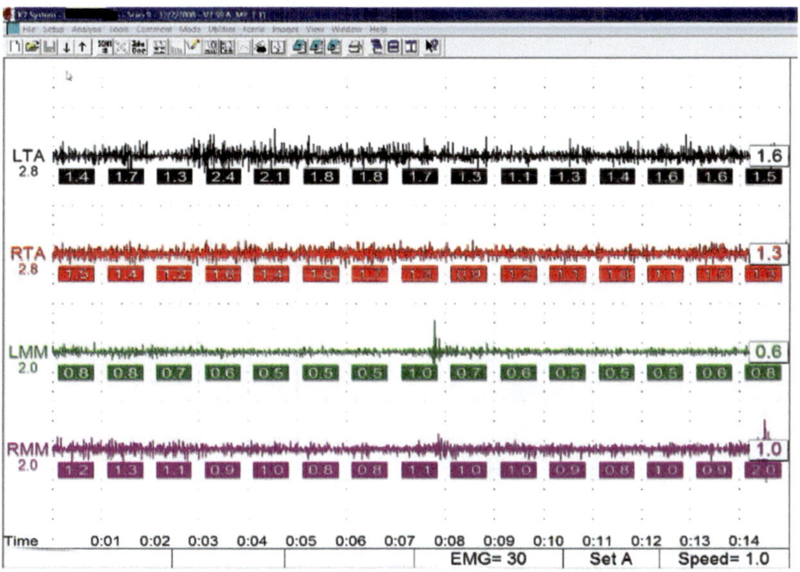

Fig. 12.21 Scan 9 (posttreatment) showing the muscle activity before relaxation with the Aqualizer and TENS. All the values were within normal limits. EMG: electromyography; LMM: left masseter muscle; LTA: left anterior temporalis; RMM: right masseter muscle; RTA: right anterior temporalis; TENS: transcutaneous electrical nerve stimulation

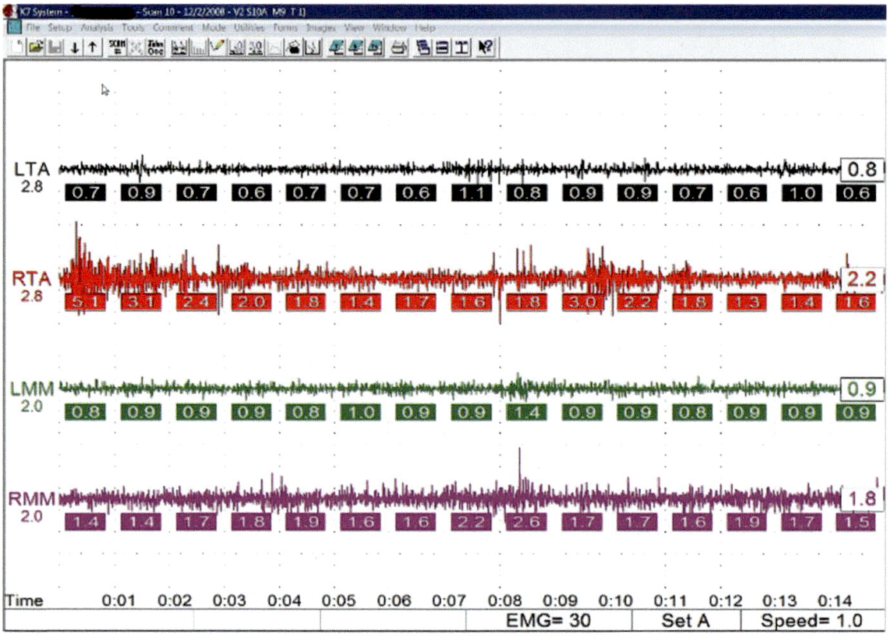

Fig. 12.22 Scan 10 (post-treatment) showing the muscle activity at rest after 45 min of relaxation with TENS. All the values were within the normal limits. EMG: electromyography; LMM: left masseter muscle; LTA: left anterior temporalis; RMM: right masseter muscle; RTA: right anterior temporalis; TENS: transcutaneous electrical nerve stimulation

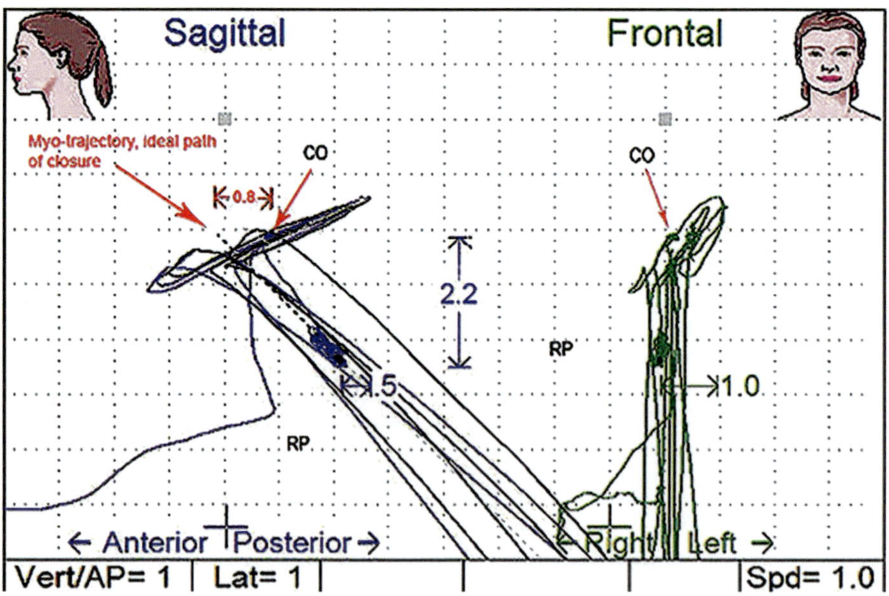

Fig. 12.23 Scan 5 (post-treatment) clarifies the slight posterior slide of the mandible at tooth contact. AP: anterior-posterior; Lat: lateral; Spd: speed; Vert: vertical

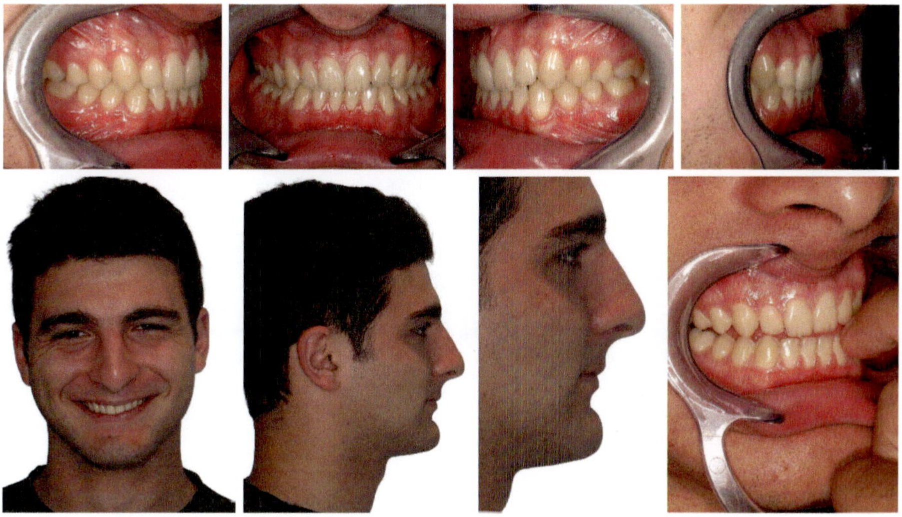

Fig. 12.24 Intra- and extraoral photographs at 7.5 years after treatment

requires additional sagittal correction. Further Freeway space correction may be possible.

Figure 12.24 depicts intra and extraoral photos taken 7.5 years post-treatment, while Fig. 12.25 displays the results of a follow-up functional analysis. The patient has been asymptomatic since 2005 and expressed satisfaction with the outcome. Upon closer examination of the CMS results, a minor general relapse was detected. Specifically, while 0.8 mm anterior to CO on HP was considered as a satisfactory result 7 years prior, the value had increased to 1.5 mm. Although seemingly insignificant, this change may be attributed to an increase in freeway space, insufficient upper incisal torquing, and non-ideal overjet. Notably, scan 11 now indicates correct masseter muscle firing during clenching, with greater activation than the temporalis muscles, which could result from postural adaptation of the cranio-cervical complex.

Together with the patient, we decided to strive for a perfect neuromuscular outcome, although I believed the likelihood of achieving it was low. In my opinion, the ideal function can only exist with perfect anatomy. In April 2020, 12.5 years after the initial treatment, we began a fixed upper orthodontic correction for the incisors and canine torque. Brackets were applied to the upper arch, and we used the Savasystem® Bracket prescription. The torque and tips were selected based on proper disocclusion results seen during my 30 years orthodontic experience, specifically studying scans 4/5. This treatment lasted for 12 months, following which a neuromuscular Positioner was fitted for a 3-month retention period, to be worn for 4 h during the day and nighttime. Intra- and extraoral photos were taken in June 2021 and can be seen in Fig. 12.26.

The neuromuscular positioner was constructed to have a vertical opening of approximately 3.5 mm, as indicated by the mandibular kinesiograph. To create this

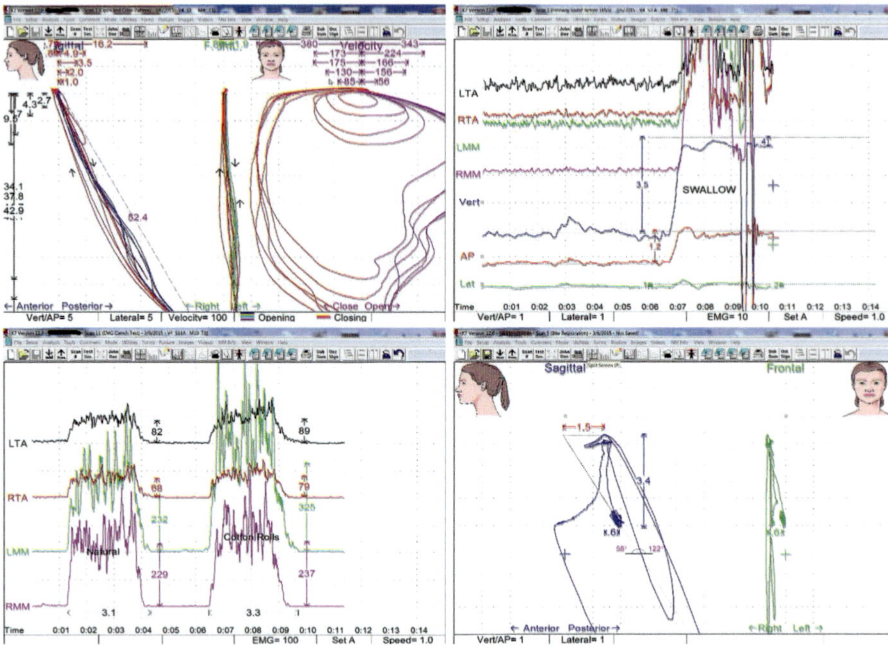

Fig. 12.25 *Upper left*: Scan 1 (post-treatment follow-up) shows that all the values were within the normal limits, the speed at tooth contact was high, and the movement was fluent. *Upper right*: Scan 21 (post-treatment follow-up) shows an improvement in the patient's swallow pattern. *Lower Left*: Scan 11 (post-treatment follow-up) showing natural clenching (ideal balanced function during clenching, with both masseters and temporalis muscles well balanced) and cotton roll clenching (no change in the general output pattern). The output of the masseters was higher than that of the temporalis muscles. *Lower right*: Scans 5 (post-treatment follow-up) shows that although the physiological rest position was 0.6 mm posterior to the CO, the neuromuscular trajectory was still projected with respect to the horizontal plane of occlusion by 1.5 mm. The incisors were too steep; this slight relapse is most probably due to incisor lingual tipping. AP: anterior-posterior; A/V: anterior/vertical EMG: electromyography; LMM: left masseter muscle; LTA: left anterior temporalis; RMM: right masseter muscle; RTA: right anterior temporalis.; CO: centric occlusion; Lat: lateral; Spd: speed; Vert: vertical. TENS: transcutaneous electrical nerve stimulation

device, it was crucial to utilize the physiological rest position, and some of the frontal elements were partially set up without altering the torque values (see Fig. 12.27). To ensure optimal results, it is imperative to employ a face bow during these procedures. This is the only way to identify any canting of the upper arch/maxilla or other significant alterations of the occlusion plane. Furthermore, if necessary, the dental setup can be fine-tuned to correct any minor canting.

Figure 12.28 shows the resulting scan 4/5 after correcting incisal torquing (on left). A 0.9-mm discrepancy is considered satisfactory, although freeway space can still be corrected to reduce the AP difference. Active retention is necessary to avoid re-intrusion of the posterior teeth. This can be achieved by bite plane removable appliances or by functional appliances. All these appliances require collaboration.

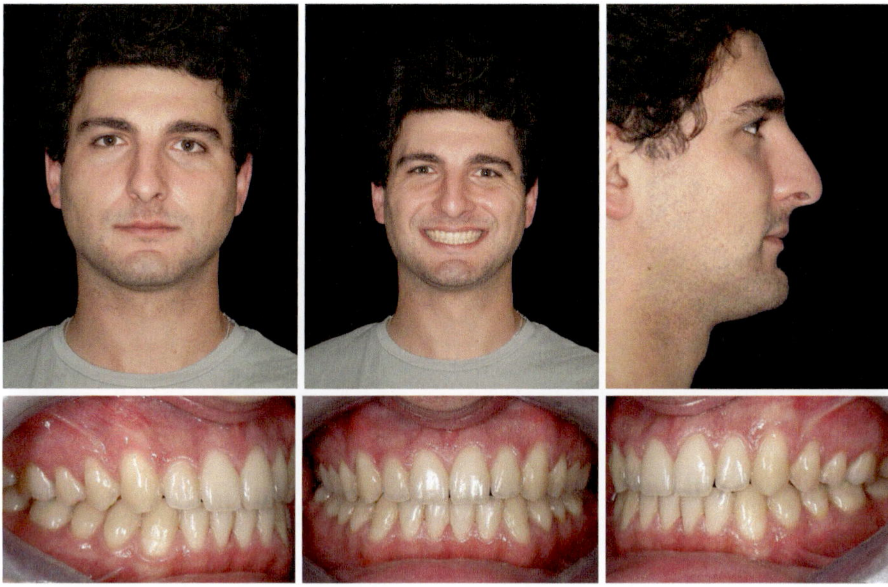

Fig. 12.26 Intra and extraoral photos at 36 months after incisor correction with Savasystem® bracket prescription and 13.5 years after initial treatment

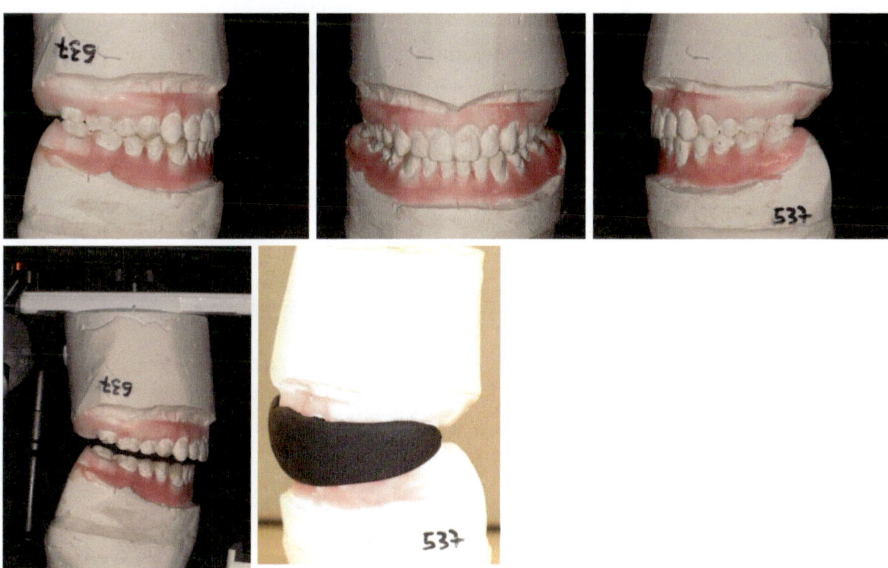

Fig. 12.27 Setup on neuromuscular recording for the fabrication of intraoral neuromuscular positioner. Lower left: mounted on Artex articulator: note the circa 3.5 mm opening (freeway space) as recorded by PRP after setup. Lower right: Positioner constructed after setup, natural rubber (Courtesy of Orthosystem®, Milan, Italy

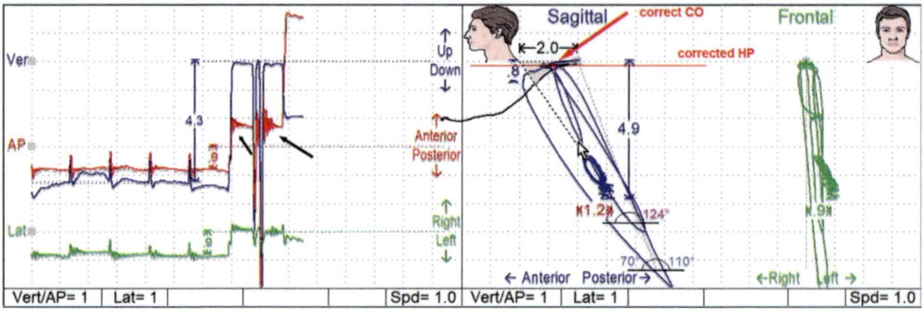

Fig. 12.28 Scan 4/5 (post-treatment at 15 years after initial treatment) clarifies the tracing correction due to vibration to the sensor array during vigorous tooth contact. AP: anterior-posterior; Lat: lateral; Spd: speed; Vert: vertical. Left: black arrows indicate vibration of AP line. Right: in red correct CO position, corrected HP. The AP discrepancy is 0.9 mm on the HP

Morphology plays a major role in these cases, and the continuous production of freeway space cannot be totally corrected. It is a physiologic characteristic of these patients.

Case 12.2

Class I Occlusion with Increased OJ and Reduced Freeway Space

Neuromuscular Consequences to Excessive Positioner Use

Summary On January 2008, an 8-year-old Caucasian girl sought orthodontic treatment for misaligned teeth (Fig. 12.29).

Pre-treatment	
Extraoral analysis (Fig. 12.29)	
Facial profile	Convex
Facial height	Slightly increased
Occlusal plane	No tipping
Facial symmetry	Symmetric
Lips	Incompetent, short upper
Mandibular posture	Neutral
Head posture	Slightly forward
Intraoral analysis (Fig. 12.29)	
Teeth	
Molar class	1 right, 2 left
Canine class	2
Overjet	6 mm
Overbite	3
Oral hygiene	Good/fair
Rotations	
Crossbite	
Diastemas	

Crowding	
Agenesis	
Missing teeth	
Intraoral functional analysis	
Swallow	Tongue thrust
Tongue tie	No
Tongue posture	
Tongue thrust	Yes
Slurred speech	No
Neuromuscular diagnosis	
Freeway space	Reduced
Skeletal class	I
Anterior Wall	No
TMJ left	
TMJ right	

Problem list

- Reduce OJ
- Align teeth in Class I
- Check respiratory problems

Neuromuscular treatment objectives

- Increase or limit the loss of freeway space
- Mandibular freedom and SMM
- Slight upper distalization

Introduction

Neuromuscular Orthodontics does not cancel clinical judgment before functional kinesiographic analysis, but rather changes it. Functional K7 evaluation can be conducted after treatment to verify treatment results. Furthermore, this case study is important because it demonstrates the effects of prolonged use of rubber positioners as semi-permanent retainers. Even if the hours per day are circa 12 (8 nightime+4 daytime), the most active part is during wake (4 h) because of clenching on the appliance. This is sufficient in the long term to determine occlusal changes mainly by determining a clockwise rotation of the occlusal plane through upper mid/posterior intrusion. The effects on the lower arch are less evident. This results in overclosure with a more forward mandibular positioning in ICP. We are discussing millimetric effects that have obvious consequences on muscle function and condylar repositioning. Open-bite morphology is even characterized by reduced anatomical tolerance to condylar positional changes.

Discussion

This young patient most probably had some breathing issues before coming to seek orthodontic treatment. Nevertheless, ENT evaluation was carried out and no pathologies were found. The increased OJ and the incompetent lips were most probably responsible for the tongue thrust. No K7 evaluation was carried out at the beginning of treatment because this case was considered clinically a ***tendency to skeletal Class II.*** Therefore, considering the probability of a normal or slightly reduced freeway

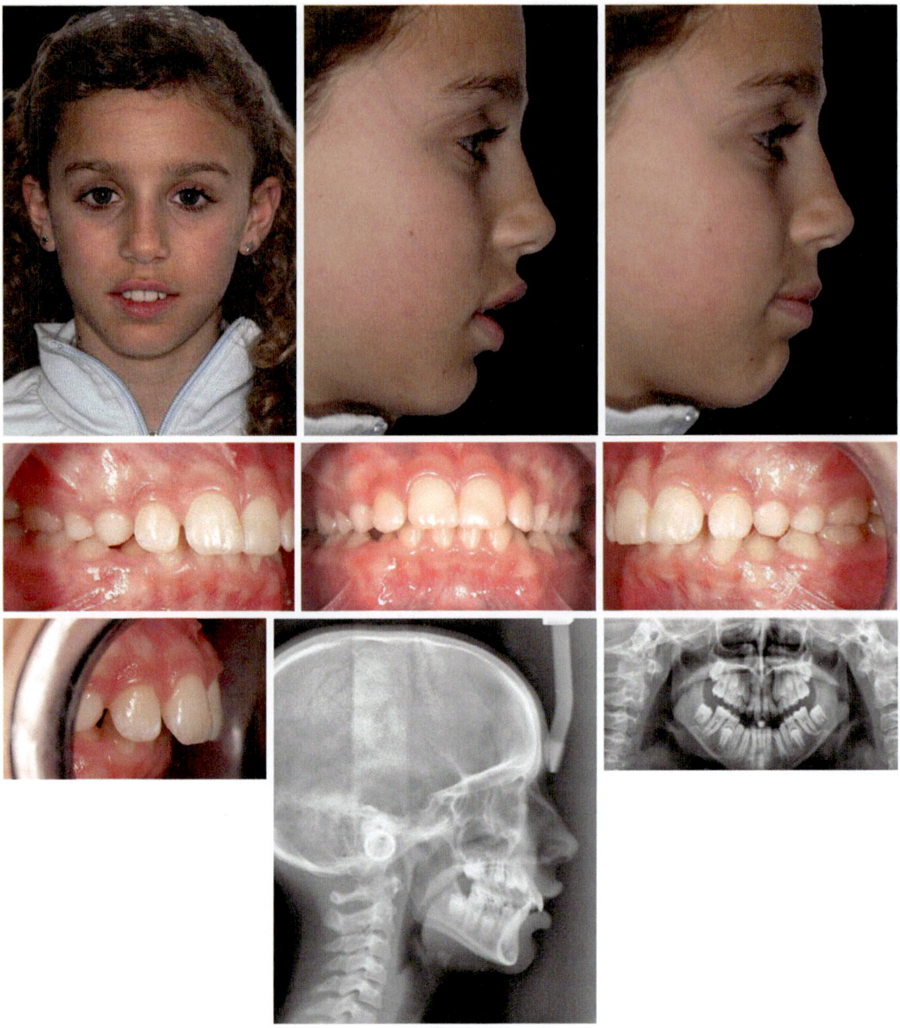

Fig. 12.29 Initial case March 2008. Extraoral, intraoral photos; Lateral cephalogram X-Ray and panoramic. Female, age 8 years, no breathing problems, short upper lip. Skeletal open-bite tendency. March 2008

space, it was decided to distalize the upper arch after initial alignment and to control vertical freeway space without reducing it.

Two jigs were used to distalized the upper arch while a lower lingual arch was applied to control anchorage and lower vertical eruption. Treatment was terminated by December 2011 and a rubber positioner was prescribed and delivered for initial retention (Fig. 12.30). Positioner treatment is usually carried out for a maximum of

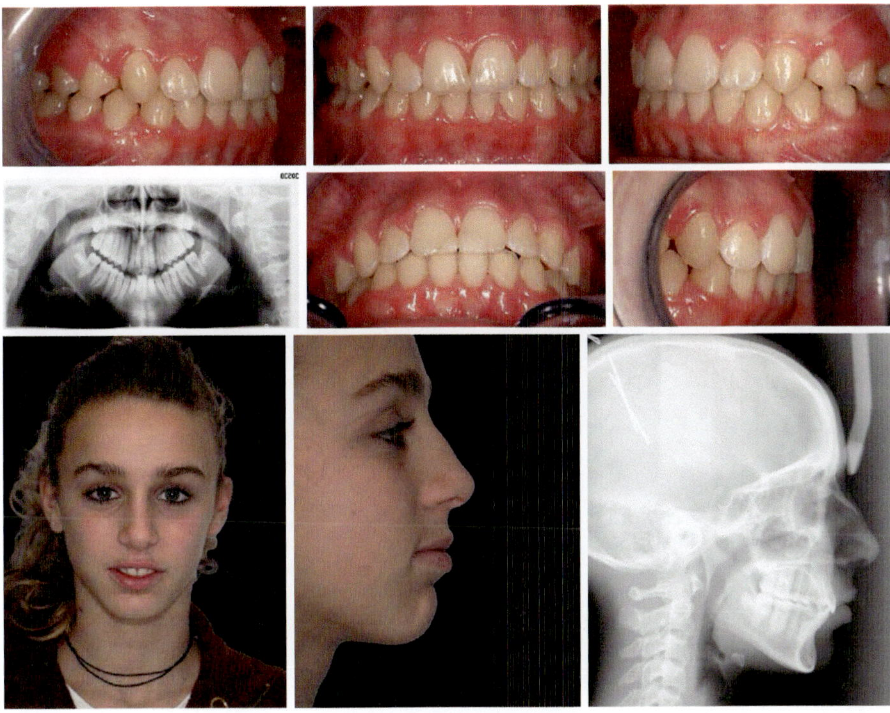

Fig. 12.30 Case finished in December 2011. Showing intra and extraoral photos and panoramic X-Ray, lateral ceph X-Ray 50 days after application of rubber positioner 4 h/day and full night-time. Note posterior occlusal spacing

30–60 days at a 12 h/day application, in which daytime application is 4 h and patient is instructed to clench lightly.

Unfortunately, the patient did not follow-up to the office for 7 years and we had no chance to interrupt positioner application Intra oral photographs were taken after 7 years from treatment and the results can be seen in Fig. 12.31. To evaluate functional consequences, a full K7 functional evaluation was carried out, and the results can be seen in Fig. 12.32.

These first kinesiographic results confirm the unhealthy effect of prolonged use of rubber positioners on occlusion and function. Scan 11 shows the resulting occlusal effect on musculature: the masseters are not activated during MVC because there is a lack of posterior support (scan 11). Gummy rubbery-like positioners determine posterior intrusion effects in the pre-molar/molar region and favor a more anterior mandibular occlusion. In other words, from a kinesiographic point of view, the HP of occlusion is positioned slightly upward of where it should be. The logical treatment is the lowering of the HP which is achieved by re-extruding the posterior sectors of the upper arch. This will result in a more balanced occlusion with greater posterior occlusal support and increased muscular activation of the masseters

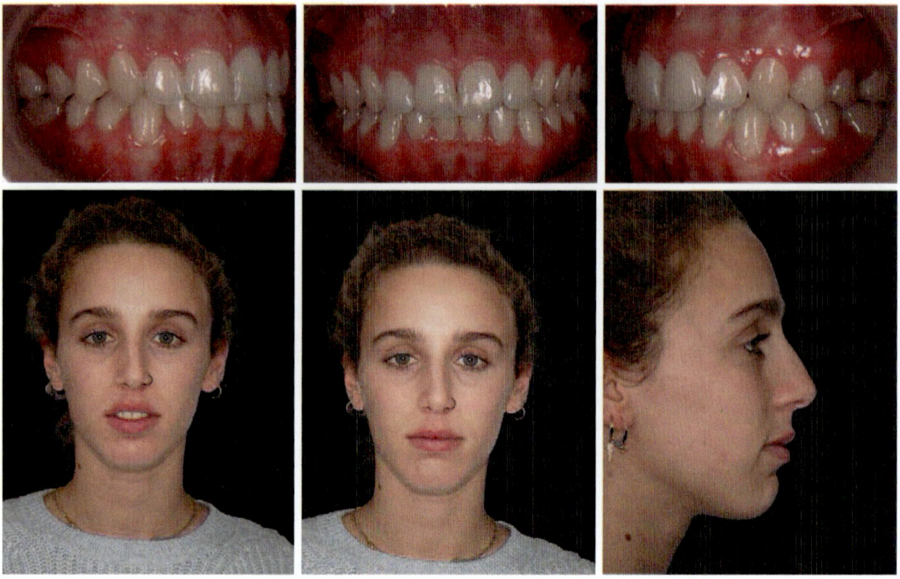

Fig. 12.31 Same patient cont. 7 years after treatment (2019). She kept wearing the positioner at nighttime even though she was told to suspend retention. There is still a visible lack of posterior support. Even though asymptomatic, a complete k7 analysis was carried out

during MVC. In this particular case, even an extrusion of 0.5 mm can make a significant difference. Even though this case is to be considered a skeletal open bite and the masseter output is never very high, there should be a greater activation of the masseter muscles during clench. There is still an excessive discrepancy of the Myotrajectory in relation to CO, as seen in scan 5 (2.1 mm, Figs. 12.32 and 12.33).

Although advised to suspend positioner treatment, nightwear was continued until 2022. Even though daytime application was suspended, night retention with the rubber positioner maintained loss of posterior support. These and other results can be confirmed in another K7 evaluation at 10 years after treatment (Figs. 12.34, 12.35, 12.36, 12.37 and 12.38).

This patient was again evaluated in 2022, but surprisingly she did not want to completely suspend positioner treatment but had progressively reduced its application (Figs. 12.32, 12.33, 12.34, 12.35, 12.36, 12.37 and 12.38). Although there is a slight improvement of the masseter output (Scan 11, Fig. 12.36), a slight AP discrepancy persists (**0.7 mm** corrected from 1.2 due to sensor array vibration and erroneous computer calculation, this is visible on scan 5, 1.2 mm). This is a satisfactory result, but it is advisable to convince the patient that excessive positioner use will affect occlusion in a negative way. So once again positioner suspension was advised properly. Final cephalograms compared to initial can be seen in Fig. 12.39. Further evaluation will be necessary to evaluate positioner suspension effects on masseter function.

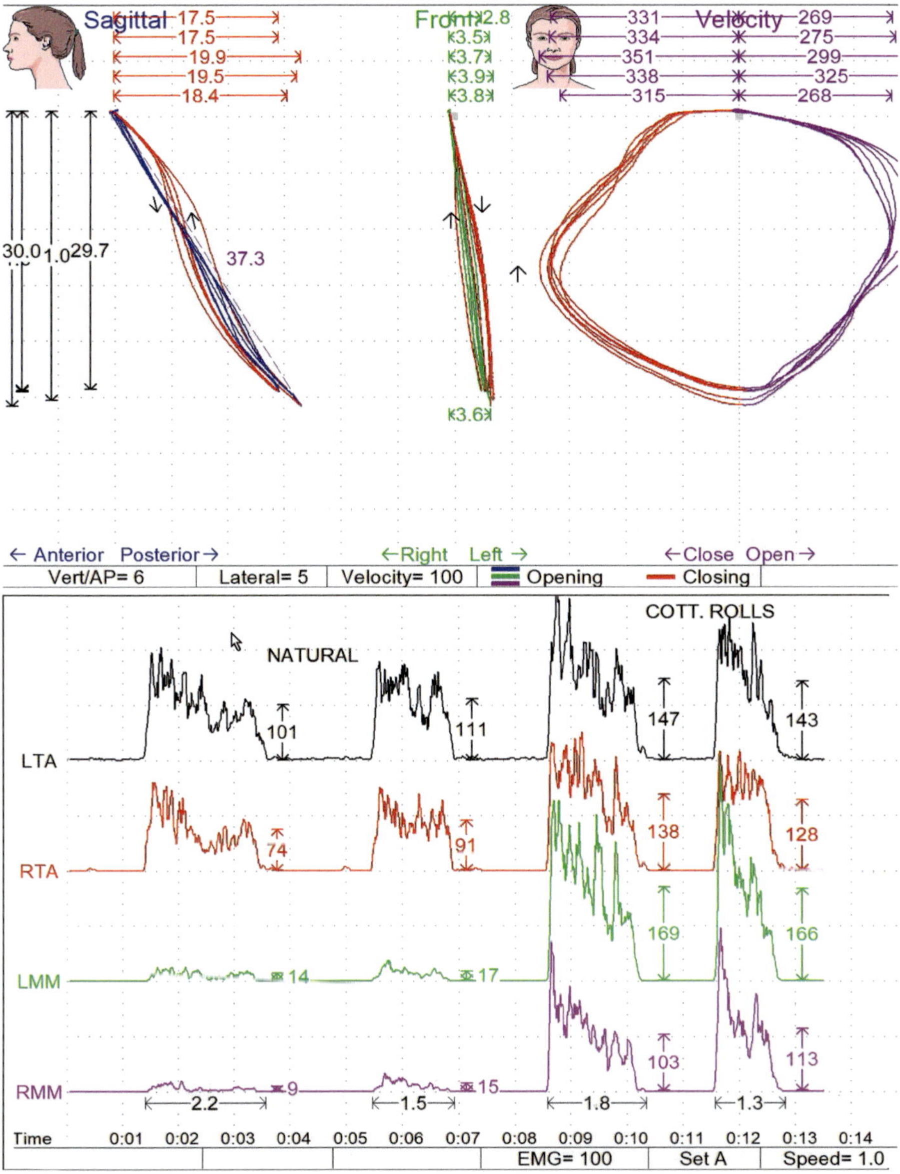

Fig. 12.32 From top to bottom, scan 1, scan 11, scan10, scan 4/5; (2019) See text for explanation

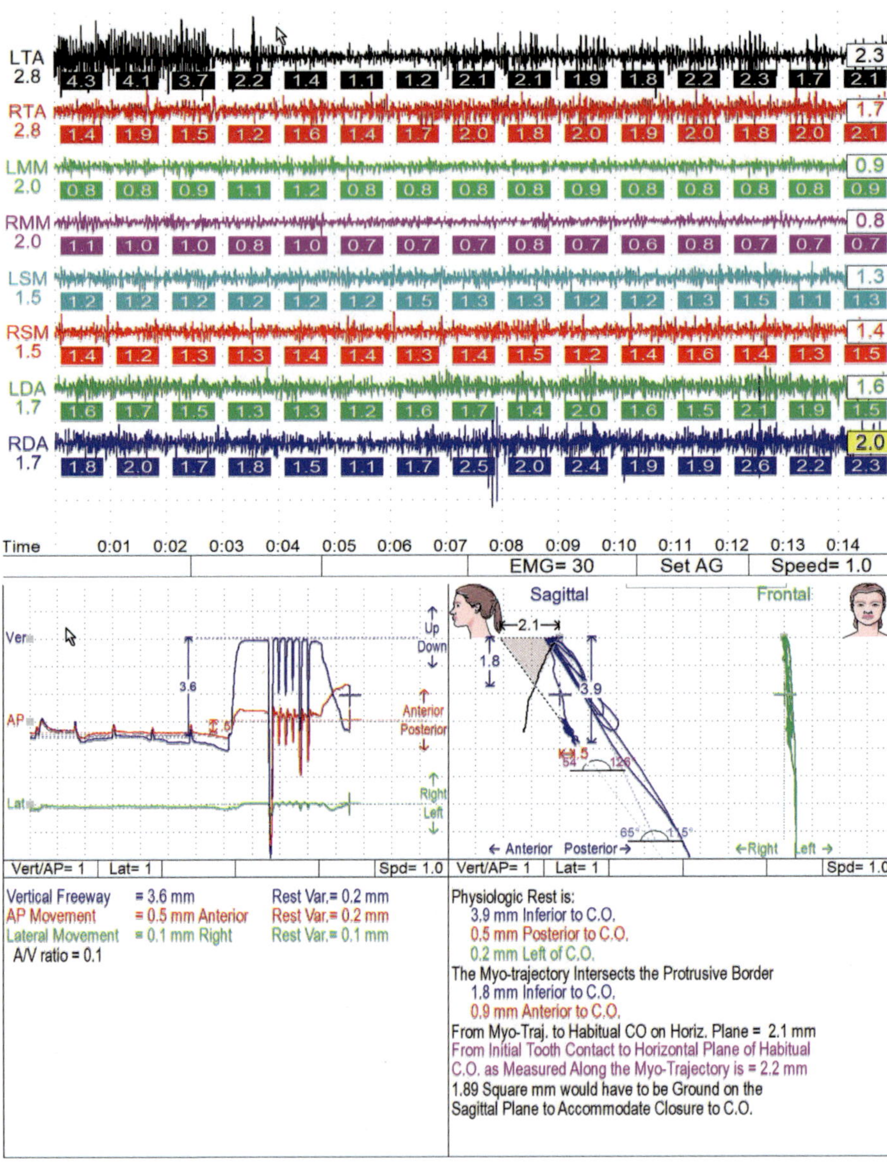

Fig. 12.32 (continued)

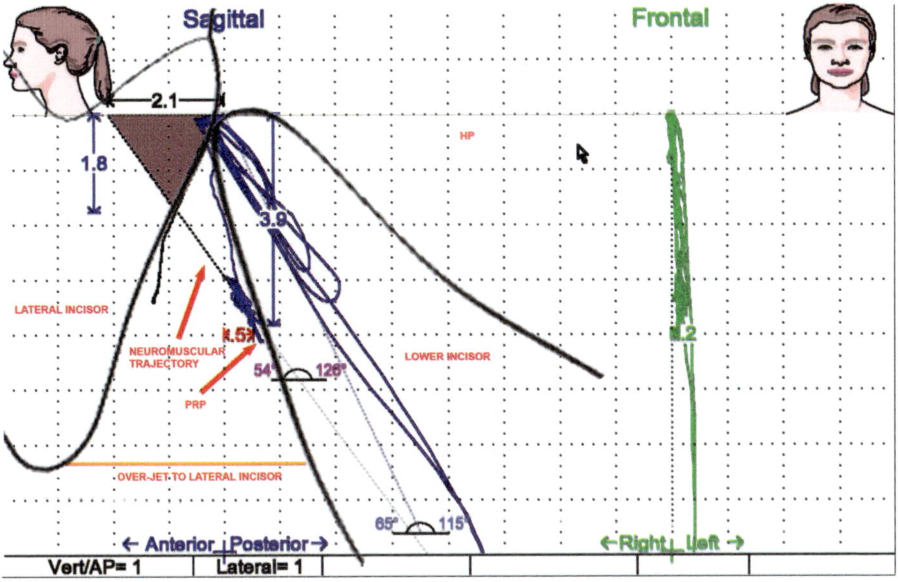

Fig. 12.33 Scan 5 as in Fig. 12.32. In red neuromuscular references are indicated

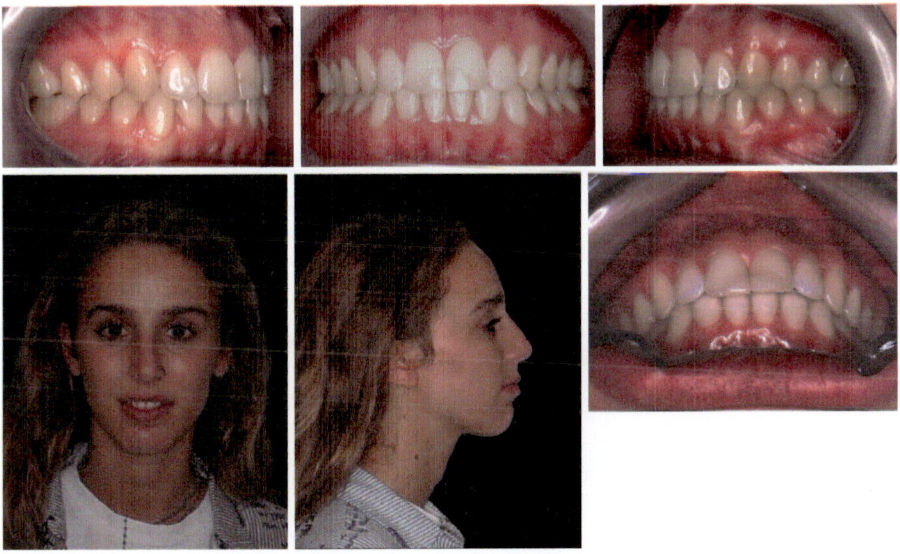

Fig. 12.34 Cont. Intra and extraoral photos at 10 years after treatment. Lower right: Anterior wall is present because of excessive positioner use

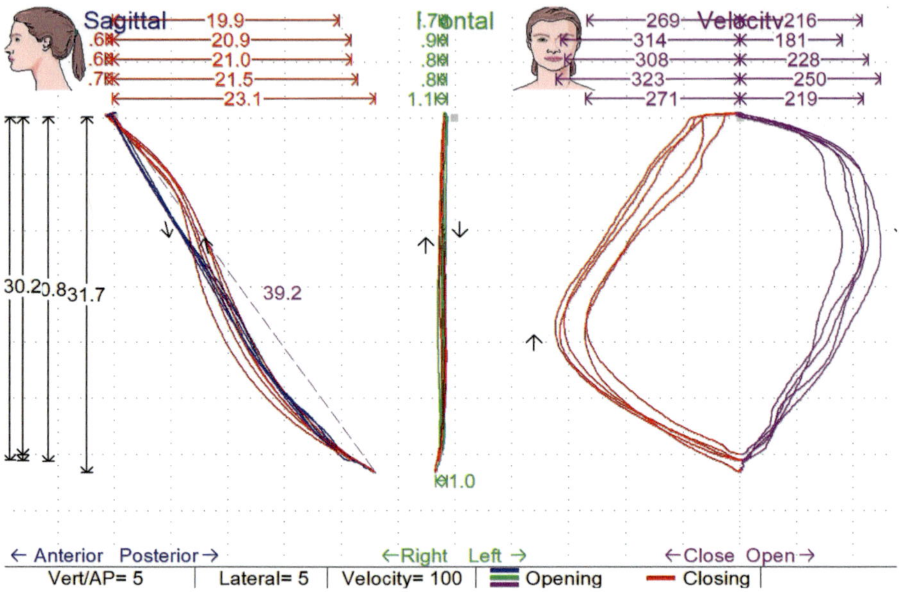

Fig. 12.35 Scan 1 (post-treatment follow-up at 10 years after treatment) showing that the degree of mouth opening was satisfactory (the total mouth aperture was approximately 39 mm), there was no significant lateral deviation upon opening (6.4 mm), and the velocity at tooth contact was also satisfactory. AP: anterior-posterior; Vert: vertical

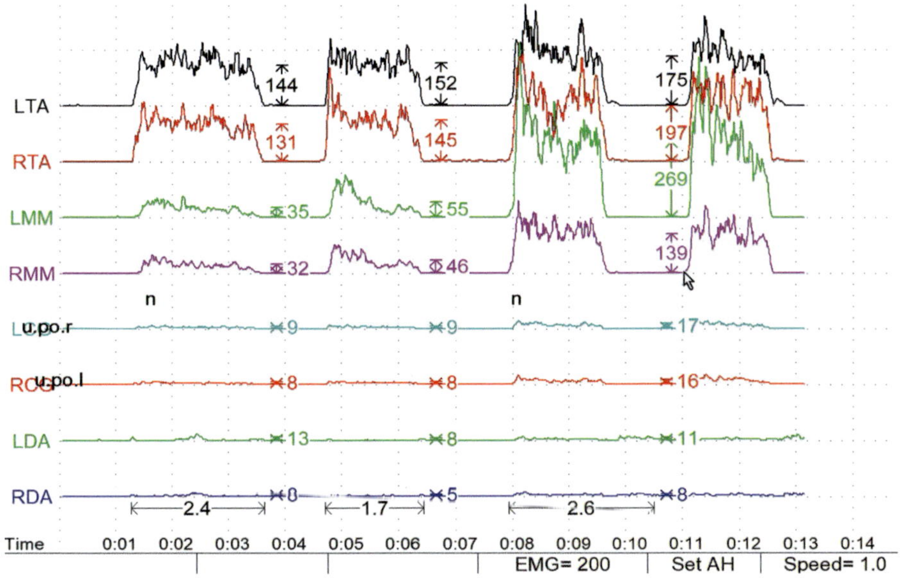

Fig. 12.36 Scan 11 post-treatment follow-up at 10 years after treatment shows the surface EMG results in sweep mode. The patient was instructed to clench in CO (first burst and second burst), and then clench with cotton rolls between the teeth, which temporarily prevented occlusion (third burst and fourth burst). Output s-EMG is satisfactory and the general there is a symmetric balancing. The Temporalis have a stronger output during clench in respect of the masseters that activate very little. CO: centric occlusion; EMG: electromyography; LMM: left masseter muscle; LTA: left anterior temporalis; RMM: right masseter muscle; RTA: right anterior temporalis

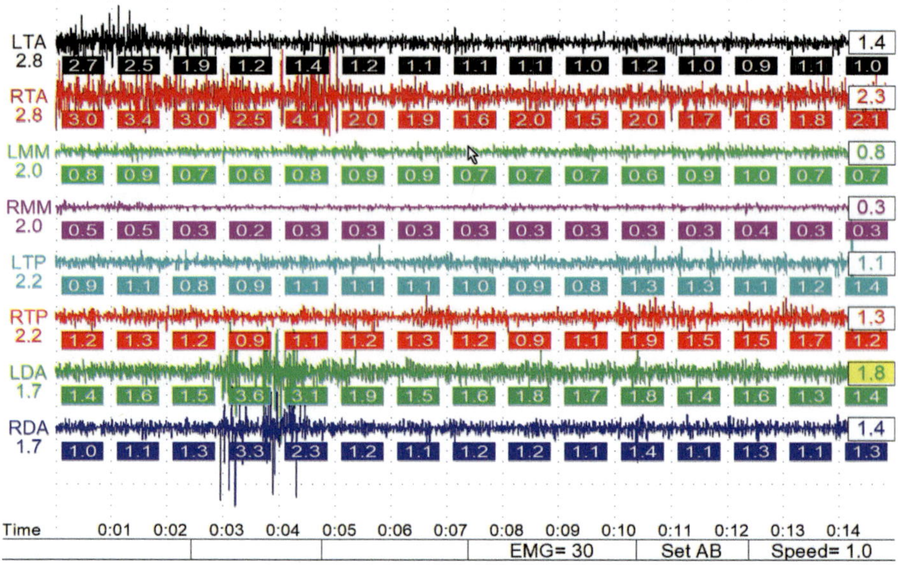

Fig. 12.37 Scan 10 (post-treatment follow-up at 10 years after treatment) shows that the muscles were relaxed (after TENS). An Aqualizer was used to avoid tooth contact for CNS deconditioning. CNS: central nervous system; LMM: left masseter muscle; LTA: left anterior temporalis; RMM: right masseter muscle; RTA: right anterior temporalis; LDA: Left Digastric Anterior; RDA: Right Digastric Anterior; LTP. Left Temporalis Posterior; RTP: Right Temporalis Posterior TENS: transcutaneous electrical nerve stimulation

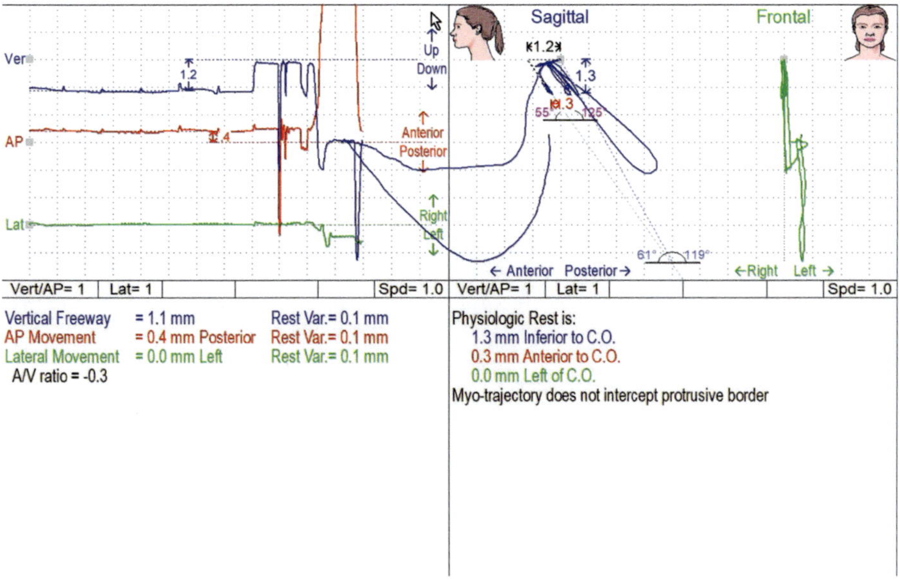

Fig. 12.38 MKG at 10 years after treatment. The effects of positioner use are still visible even if there has been a reduction of time wear. (10/2022) Showing scan 4/5 in split screen modality. On the left sweep of V, AP, and Lat lines. The patient is instructed to rest mandibular posture and the instructed to close to Centric Occlusion. Note the TENS spikes on V and AP lines. On the right, the corresponding Sagittal/frontal scan 5 shows a 0.7-mm. AP discrepancy on HP (Horizontal Plane of Occlusion, corrected due to sensor array tremble). Vertical freeway space is 1.3 mm. AP: anterior-posterior; CO: centric occlusion; Lat: lateral; Spd: speed; Vert: vertical

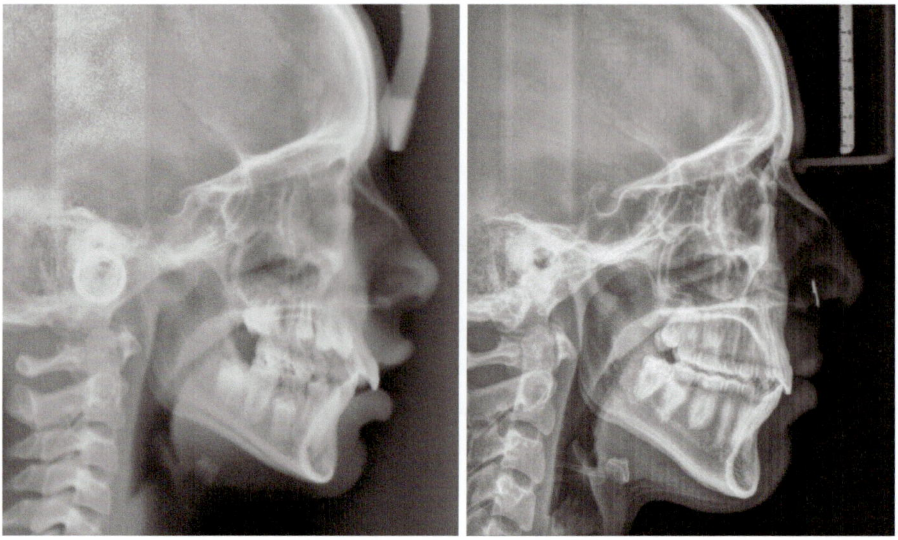

Fig. 12.39 Before and post-treatment lateral cephalograms

Case 12.3

Class III Occlusion with Negative OJ and Increased Freeway Space

Summary An 8-year-old Caucasian girl sought orthodontic treatment for misaligned teeth lamenting reverse OJ.

Pre-treatment	
Extraoral analysis (Fig. 12.40)	
Facial profile	Flat
Facial height	Normal
Occlusal plane	Normal
Facial	Symmetry
Lips	Competent
Mandibular posture	
Head posture	Suspected ocular torticollis
Intraoral analysis (Fig. 12.40)	
Teeth	
Molar class	III
Canine class	III
Overjet	Negative
Overbite	
Oral hygiene	Fair
Rotations	
Crossbite	
Diastemas	

Crowding	Slight upper
Agenesis	
Missing teeth	
Intraoral functional analysis	
Swallow	Good
Tongue tie	No
Tongue posture	Low, forward
Tongue	Thrust, transitional
Slurred speech	
Cephalometrics	
Neuromuscular diagnosis	
Freeway space excess	
Skeletal class	III
Anterior wall	No
TMJ left	
TMJ right	

Problem list

- Correct OJ without distalizing condyle.
- Reduce AP discrepancy.

Neuromuscular treatment objectives

- Correct freeway space, extrusion.
- Correct tongue posture and swallow.

Introduction

The main difficulty of all Class III occlusions is the correction of the OJ and the lower incisor tip/torque. The risk related to condyle misplacement is persistent throughout the orthodontic treatment. Probably the only valuable tool to objectively measure the skeletal discrepancy and evaluate proper treatment alternatives, lies in the use of ULF-TENS and CMS.

This case describes the treatment and follow-up of a skeletal Class III and occlusal Class III patient and how the neuromuscular procedure should be applied to avoid iatrogenic TMD. A selection of scans during the treatment period and at 20-year follow-up are commented.

Discussion

Figure 12.40 depicts the intraoral and extraoral photographs taken at the outset of interceptive treatment in July 1998. It is worth noting that there appears to be a postural issue that may be related to the patient's visual system, potentially indicating an ocular torticollis. Additionally, the intraoral photographs reveal a reverse overjet and Class III occlusion. Figure 12.41 illustrates the panoramic and lateral head cephalogram radiographs taken with the patient in centric occlusion.

Upon initial examination, the patient was referred to both an ear, nose, and throat (ENT) specialist for a breathing evaluation and an eye specialist for further evaluation of the potential visual system involvement. However, despite their efforts, none of the specialists identified any pathological conditions or concerns with the patient.

Following the completion of interceptive therapy, which included upper expansion and premaxilla correction, it was deemed necessary to perform a detailed

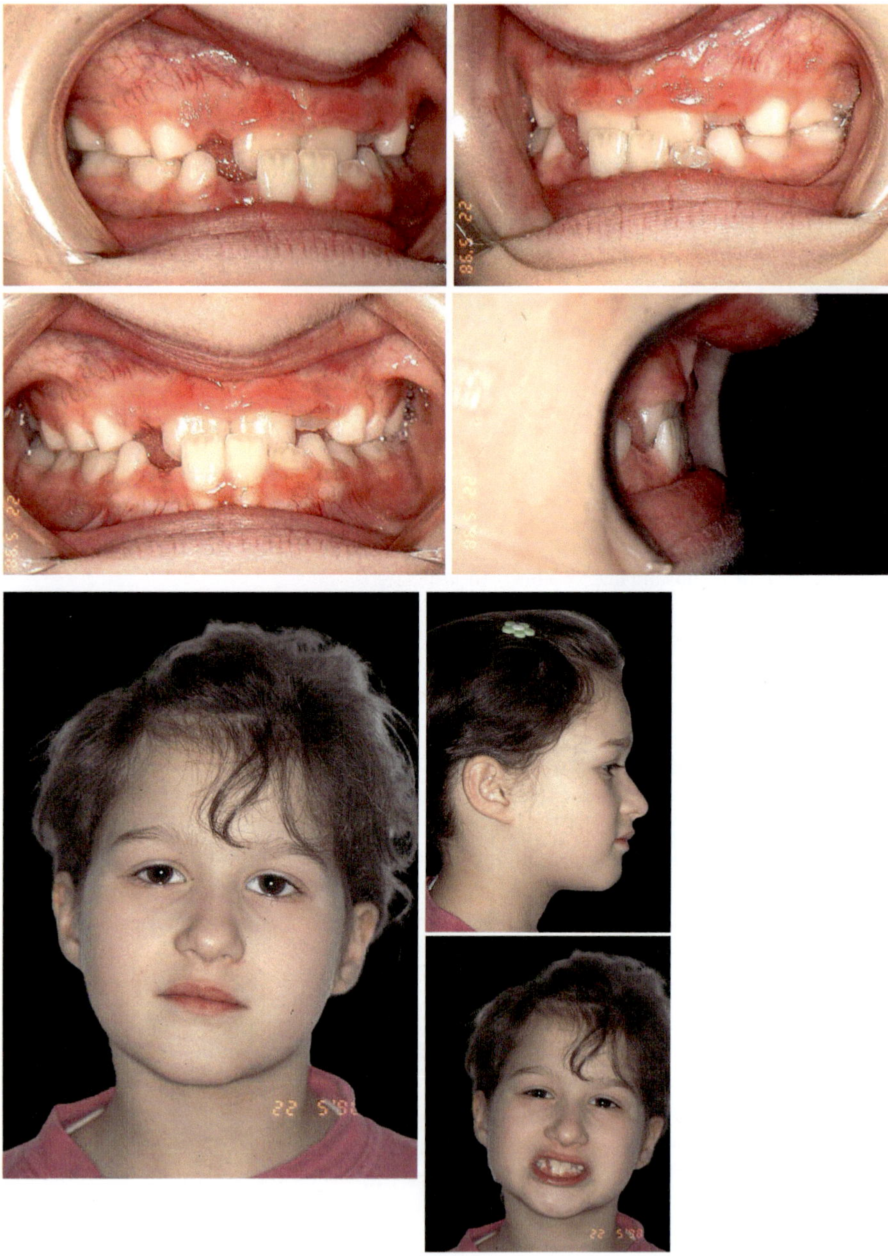

Fig. 12.40 Intra and extraoral photos, before treatment

analysis of the Class III discrepancy using Kinesiography. This functional evaluation was conducted in July 2001, and the results are presented in Figs. 12.42, 12.43, 12.44, 12.45, 12.46 and 12.47 for reference. It is important to note that the purpose

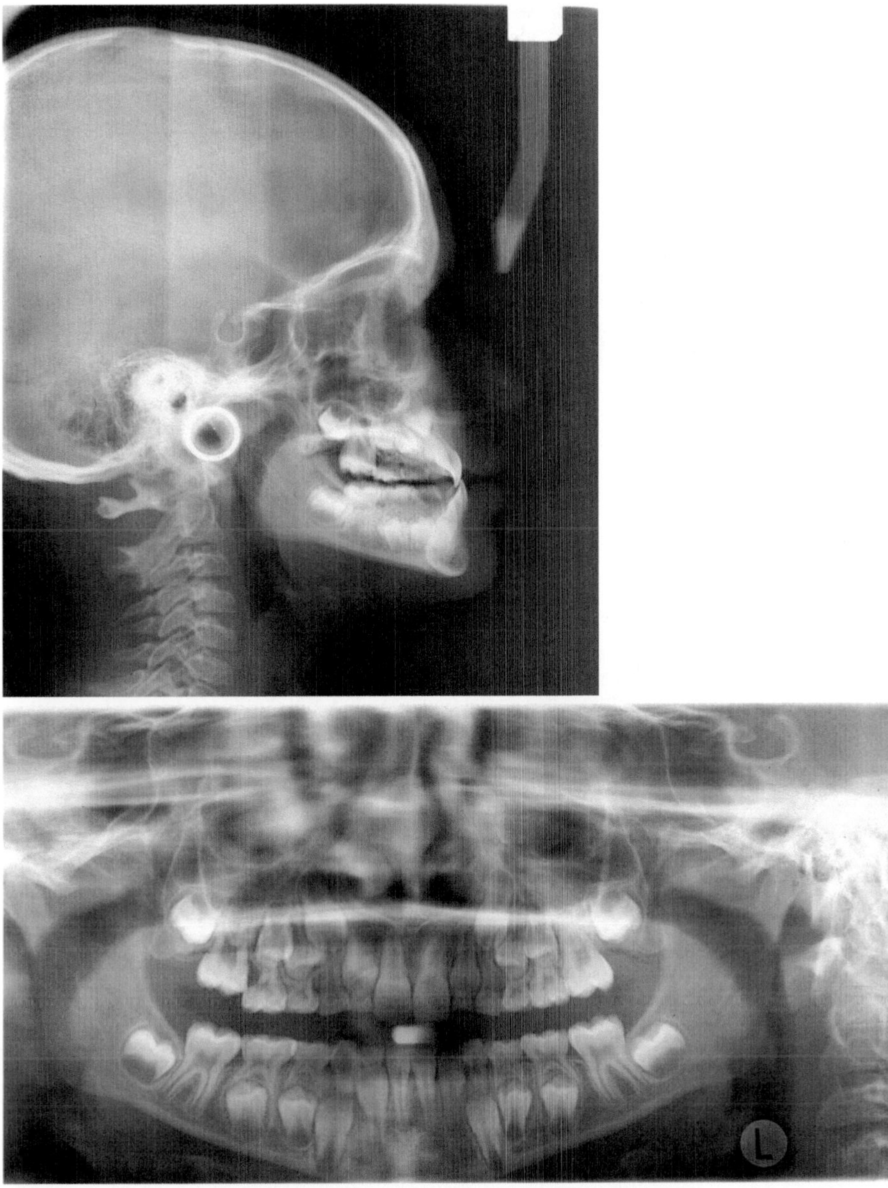

Fig. 12.41 Lateral cephalogram and panoramic X-ray before treatment

of the kinesiographic assessment was to develop an optimal treatment plan that could address the patient's unique muscular requests and to gain valuable insights into the underlying factors contributing to the malocclusion.

Figure 12.46 depicts scan 10, and the values obtained from this scan should fall within the normal range before proceeding to scan 4/5. Unfortunately, it is often

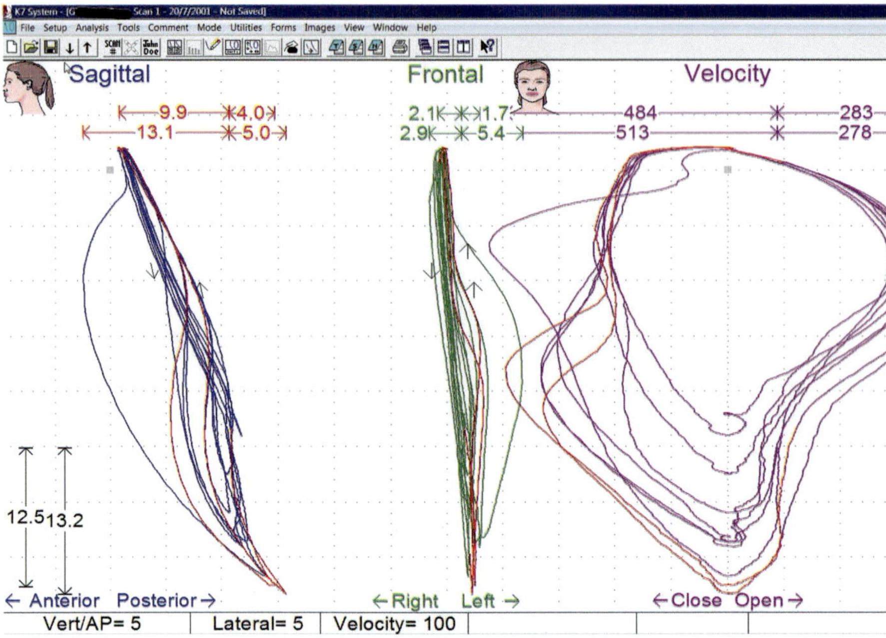

Fig. 12.42 Scan 1 (post interceptive treatment) shows that the sagittal, frontal, and velocity tracings were within the normal limits. The sagittal tracing shows that during the first half of closure there is an increment in speed that corresponds to anterior trajectory of closure. The second half of closure tracing shows a reduction of speed as dental occlusion gets closer. This pattern can be significant for anterior wall. The speed at tooth contact to CO is good. AP: anterior-posterior; CO: centric occlusion; Vert:vertical

challenging to relax the musculature within a 45-min period of tensing, especially for an 11-year-old girl. Scan 10 was taken 33 min after the deconditioning started, as the child could no longer tolerate TENS application. Therefore, even though scan 4/5 is compromised, we can still gather useful information for our neuromuscular orthodontic diagnosis.

Figure 12.47 shows scan 4/5 post-interceptive treatment. There is a large freeway space and anterior/posterior discrepancy. This case has a positive outlook because the RP is well behind the vertical line through CO. This means that vertical correction through extrusion procedure can produce the best physiological correction. Incisor correction is necessary (torque) because the protrusion as seen in scan 5 is certainly very steep. Any forward movement of CO on HP is well accepted. These measurements show that the physiological requests are certainly excessive, so an aggressive orthopedic treatment was advisable.

The treatment began in July 2001 with a fixed appliance that emphasized expansion and extrusion mechanics. Once the lower arch was engaged with a stainless steel archwire (0.019 × 0.025), class III elastics were applied continuously ¼ in. 4.5 oz. In addition, a facemask with 400-gram elastics was attached to soldered hooks on the upper arch. Back bends were applied to the upper archwire to increase

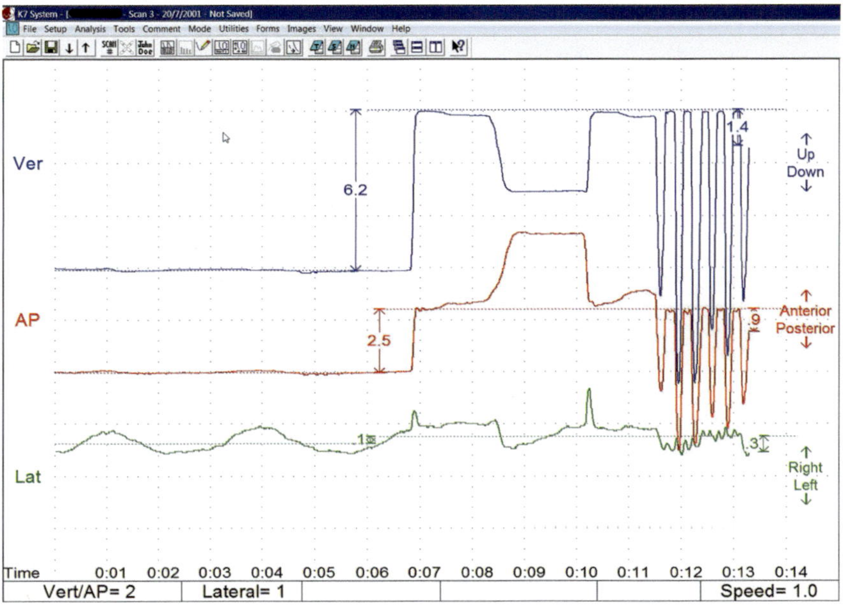

Fig. 12.43 Scan 3 (post interceptive treatment) shows the vertical, anterior-posterior, and lateral movements of the mandible in sweep mode. The patient was instructed to maintain the mandible in the rest position and then to close it to CO. There was an excess in freeway space (6.2 mm). When closing, there was an anterior, forward movement (2.5 mm). AP: anterior-posterior; Lat: lateral; Ver: vertical

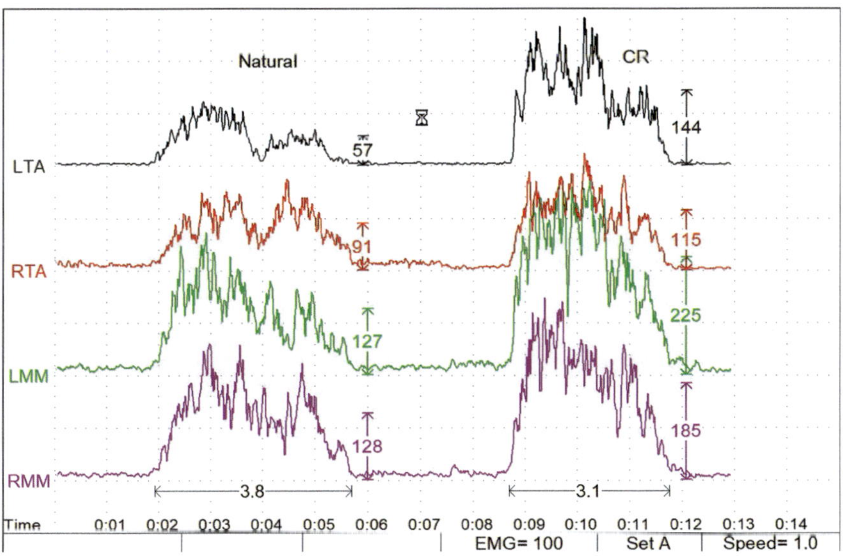

Fig. 12.44 Scan 11 (post-interceptive treatment) showing muscle function during clench (MVC) was with balanced masseters and unbalanced temporalis muscles and the overall output was good.; LMM: left masseter muscle; LTA: left anterior temporalis; RMM: right masseter muscle; RTA: right anterior temporalis

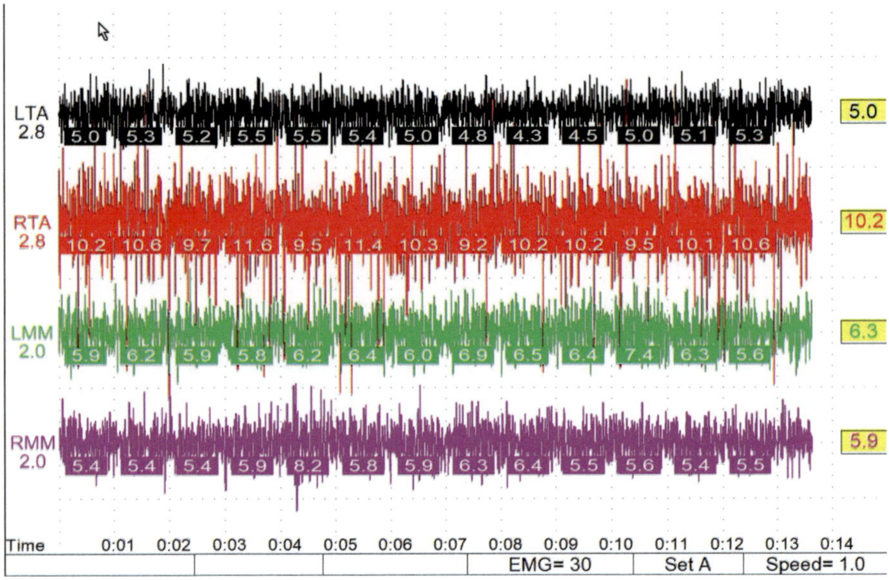

Fig. 12.45 Scan 9 (post-interceptive treatment) shows that the muscles were not relaxed (pre-TENS). LMM: left masseter muscle; LTA: left anterior temporalis; RMM: right masseter muscle; RTA: right anterior temporalis; TENS: transcutaneous electrical nerve stimulation

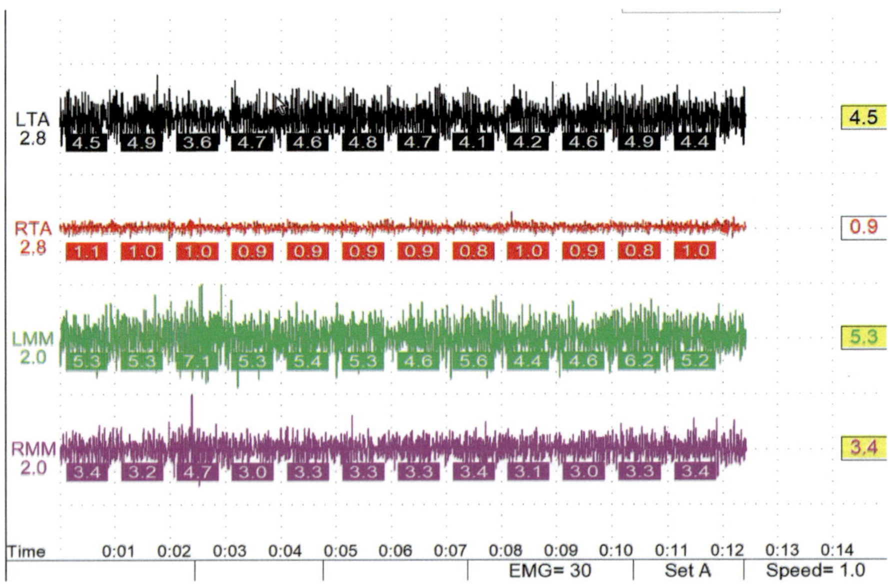

Fig. 12.46 Scan 10 (post-interceptive treatment) shows that the muscles were not fully relaxed(after TENS). An Aqualizer was used to avoid tooth contact for CNS deconditioning. CNS: central nervous system; LMM: left masseter muscle; LTA: left anterior temporalis; RMM: right masseter muscle; RTA: right anterior temporalis; TENS: transcutaneous electrical nerve stimulation

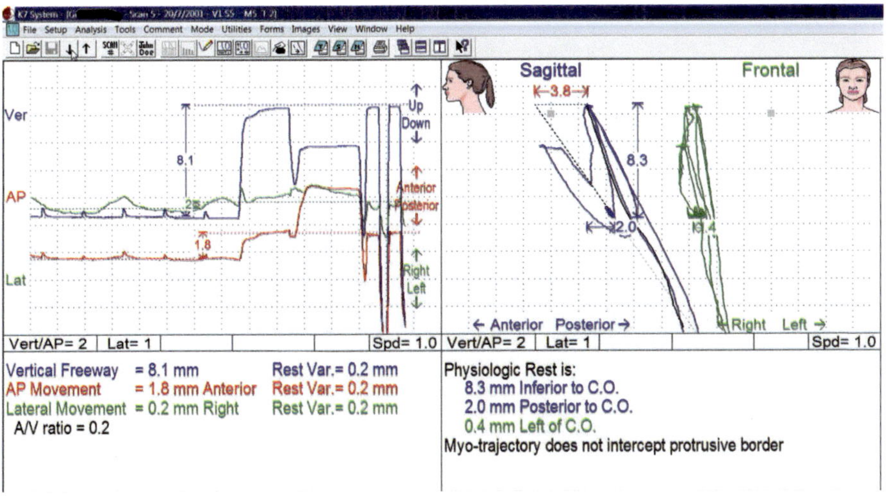

Fig. 12.47 Scan 4/ 5 ((post-interceptive treatment) Showing a 3.8-mm. AP discrepancy on HP and an excess of freeway space (8.3 mm). RP is behind the vertical line passing through CO. AP: anterior-posterior; Lat: lateral; Spd: speed; Vert: vertical. Left: black arrows indicate vibration of AP line. Right: in red correct CO position, corrected HP. The AP discrepancy is actually 0.9 mm on the HP

anchorage. The patient was instructed to wear the facemask only at home, during which time class III elastics were suspended.

After 21 months of fixed orthodontic therapy, the patient expressed satisfaction with the results and the treatment was terminated in May 2003. An upper removable retention appliance was given to be worn for 18 h/day, while lower fixed 3–3 retention was applied. The final results of this treatment can be seen in Fig. 12.48 from June 2003.

Figure 12.48 depicts extraoral photographs that reveal a noticeable lateral head tilt. It is possible that this positioning is a result of a habitual or attitudinal inclination. This finding is important to note as it can impact the evaluation and interpretation of the patient's facial and dental features. Further investigation and consideration may be required to accurately assess and address this characteristic. Final X-rays, the lateral cephalogram and panoramic show characteristic skeletal deep bite with excess freeway space.

Follow-Up

Figures 12.49 and 12.50 show the follow-up intra- and extra-oral photos 20 years after treatment.

The patient has been without retention for 18 years, is asymptomatic and still satisfied with occlusal aesthetics. A complete K7 functional examination was conducted in 2/2023 to evaluate treatment outcome. A selection of the resulting scans is reported in Figs. 12.51, 12.52, 12.53, 12.54 and 12.55.

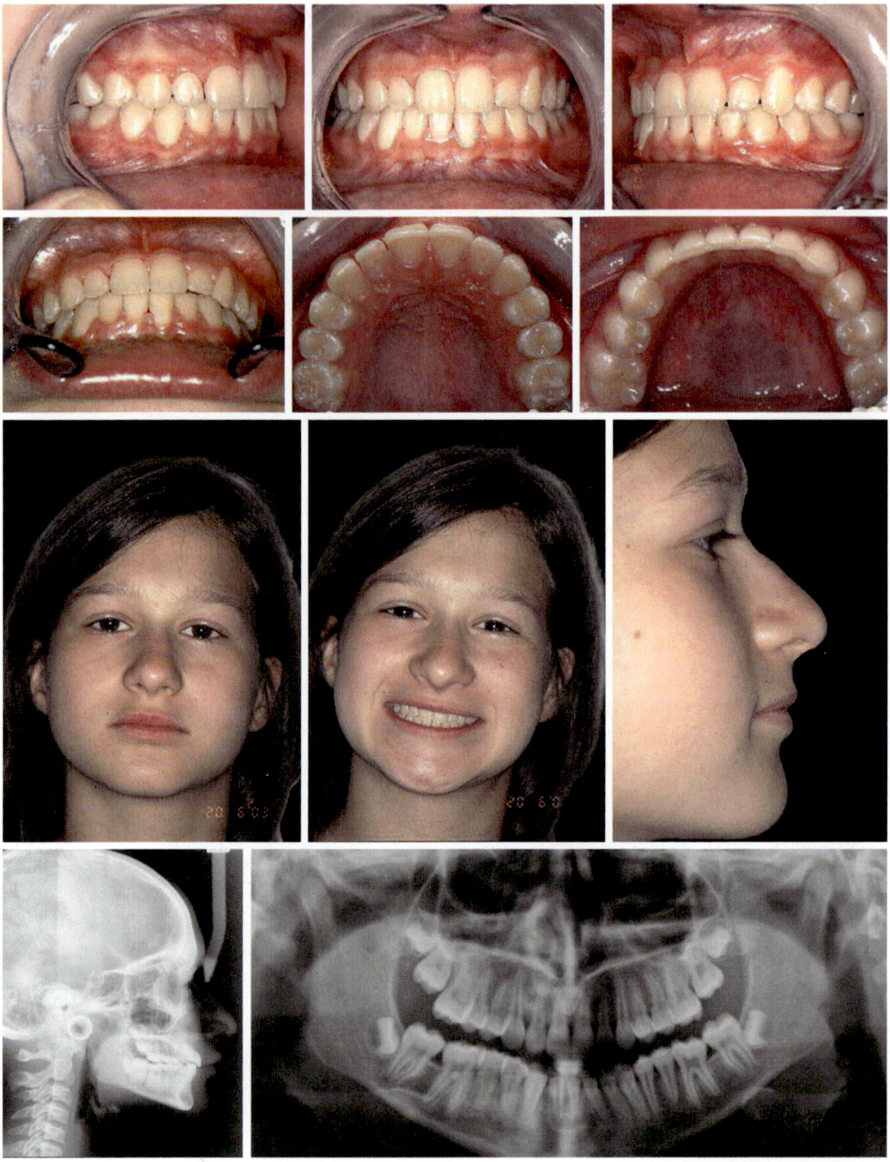

Fig. 12.48 Intra-and extraoral post-treatment photos, June 2003. Lateral cephalogram and panoramic X-rays

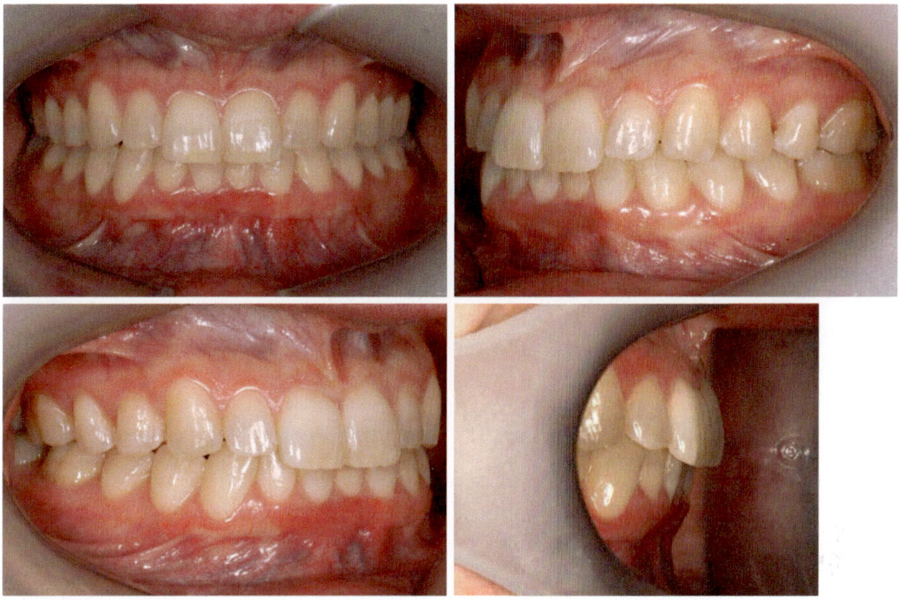

Fig. 12.49 Intraoral photos at 20 years after treatment

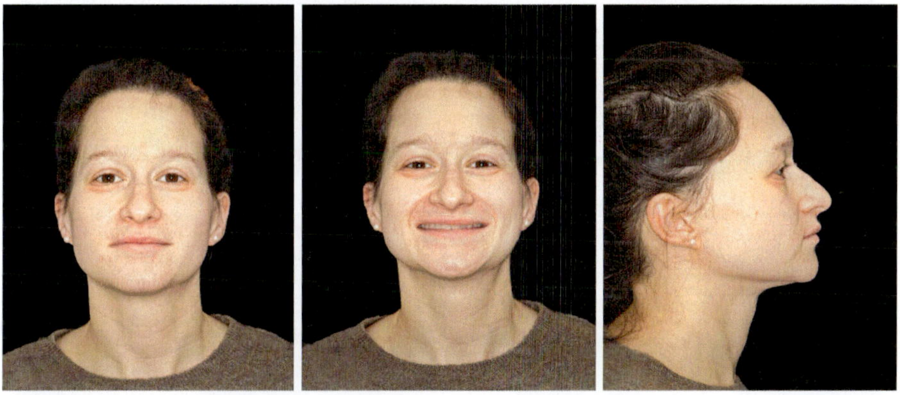

Fig. 12.50 Extraoral photos at 20 years after treatment

The primary aim of neuromuscular Orthodontics is not simply the end result of treatment, but rather the lifelong benefits it provides. This case, along with others, serves as evidence that the application of neuromuscular theory is a valid approach to preventing TMD and related occlusal disharmonies in orthodontics. It is important to monitor and establish the individual's dynamic occlusion's vertical and

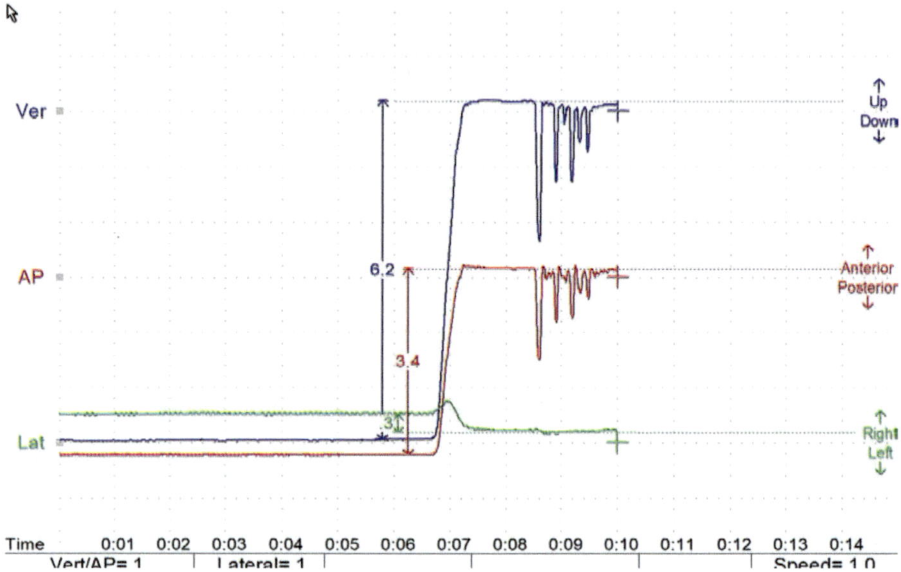

Fig. 12.51 Scan 3 at follow-up after 20 years from treatment, showing the vertical, anterior-posterior, and lateral movements of the mandible in sweep mode. The patient was instructed to maintain the mandible in the rest position and then to close it to CO. There was an excess in free-way space (6.2 mm). AP: anterior-posterior; Lat: lateral; Ver: vertical

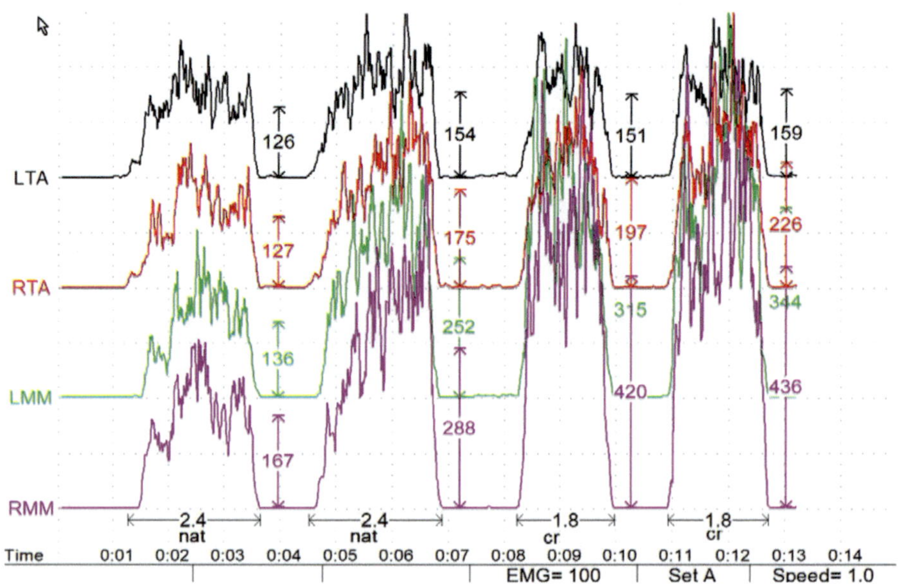

Fig. 12.52 Scan 11 (follow-up after 20 years from treatment) showing the surface EMG results in sweep mode. The patient was instructed to clench in CO (first burst and second burst), and then clench with cotton rolls between the teeth, which temporarily prevented occlusion (third burst and fourth burst). Output s-EMG is satisfactory and the general output is high. CO: centric occlusion; EMG: electromyography; LMM: left masseter muscle; LTA: left anterior temporalis; RMM: right masseter muscle; RTA: right anterior temporalis

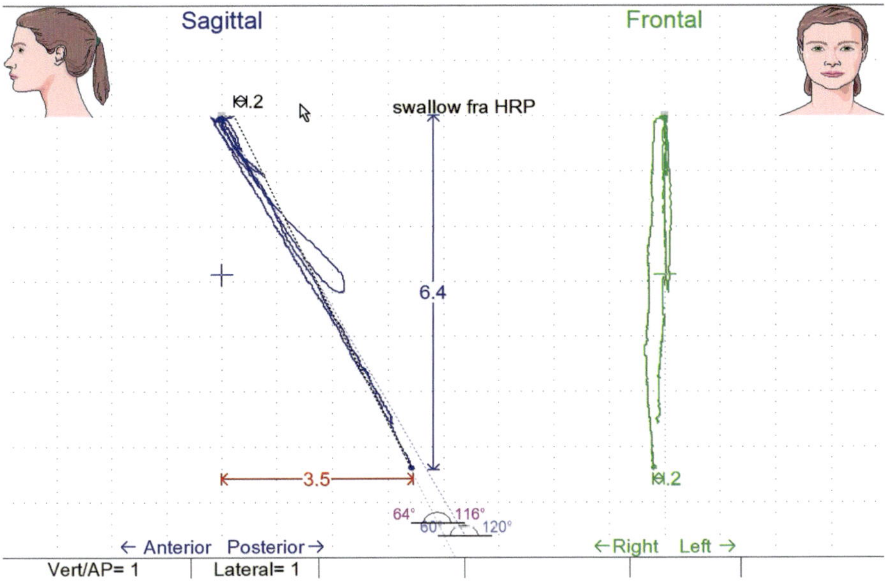

Fig. 12.53 (Follow-up after 20 years from treatment) Sagittal/Frontal swallow pattern from HRP. HRP before swallowing and with a projected trajectory is overlapping the habitual path of closure. This is a positive feature that can anticipate a positive scan 5 result

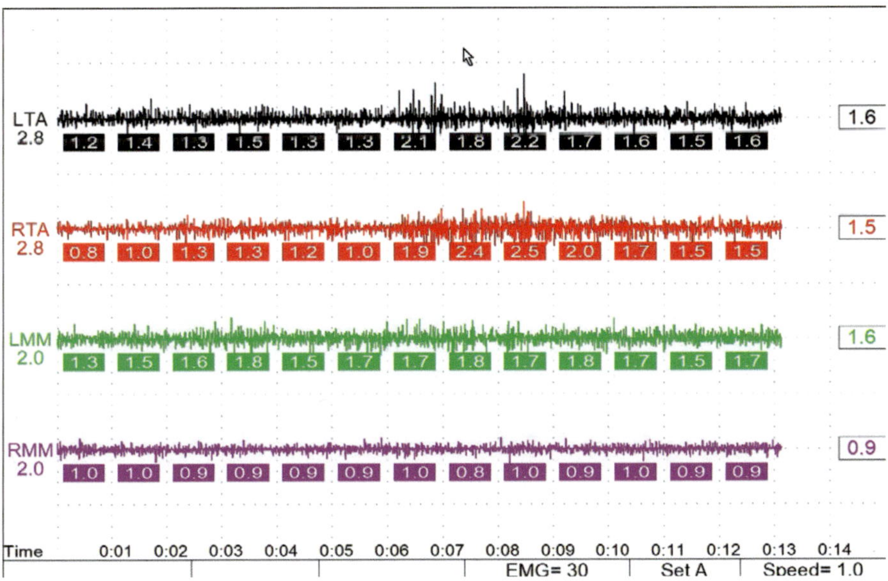

Fig. 12.54 (Follow-up after 20 years from treatment) Scan 10 shows that the muscles were relaxed (after TENS). An Aqualizer was used to avoid tooth contact for CNS deconditioning. CNS: central nervous system; LMM: left masseter muscle; LTA: left anterior temporalis; RMM: right masseter muscle; RTA: right anterior temporalis; TENS: transcutaneous electrical nerve stimulation

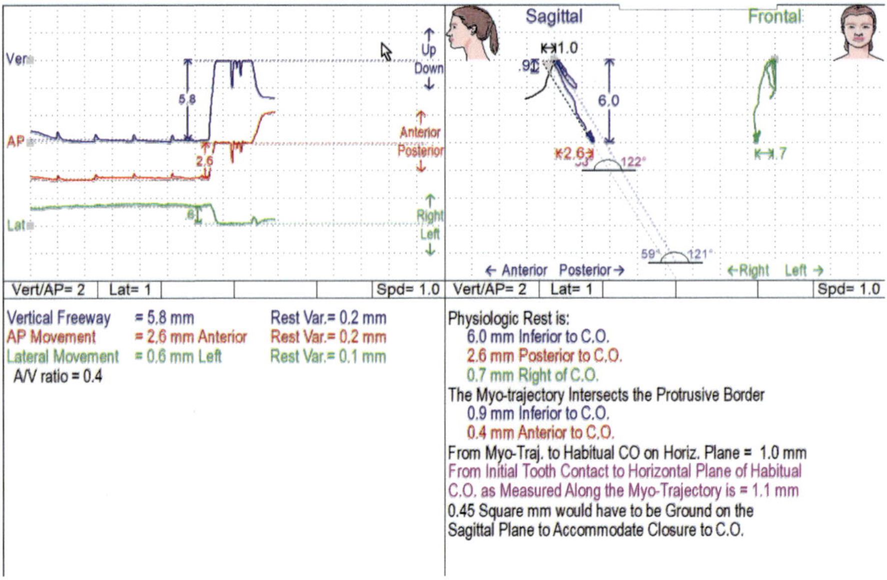

Fig. 12.55 (Follow-up after 20 years from treatment) Scan 4/5 in split screen modality. On the left sweep of V, AP, and Lat lines. The patient is instructed to rest mandibular posture and the instructed to close to Centric Occlusion. Note the TENS spikes on V and AP lines. On the right, the corresponding Sagittal/frontal scan 5 shows a 1-mm. AP discrepancy on HP. AP: anterior-posterior; CO: centric occlusion; Lat: lateral; Spd: speed; Vert: vertical. HP: Horizontal Plane of Occlusion

sagittal requests objectively to anticipate a stable functional outcome for the patient's future. While orthodontic treatment can be aggressive in extruding dentures in severe deep bite individuals, there are limits to what it can achieve. Scan 5 taken in 2023 shows that the freeway space is 6 mm. Unfortunately, severe deep bites lead to freeway space increase as a natural outcome of counterclockwise mandibular rotation during growth and development. Thus, limiting or slowing down this physiological trend is one of the primary technical objectives of this treatment.

Case 12.4

Class I Occlusion with TMD Symptoms

Summary A 40-year-old Caucasian woman presented with a concern regarding misaligned teeth and sought orthodontic treatment. Upon further inquiry, it was discovered that she had a history of cervical pain and pain in the left temporomandibular joint (TMJ).

Pre-treatment	
Extraoral analysis	
Facial profile	Flat
Facial height	Normal
Occlusal plane	Normal
Facial symmetry	
Lips	Competent
Mandibular posture	
Head posture	
Intraoral analysis (Fig. 12.56)	
Teeth	
Molar class	I
Canine class	I
Overjet	Negative
Overbite	
Oral hygiene	Fair
Rotations of lower and upper canines	
Crossbite	
Diastemas	
Crowding	Slight upper/lower
Agenesis	
Missing teeth	
Intraoral analysis (Fig. 12.57)	
Swallow	Tongue thrust
Tongue tie	No
Tongue posture	Normal
Tongue thrust	
Slurred speech	
Cephalometrics	
Neuromuscular diagnosis	
Freeway space norm	
Skeletal class	I
Anterior wall	Yes
TMJ left pain during aperture (functional pain), click during opening	
TMJ right	
Problem list • Mandible is blocked posteriorly from anterior wall. • Lower crowding.	
Neuromuscular treatment objectives • Mandibular freedom. • Increase OJ to align the lower arch. • Correct tongue posture and swallow.	

Introduction

Upon reviewing the anamnestic records, it was found that the patient had no history of physical traumas, sleeping or dietary problems, or chronic diseases. Additionally, the patient reported being very happy with a pleasant life, good sleep quality, and no bad habits. However, it was noted that she is currently experiencing cervical pain and TMJ pain which affects her daily routine. Alignment issues were also identified, and the patient requested orthodontic treatment in the hope of reducing the symptoms in the cervical area as well as alleviating the pain on the left TMJ.

Figures 12.56 and 12.57 show the intra- and extraoral photos before treatment.

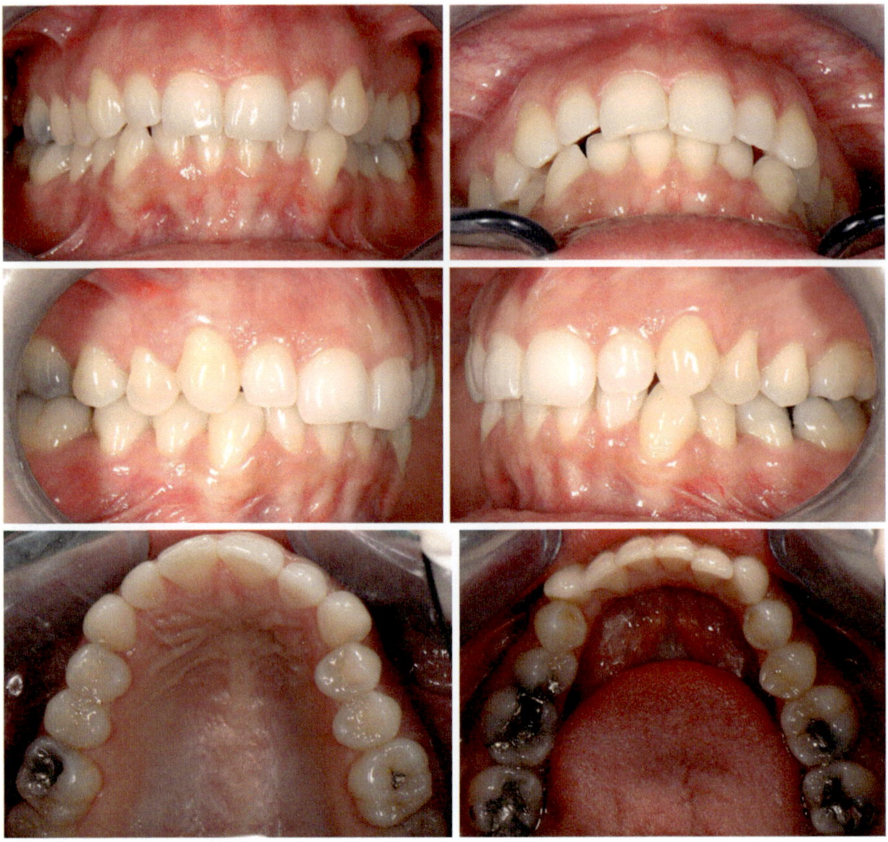

Fig. 12.56 Pre-treatment intraoral photos

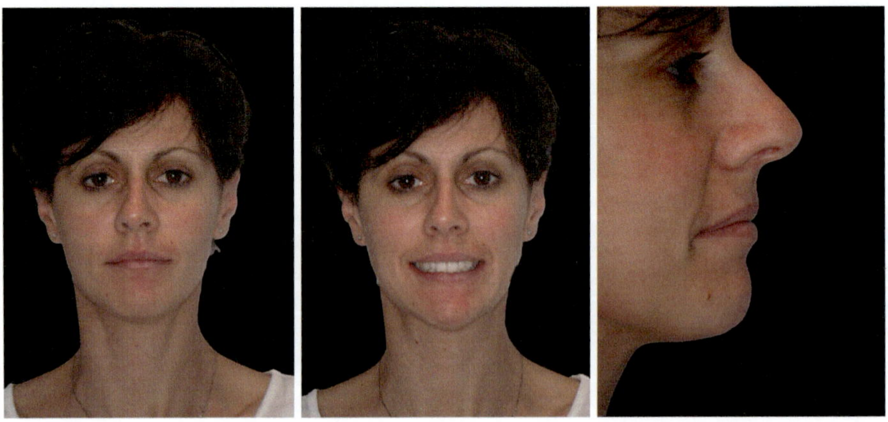

Fig. 12.57 Pretreatment extraoral photos

Orthodontic treatment with the fixed appliance commenced in July 2015, using the Savasystem® bracket prescription. Initially, the appliance was applied to the upper arch and maintained solely on the upper dentition for 12 months. As expected, a significant reduction of 90% in symptomatology was observed within 4 months, which corresponded to the upper expansion and alignment achieved. The procedure for aligning the upper arch and correcting the torque of the upper incisors enabled the attainment of mandibular freedom (MF) with ease. Only after 13 months of treatment, the lower arch was included in the fixed appliance therapy.

This is a typical case of mild temporomandibular disorder (TMD), in which the posterior displacement of the condylar is caused by the upper front wall. A complete K7 diagnostic procedure was conducted to diagnose this condition, and the results are shown in Fig. 12.58.

In Fig. 12.58, a significant lateral deviation is observed on the affected side, where the patient experiences pain and discomfort. Figs. 12.59 and 12.60 Show Scan 11 with MVC and balanced muscular output. Scan 3 is within normal limits, with a slight excess of freeway space (3.8 mm). This deviation is likely due to a disk interference that results from posterior condylar displacement on the left. Figure 12.61 presents the most crucial finding, as it measures the sagittal and vertical requests from the neuromuscular system. Scan 5, in particular, shows a significant discrepancy in the horizontal plane of the projected Myotrajectory (≥4.1 mm) and an increase in freeway space (4.4 mm). This indicates that our orthodontic

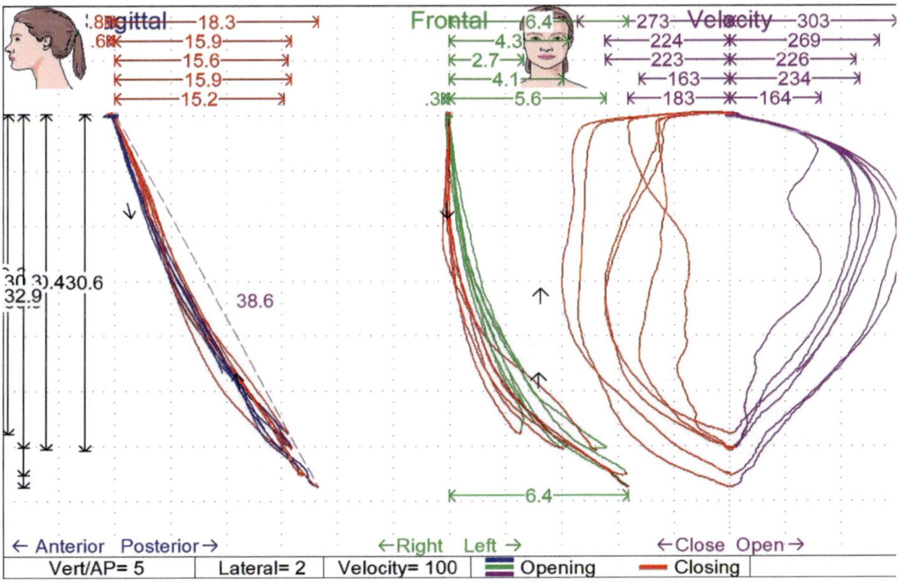

Fig. 12.58 Scan 1 (pre-treatment) shows that the degree of mouth opening was satisfactory (the total mouth aperture was approximately 38 mm), there was a significant lateral deviation to the left upon opening (6.4 mm), and the velocity at tooth contact was also satisfactory. AP: anterior-posterior; Vert: vertical

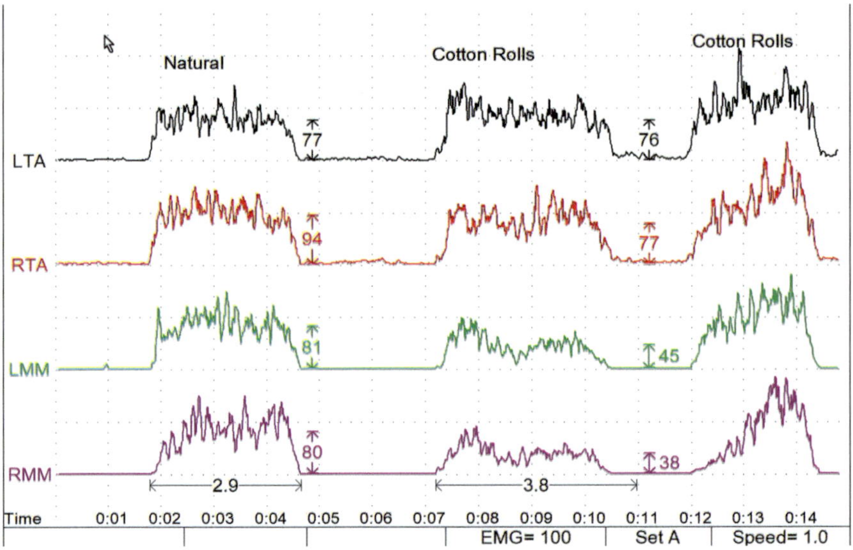

Fig. 12.59 Scan 11 (pre-treatment) shows the surface EMG results in sweep mode. The patient was instructed to clench in CO (first burst and second burst), and then clench with cotton rolls between the teeth, which temporarily prevented occlusion (third burst). The general s-EMG output is slightly low but shows some balancing between muscle groups. CO: centric occlusion; EMG: electromyography; LMM: left masseter muscle; LTA: left anterior temporalis; RMM: right masseter muscle; RTA: right anterior temporalis

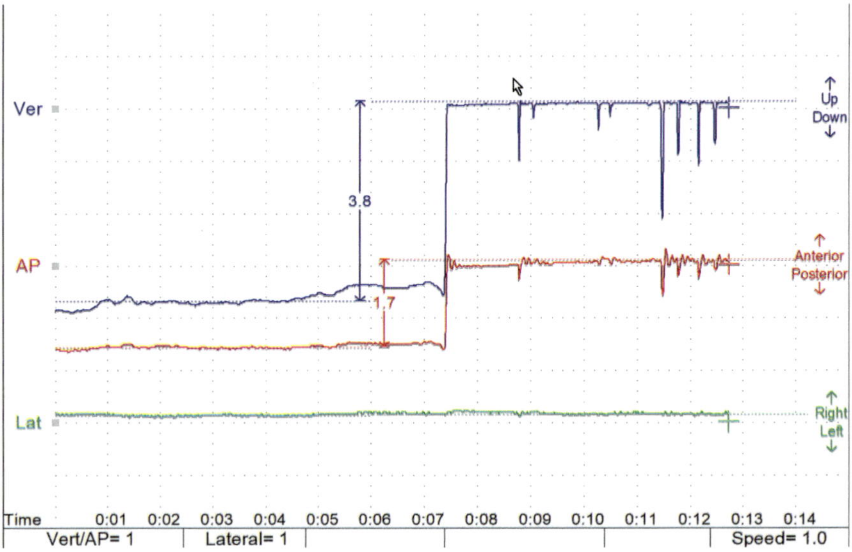

Fig. 12.60 Scan 3 (pre-treatment) showing the vertical, anterior-posterior, and lateral movements of the mandible in sweep mode. The patient was instructed to maintain the mandible in the rest position and then to close it to CO. There was an excess in freeway space (3.8 mm). When closing, there was an anterior, forward movement (1.7 mm). AP: anterior-posterior; Lat: lateral; Ver: vertical

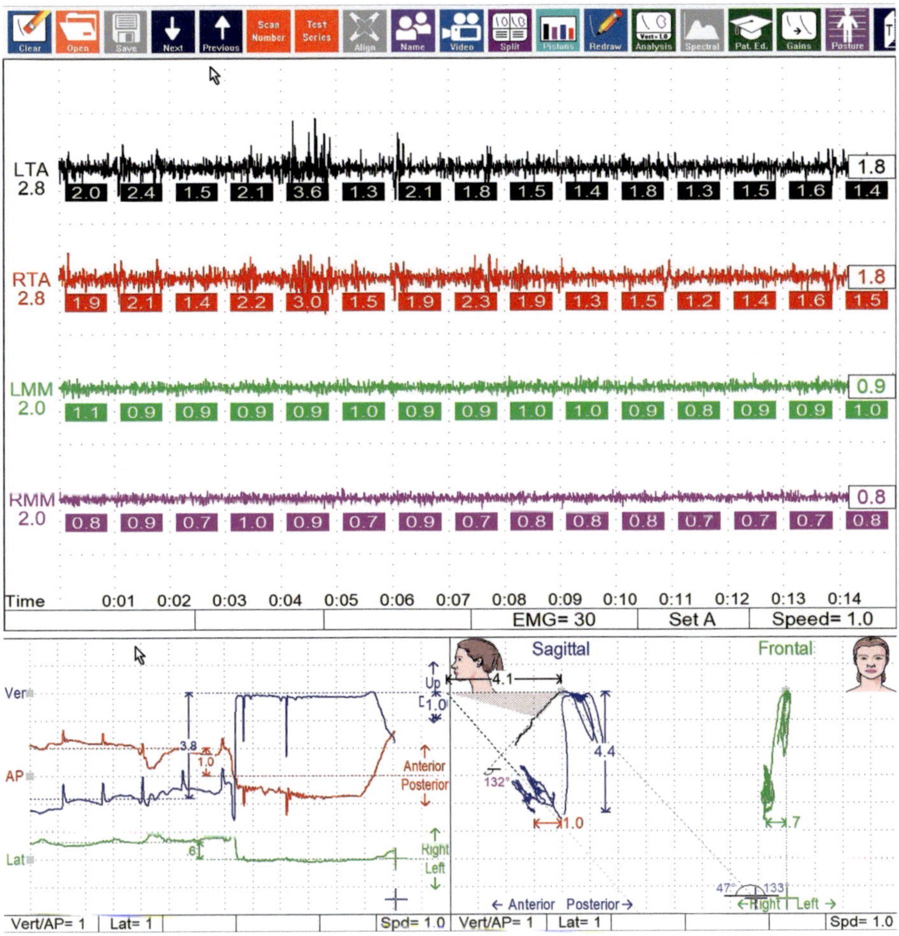

Fig. 12.61 Pre-treatment scans: upper: Scan 10 shows that the muscles were relaxed (after TENS). An Aqualizer was used to avoid tooth contact for CNS deconditioning. CNS: central nervous system; LMM: left masseter muscle; LTA: left anterior temporalis; RMM: right masseter muscle; RTA: right anterior temporalis; TENS: transcutaneous electrical nerve stimulation. Lower: Showing scan 4/5 in split screen modality. On the left sweep of V, AP, and Lat lines. The patient is instructed to rest mandibular posture and the instructed to close to Centric Occlusion. Note the TENS spikes on V and AP lines. On the right, the corresponding Sagittal/frontal scan 5 shows a 4.1-mm. AP discrepancy on HP and a vertical freeway space of 4.4 mm. AP: anterior-posterior; CO: centric occlusion; Lat: lateral; Spd: speed; Vert: vertical. HP: Horizontal Plane of Occlusion

therapy must create an overjet (OJ) of at least 4.1 mm to accommodate postural mandibular repositioning. Additionally, extra OJ will be required to align the lower incisors ***on that horizontal plane of occlusion (HP). Extrusion lowers the HP and can reduce sagittal functional requests***. However, the PRP is located in front of the V line, making it imperative to bring the CO point forward. For this reason, it is essential to avoid lower alignment until adequate room is available. Premature

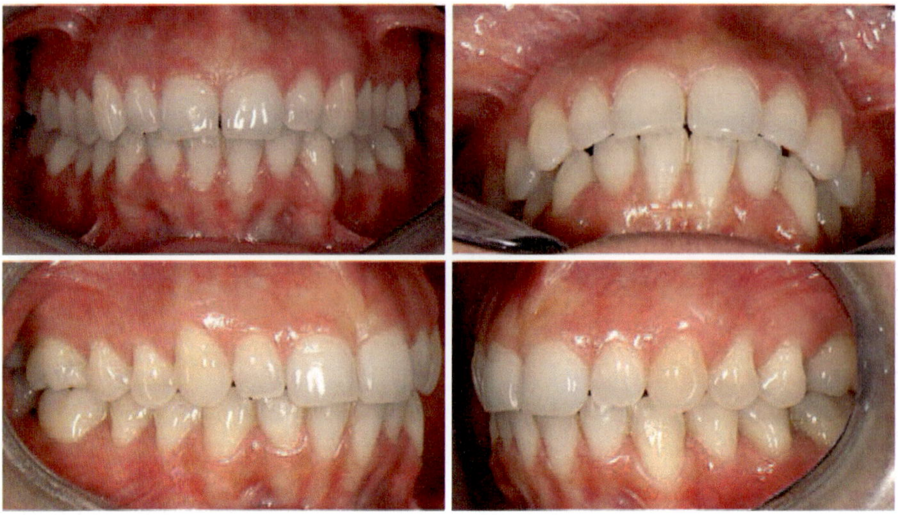

Fig. 12.62 Intraoral photos, at 5 years post-treatment

alignment of lower front incisors can cause condylar distalization in the glenoid fossa. In this case, expansion of the upper arch focuses on the premaxilla, while low force class III elastics (1/4 4.5 oz.) are worn for 24 h. Class III elastics promote lower distal crown tipping, which favors anterior positioning of the condyle and reduces the anterior space required for lower alignment. The extrusion effect is highly beneficial in reducing freeway space and, as a result, reducing the AP discrepancy.

The sagittal discrepancy is severe and can explain TMD symptoms. The RP after TENS is anterior to the V line, indicating a very challenging treatment procedure.

Treatment was terminated in September 2017 and a removable upper appliance was delivered for retention. Fixed lower 3–3 retention was applied. Follow-ups were every 3 months, and a full K7 evaluation, X-rays, and photos were performed in January 2023. The results can be seen with the intra- and extraoral photos in Figs. 12.62 and 12.63.

Discussion

At 5 years, post-treatment the patient refers to be asymptomatic since orthodontic treatment. The resulting Kinesiographic scans showed the results obtained through orthodontic therapy. Scan 13 (Fig. 12.64) showed a decrease in lateral left deviation upon aperture. Since there was no appreciation of any particular TMJ noise, most likely the condylar repositioning favored a correct articular function. Scan 3 (Fig. 12.65) showed a vertical freeway space of 2.5 mm and a forward movement of 2.1 mm. Even though this ratio is not ideal, it is an indication that HRP is behind the V line. This is a positive feature because we have now permitted the mandible to assume a more anterior position and if we had not corrected sagitally with decision,

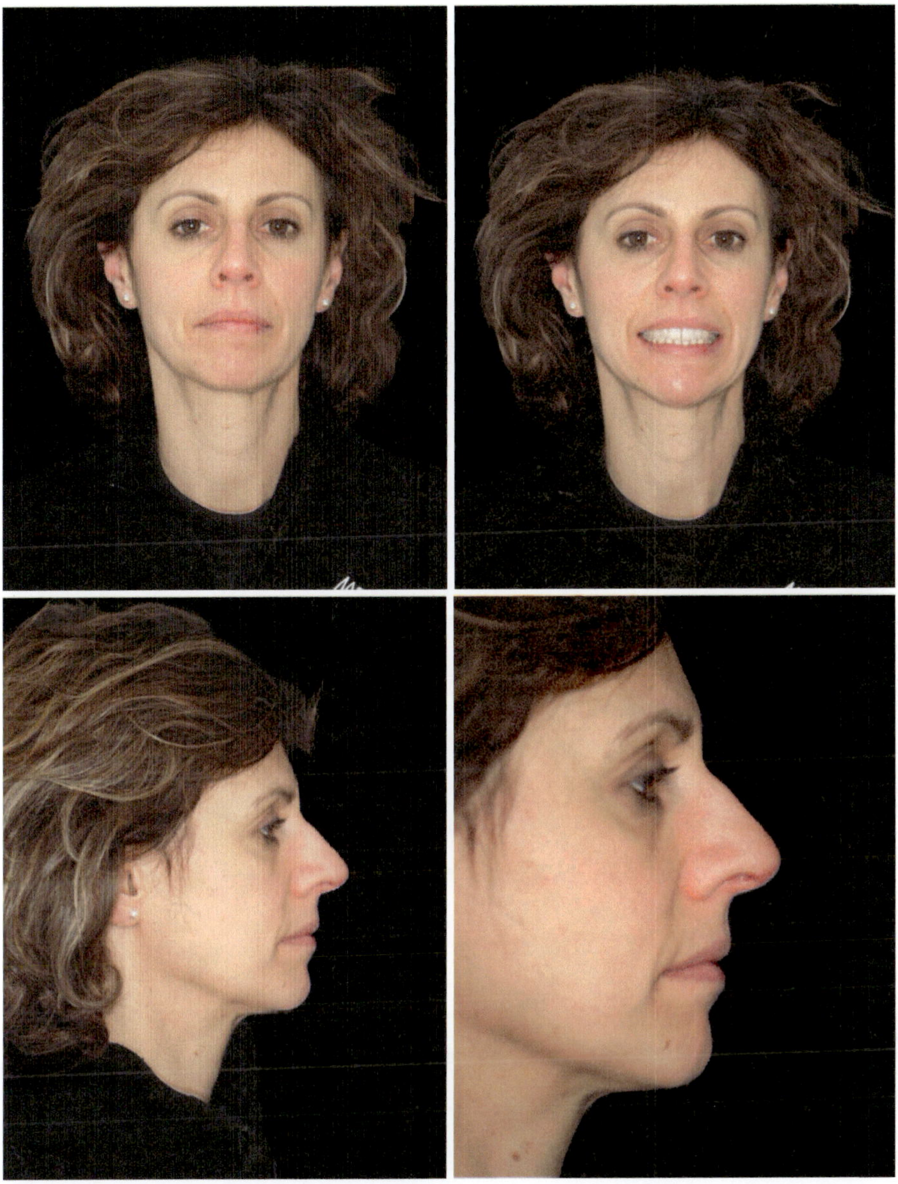

Fig. 12.63 Extraoral photos, 5 years post-treatment

we could have seen an anterior movement well inferior to 1 mm during closure. Scan 9 (Fig. 12.66) shows a good muscle rest output in habitual posture. Scan 11 (Fig. 12.67) shows a balanced output from a symmetric point of view. There is a favoring of the Temporalis output in respect of the Masseter output. In general, this can be considered a satisfactory result, because the differences are rather limited.

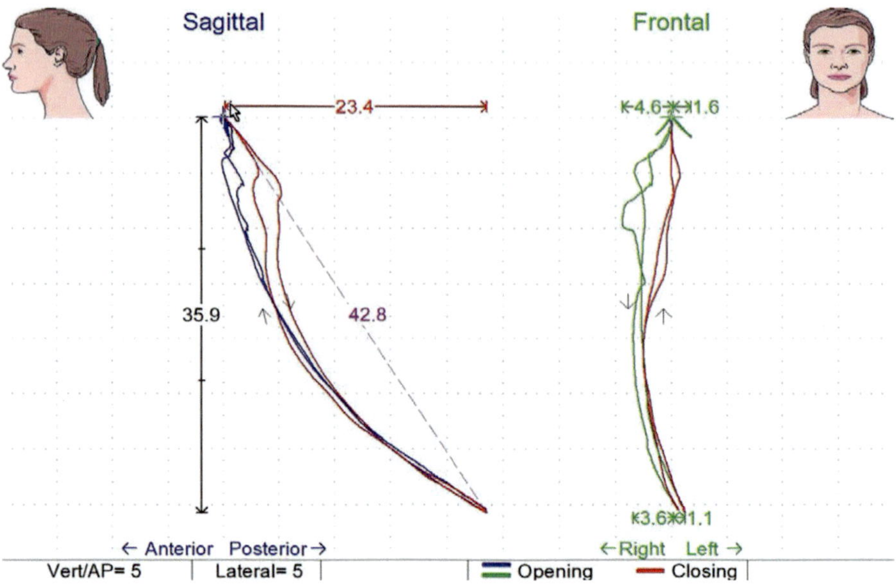

Fig. 12.64 (5 years post-treatment) Scan 13, range of motion with lateral canine disocclusion. AP: anterior-posterior

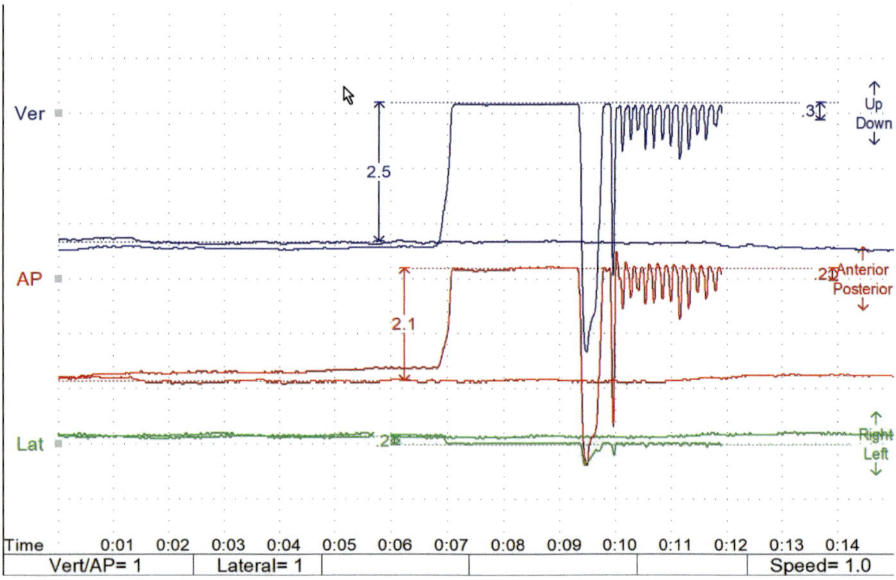

Fig. 12.65 (5 years post-treatment Scan 3 (post-treatment) showing the vertical, anterior-posterior, and lateral movements of the mandible in sweep mode. The patient was instructed to maintain the mandible in the rest position and then to close it to CO. There was a very slight excess in freeway space (2.5 mm). When closing, there was an anterior, forward movement (2.1 mm). AP: anterior-posterior; Lat: lateral; Ver: vertical

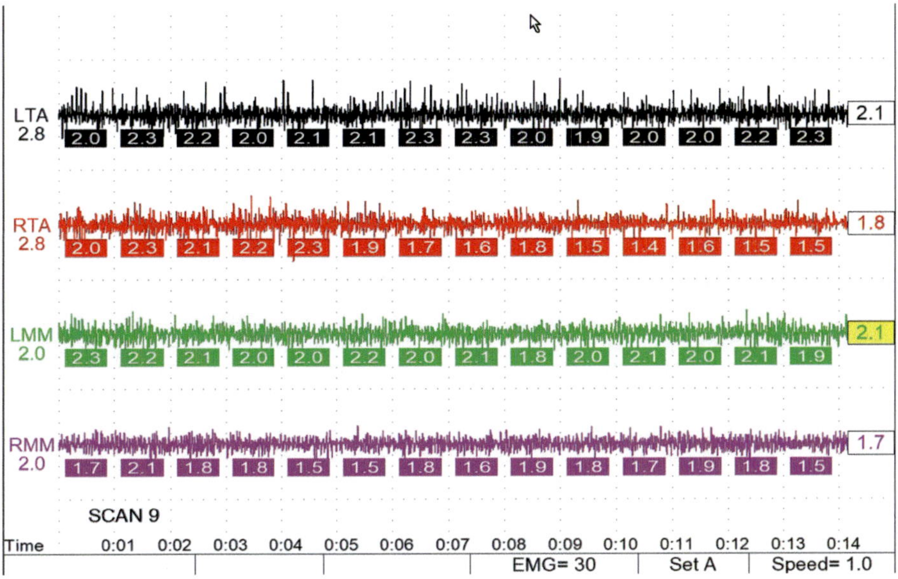

Fig. 12.66 (5 years post-treatment) Scan 9 showing that the muscles were relaxed (pre-TENS). LMM: left masseter muscle; LTA: left anterior temporalis; RMM: right masseter muscle; RTA: right anterior temporalis; TENS: transcutaneous electrical nerve stimulation

Swallow Assessement

Figures 12.68 and 12.69 show two polygraphic scans (Scan 21) to study swallow function in this patient. Figure 12.68 shows a VSS (Voluntary Swallow of Saliva) that starts from "D" point. Note the activation of the masseters prior to that of the Temporalis muscles, indicating that swallow starts with the tongue between the dental arches. Figure 12.69 shows capture of a SSS (Spontaneous Saliva Swallow). Note that here again the masseters are activated prior to the temporalis but a closer look at the mandibular movements reveals that CO is recorded for a very short period of time. During swallowing, a probable anterior tongue thrust is responsible for the loss of CO and the application of a distalizing action on the mandible by tongue dysfunction. This analysis shows that a modest tongue thrust is probably not sufficient in creating an anterior open-bite if no low anterior tongue posture is present. See Fig. 12.69 for explanation.

The patient has been instructed to correct swallow with several OMT exercises but without success. Unfortunately, there is no possible solution to treat these habits without intensive collaboration.

Figure 12.70 shows resting muscle output after 45′ tensing. These results indicate that the resulting scan 4/5 will be highly diagnostic.

Figure 12.71 includes the split screen of scan 4/5. When looking at scan 5 to assess progress achieved with orthodontic/orthopedic therapy, it is notable that now CO and vertical V line are in front of RP. Furthermore, there has been a reduction of freeway space of about 1.1 mm. This extrusive effect has been gained using Class

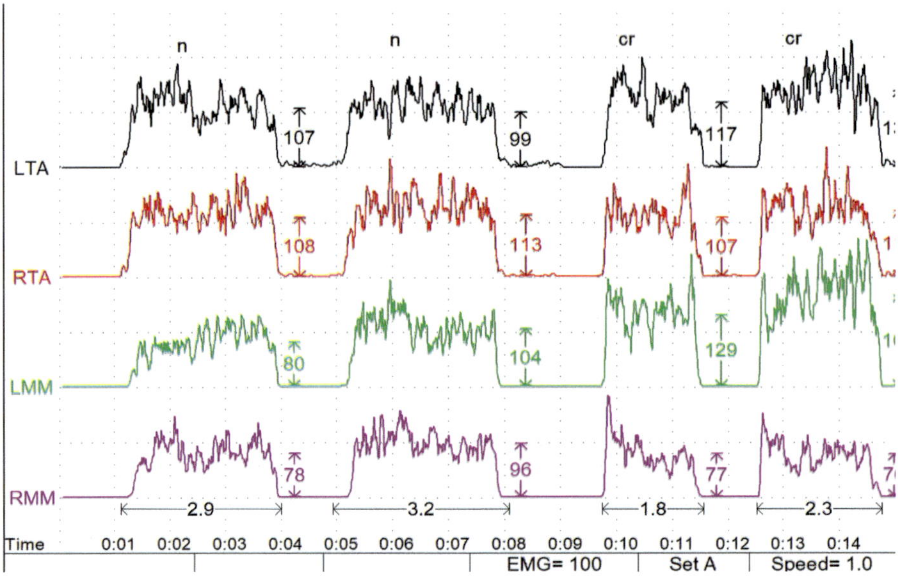

Fig. 12.67 (5 years post-treatment) Scan 11 shows the surface EMG results in sweep mode. The patient was instructed to clench in CO (first burst and second burst), and then clench with cotton rolls between the teeth, which temporarily prevented occlusion (third burst and fourth burst). Output s-EMG is satisfactory. and the general there is a symmetric balancing. The Temporalis have a slightly stronger output during clench in respect of the masseters. CO: centric occlusion; EMG: electromyography; LMM: left masseter muscle; LTA: left anterior temporalis; RMM: right masseter muscle; RTA: right anterior temporalis

III elastics. The other benefit obtained by this type of mechanics, is a counterclockwise rotation of the occlusal plane [5]. Even a small adjustment in a counterclockwise fashion should be considered physiological because it mimics the natural growth and development of the maxillary-mandibular complex [5].

Figure 12.72 shows cephalograms before and at follow-up at 5 years.

Figure 12.73 shows panoramic X-rays before and at 5-year follow-up.

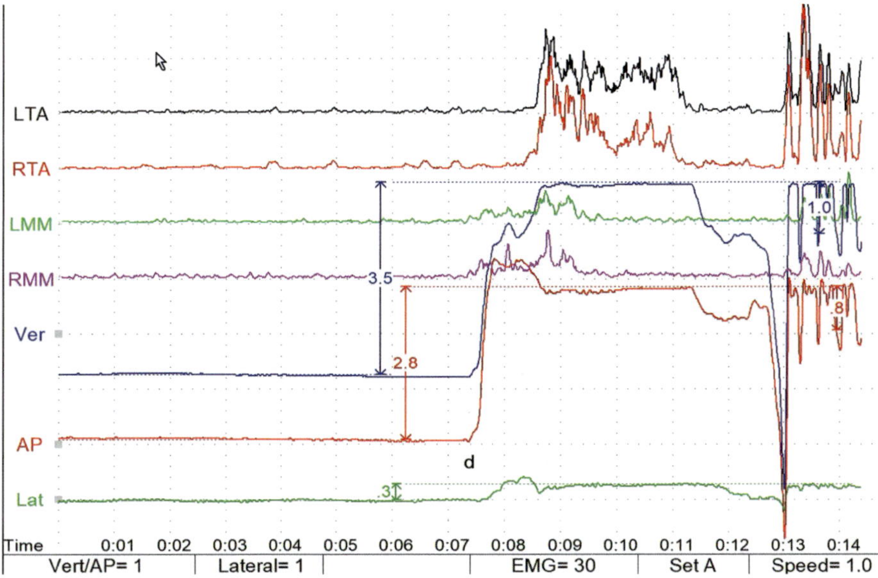

Fig. 12.68 (5 years post-treatment) Polygraphic scan (scan 3 + S-EMG filtered, scan 21) shows a VSS (Spontaneous Swallow of Saliva, indicated with "D"). The vertical blue line shows mandibular closure (upward) when swallow starts. There is a premature activation of the masseter muscles at the start of deglutition sequence indicating that the patient swallows with tongue between the teeth.). LMM: left masseter muscle; LTA: left anterior temporalis; RMM: right masseter muscle; RTA: right anterior temporalis.). AP: anterior-posterior; Lat: lateral; Ver: vertical

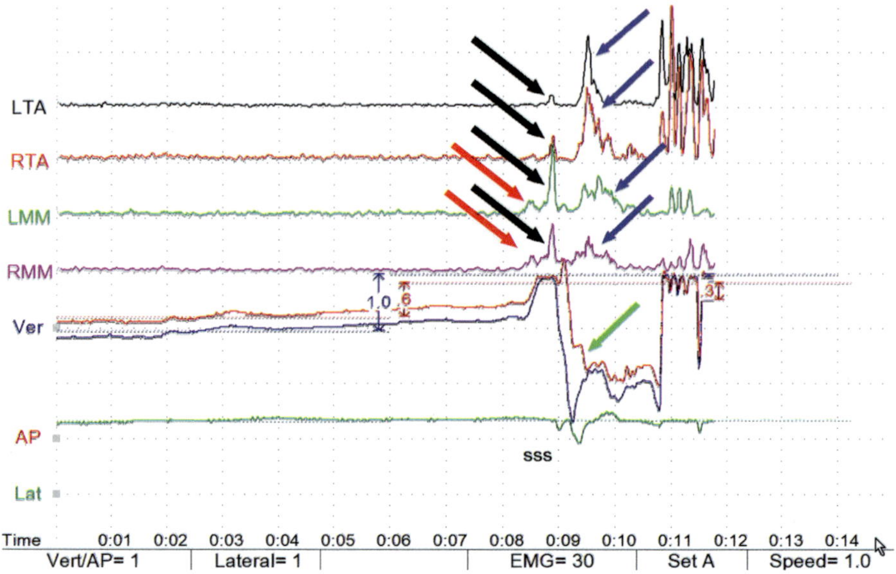

Fig. 12.69 Polygraphic scan (scan 3 + S-EMG filtered, scan 21) (5 years post-treatment) shows a SSS (Spontaneous Swallow of Saliva). The (vertical) blue line shows mandibular closure (upward) when swallow starts. The first muscles that activate are the Masseter muscles (red arrows) showing that patient starts swallowing with tongue between the teeth. The duration of ICP (Inter Cuspal Position) lasts only 0.25 seconds during which masseters and temporalis muscles are well activated (black arrows). During the swallow sequence, the blue (vertical) and red (Anterior/Posterior) lines show mouth opening (green arrow). The strongest muscular reaction is thus elicited at this point of the swallow sequence: the blue arrows indicate a strong effort to avoid mandibular displacement due to tongue activity. The green arrow indicates the exact time frame in which the mandible is finally closing (blue line upward) but red line indicates (going down) that the mandible is moved backward.). LMM: left masseter muscle; LTA: left anterior temporalis; RMM: right masseter muscle; RTA: right anterior temporalis.). AP: anterior-posterior; Lat: lateral; Ver: vertical

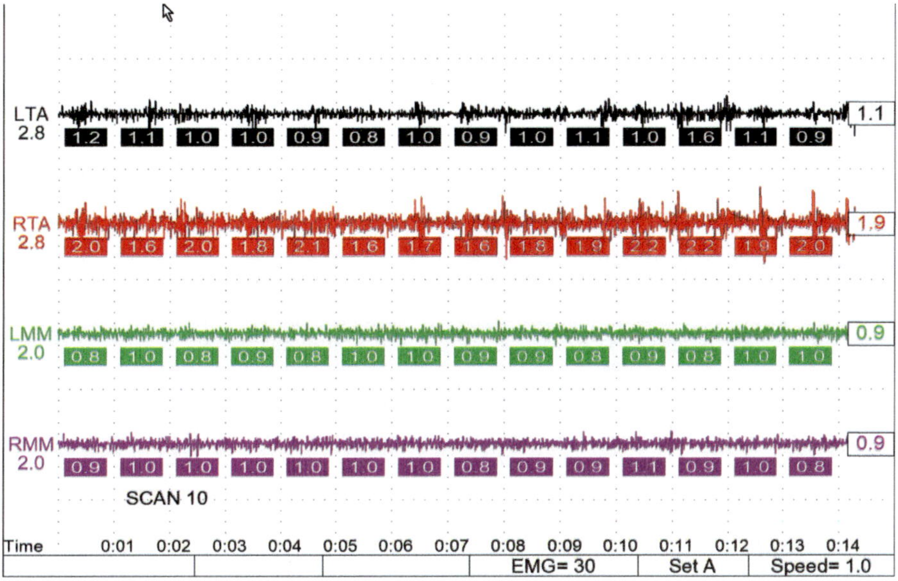

Fig. 12.70 Scan 10 (5 years post-treatment) shows that the muscles were relaxed (after TENS). An Aqualizer was used to avoid tooth contact for CNS deconditioning. CNS: central nervous system; LMM: left masseter muscle; LTA: left anterior temporalis; RMM: right masseter muscle; RTA: right anterior temporalis; TENS: transcutaneous electrical nerve stimulation

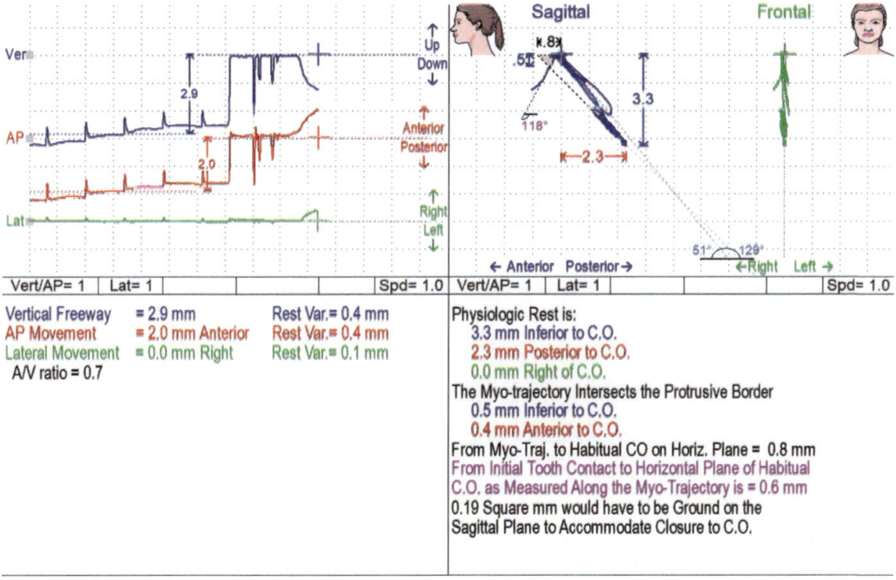

Fig. 12.71 (5 years post-treatment) Scan 4/5 in split screen modality. On the left sweep of V, AP, and Lat lines. The patient is instructed to rest mandibular posture and the instructed to close to Centric Occlusion. Note the TENS spikes on V and AP lines. On the right, the corresponding Sagittal/frontal scan 5 shows a 0.8-mm. AP discrepancy on HP (Horizontal Plane of Occlusion). Vertical freeway space is 3.3 mm. AP: anterior-posterior; CO: centric occlusion; Lat: lateral; Spd: speed; Vert: vertical

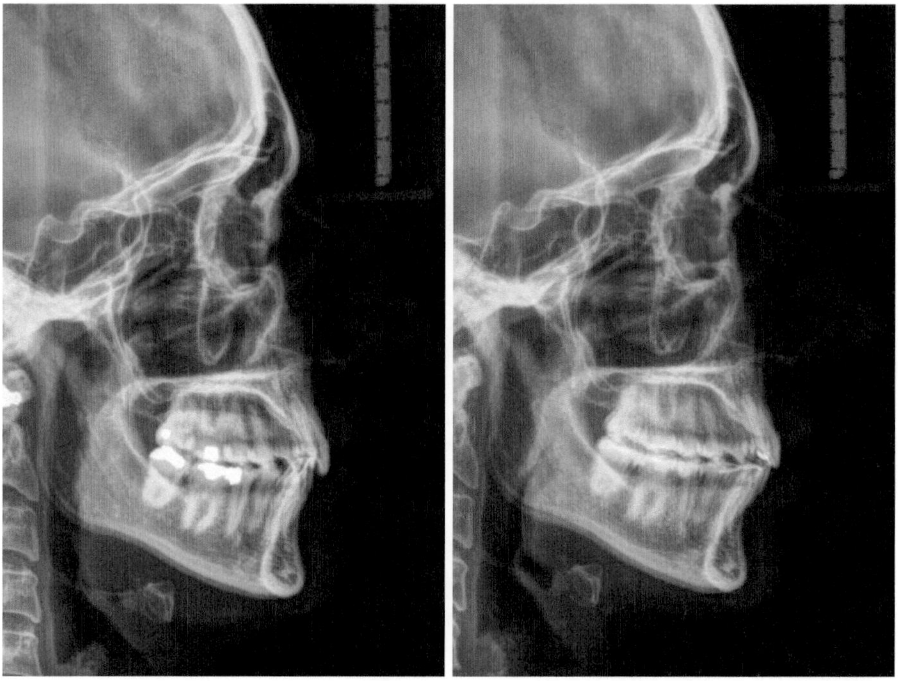

Fig. 12.72 Lateral cephalograms before (left) and at 5-year follow-up (right)

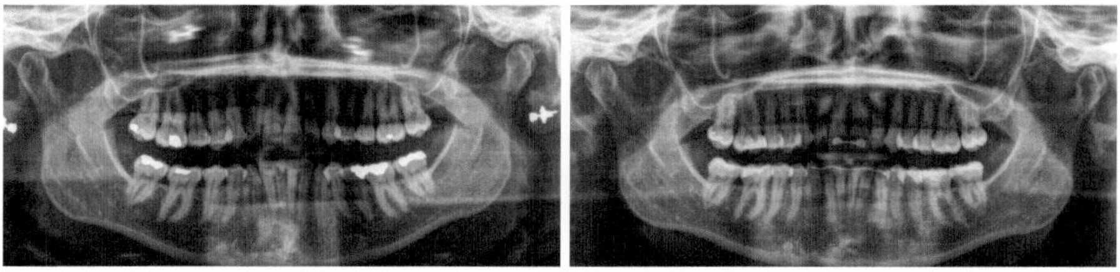

Fig. 12.73 Panoramic X-rays before and at 5-year follow-up

Case 12.5

Class III Occlusion with Excess Freeway Space. Think the Neuromuscular Way

Summary A 10-year-old Caucasian child presented with a concern regarding misaligned teeth and sought orthodontic treatment. The main reason for the orthodontic consultation was the mother's concern for mandibular prognathism.

Pre-treatment	
Extraoral analysis (Fig. 12.74)	
Facial profile	Orthognathic
Facial height	Reduced
Occlusal plane	Normal
Facial symmetry	
Lips	Competent
Mandibular posture	
Head posture	
Intraoral analysis (Fig. 12.74)	
Teeth	
Molar class	III
Canine class	III
Overjet	Positive
Overbite	3
Oral hygiene	Fair
Rotations of lower and upper canines	
Crossbite	
Diastemas: Upper lateral, lower lateral/canine	
Crowding	
Agenesis	
Missing teeth	
Intraoral functional analysis (Fig. 12.74)	
Swallow	Tongue thrust
Tongue tie	No
Tongue posture	Low
Slurred speech	
Neuromuscular diagnosis	
Freeway space increased	
Skeletal class	III
Anterior wall	Yes
TMJ	
TMJ	

Problem list

- Mandible is blocked posteriorly from anterior wall.
- Lower spacing is the result of mandibular posture.

Neuromuscular treatment objectives

- Mandibular freedom.
- Reduce sagittal functional discrepancy.
- Reduce freeway space.
- Correct tongue posture and swallow.

Introduction

Class III malocclusion can be of particular concern from both a functional and facial aesthetic standpoint. From a facial aesthetic point of view, Class III malocclusion can cause noticeable changes to the appearance of the face. Firstly, the typical maxillary insufficiency associated with Class III malocclusion can alter facial aesthetics by reducing the prominence of the zygomatic processes, which can result in a flatter-looking upper half of the face. This can have a significant impact on the overall harmony of the face, particularly in profile view.

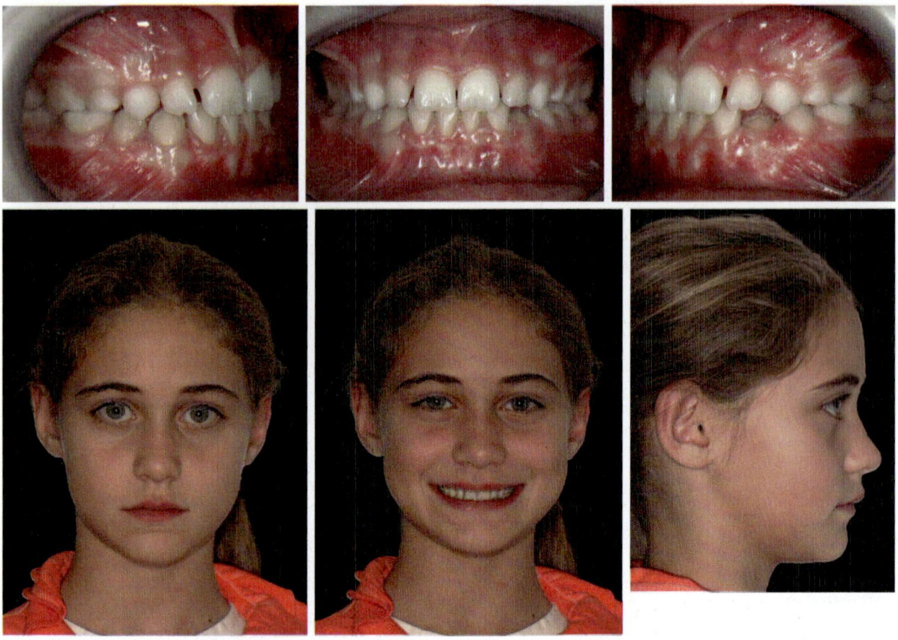

Fig. 12.74 Intra- and extraoral photos before treatment

Moreover, the lower half of the face may also present several variations depending on the typology of vertical growth. Individuals with a deep bite are more likely to notice sagittal discrepancies, which can cause the lower half of the face to look shorter and wider than usual. This can further impact facial aesthetics, particularly when viewed from the front.

This case study involves a young girl with both skeletal and occlusal Class III malocclusion. Despite having no apparent symptoms of mandibular entrapment, she experiences occasional articular clicking during mouth opening. While this may not be a significant issue at present, it could potentially cause problems in the future and highlights the importance of addressing Class III malocclusion early on.

Figure 12.74 shows intra- and extraoral photos before treatment.

Figure 12.75 shows pre-treatment lateral cephalogram and panoramic X-ray.

Clinical assessment considered this patient with an excess of freeway space. Treatment started in November 2014 with RPE and facemask, worn during home hours with a total 400-gram elastic pull. This treatment lasted until September 2015.

In March 2016, intra- and extraoral photos were taken, to assess orthopedic phase therapy results (Figs. 12.76 and 12.77).

A complete K7 functional analysis was taken to assess the vertical and sagittal physiological requests and to plan a neuromuscular orthodontic treatment; a selection of the scans can be seen in Figs. 12.78, 12.79, 12.80 and 12.81.

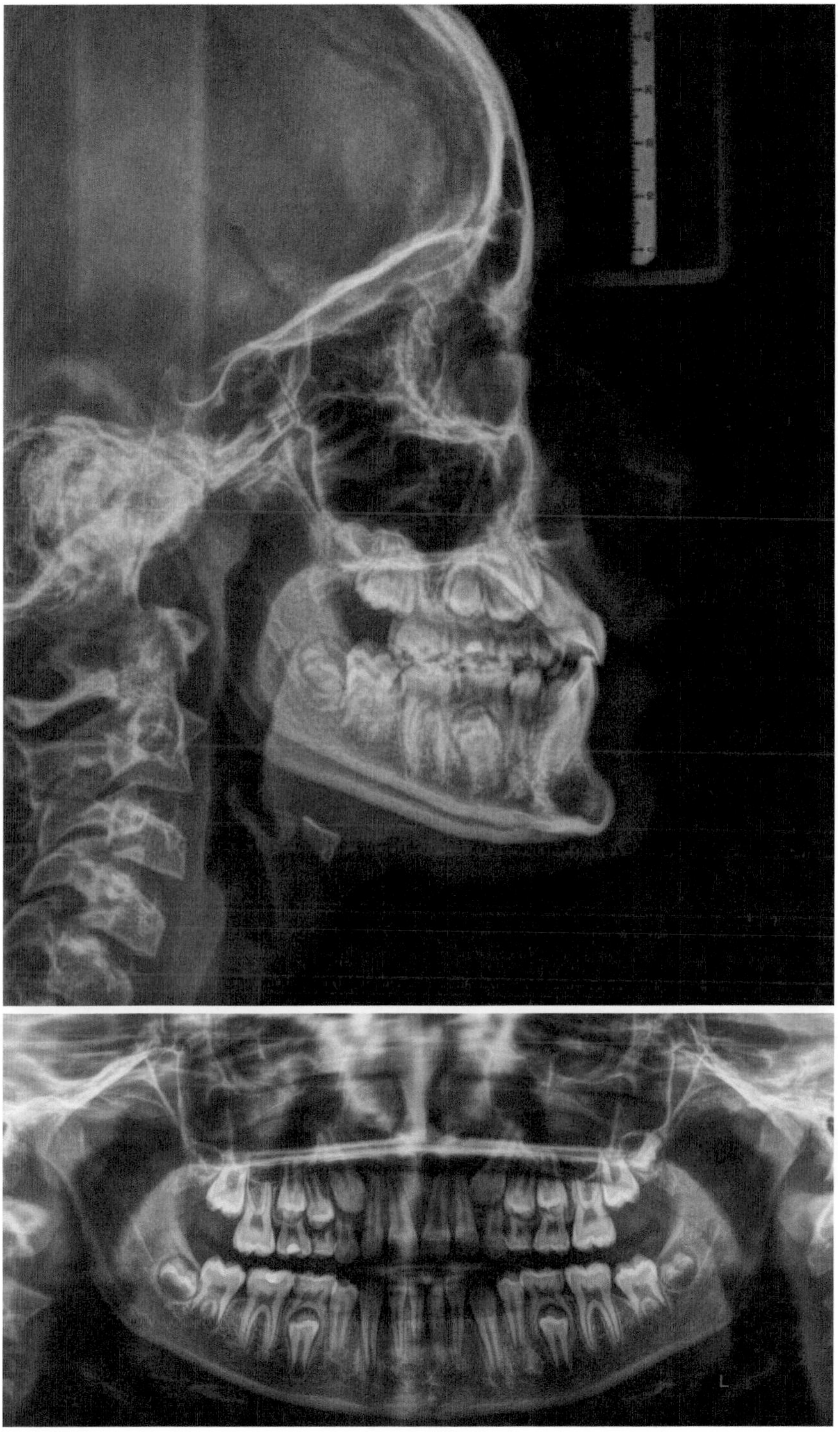

Fig. 12.75 Pre-treatment lateral cephalogram and panoramic X-ray

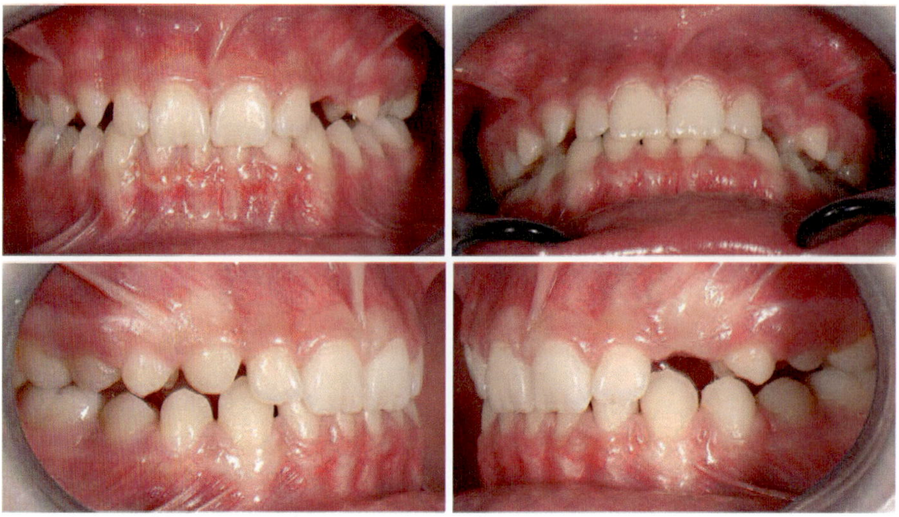

Fig. 12.76 Intraoral photos after RPE and facemask (3/2016)

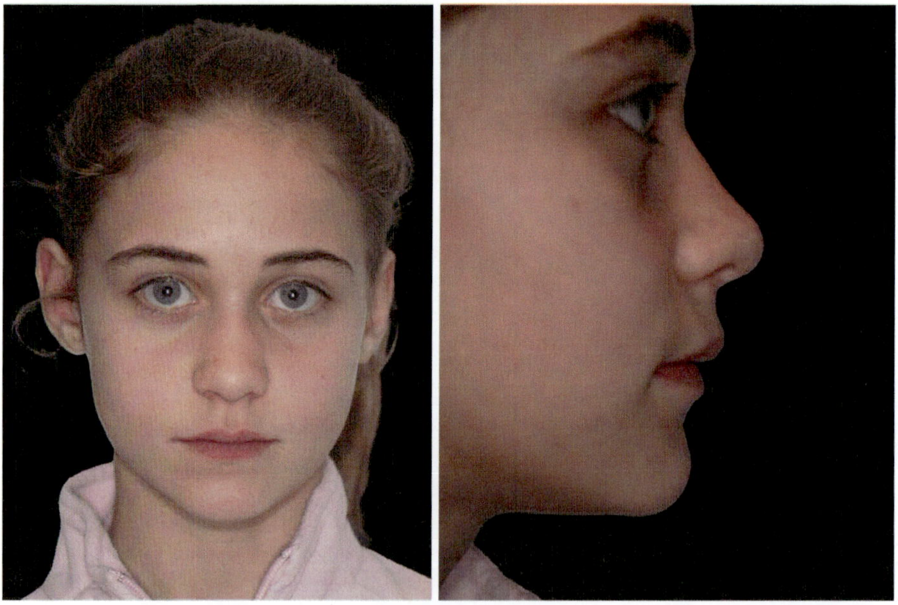

Fig. 12.77 Extraoral photos after RPE and facemask (3/2016)

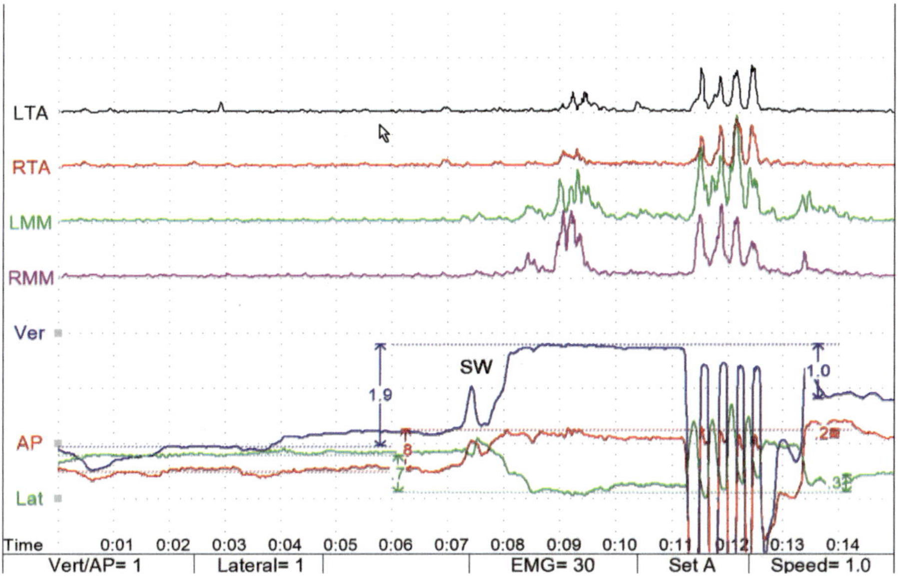

Fig. 12.78 Polygraphic scan (scan 3 + S-EMG filtered, scan 21) Post-interceptive therapy treatment showing a VSS (Voluntary Swallow of Saliva, indicated with "SW"). The blue line (vertical) shows mandibular closure (upward) when swallow starts. There is a premature activation of the masseter muscles at the start of deglutition sequence indicating that the patient swallows with tongue between the teeth.). LMM: left masseter muscle; LTA: left anterior temporalis; RMM: right masseter muscle; RTA: right anterior temporalis.). AP: anterior-posterior; Lat: lateral; Ver: vertical

Discussion

The results of the bioelectric analysis are intriguing. Scan 4/5 might not accurately represent the true freeway space due to the young age of the patient and the possibility of fear and muscle contraction during TENS application in the presence of the operator. Nonetheless, the skeletal morphology suggests a typical *freeway producer* as the mandible exhibits a counterclockwise developmental rotation, which increases deep bite (and freeway space) during growth. Scan 11 indicates discomfort with the current occlusion, which may be due to compromised muscle output resulting from malocclusion and/or excessive freeway space. Other polygraphic scans exhibit the expected activation of the masseter muscles at the start of deglutition, which suggests that the patient initiates swallowing with the tongue between the teeth. This tongue posture might also be habitual, explaining the lower diastemas observed in the pre-treatment intraoral photos.

For these reasons, it was planned to aggressively reduce freeway space by extrusion, starting from the upper pre-molar area. This would have resulted in a reduction of the sagittal discrepancy. During the month of March 2016, a Fixed appliance was applied to the upper arch and levelling was gradually achieved. Lower fixed appliance was applied in August 2016.

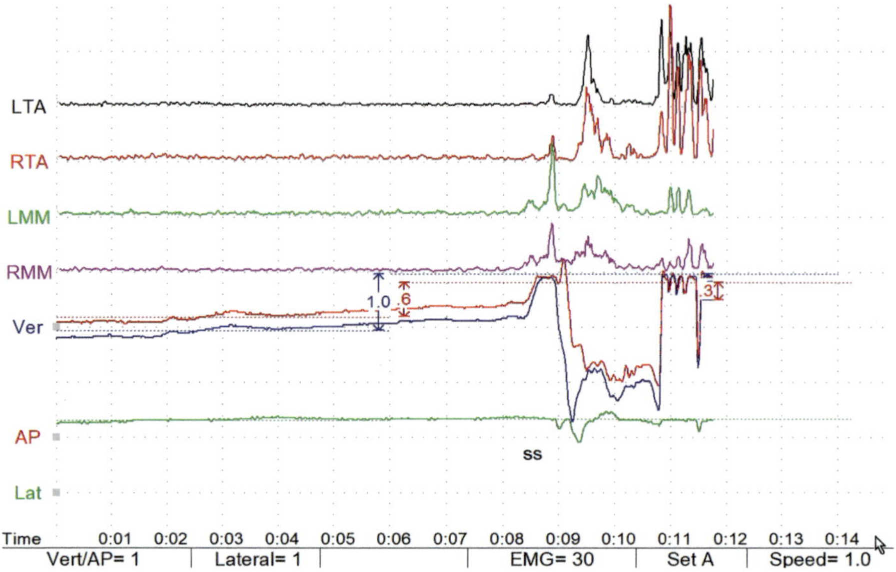

Fig. 12.79 Polygraphic scan (scan 3 + S-EMG filtered, scan 21) Post-interceptive therapy treatment shows a SSS (Spontaneous Swallow of Saliva, indicated with "ss"). The vertical blue line shows mandibular closure (upward) when swallow starts. There is a premature activation of the masseter muscles at start of deglutition sequence indicating that the patient swallows with tongue between the teeth. (LMM: left masseter muscle; LTA: left anterior temporalis; RMM: right masseter muscle; RTA: right anterior temporalis.). AP: anterior-posterior; Lat: lateral; Ver: vertical

By May 2017, Upper and lower arches were engaged in fixed bracket appliances with upper 017 x 025 NiTi wire, and lower 018 x 025 stainless steel. Upper arch turbos were applied, and intraoral vertical elastics were applied as shown in Fig. 12.82.

Treatment was terminated in October 2017 and the results can be seen in Figs. 12.83 and 12.84.

To check if the required neuromuscular objectives had been reached, by February 2018, a complete K7 evaluation was achieved and some of the acquired scans can be seen in Figs. 12.85 and 12.86.

Figure 12.85 shows scan 11 testing with an increase in overall muscular output.

Follow-up checks confirmed long-term positive results of neuromuscular orthodontic therapy. The results can be seen in Figs. 12.87 and 12.88 and represent a check-up at 5 years after treatment.

Complete scans according to the basic neuromuscular orthodontic protocol were completed by March 2023. Scans 11, 10, and 4/5 can be seen in Figs. 12.89, 12.90 and 12.91.

Figure 12.92 shows Initial lateral cephalogram and post-treatment lateral cephalogram.

The lateral cephalogram X-rays presented here serve as a structural representation of the physiological objectives that have been successfully achieved and

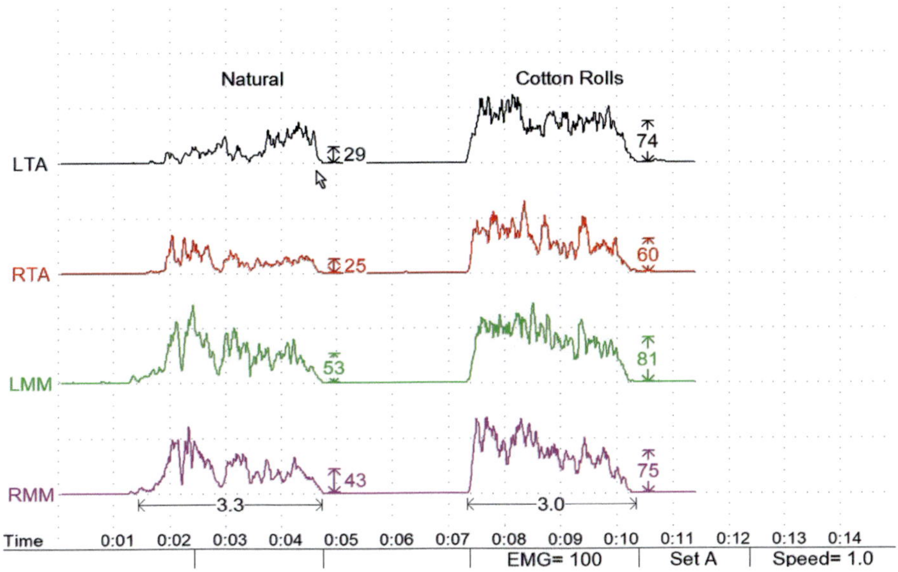

Fig. 12.80 Scan 11 Post-interceptive therapy treatment shows the surface EMG results in sweep mode. The patient was instructed to clench in CO (first burst), and then clench with cotton rolls between the teeth, which temporarily prevented occlusion (second burst). Output s-EMG is low indicating muscle fatigue/malocclusion

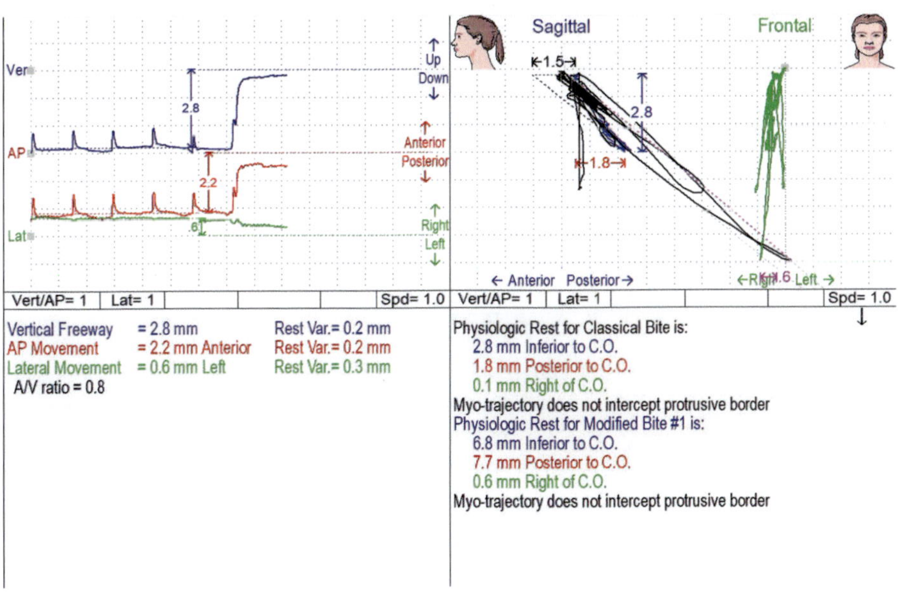

Fig. 12.81 Post-interceptive therapy treatment shows scan 4/5 in split screen modality. On the left sweep of V, AP, and Lat lines. The patient is instructed to rest mandibular posture and the instructed to close to Centric Occlusion. Note the TENS spikes on V and AP lines. On the right, the corresponding Sagittal/frontal scan 5 shows a 1.5-mm. AP discrepancy on HP (Horizontal Plane of Occlusion). Vertical freeway space is 2.8 mm. AP: anterior-posterior; CO: centric occlusion; Lat: lateral; Spd: speed; Vert: vertical

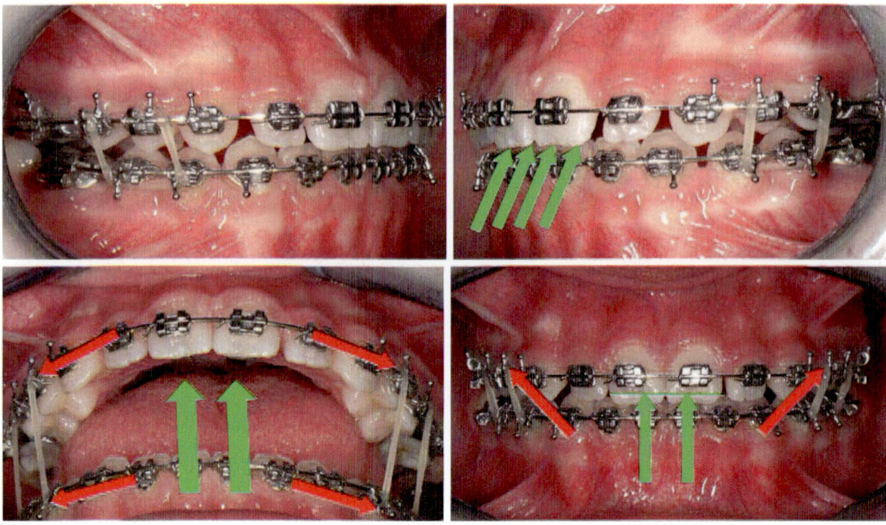

Fig. 12.82 Intraoral photo during treatment, May 2017. Vertical lateral "box "elastics are applied between upper and lower pre-molars, each side, red arrows. Bite turbos are applied to increase VD and permit extrusion, green arrows

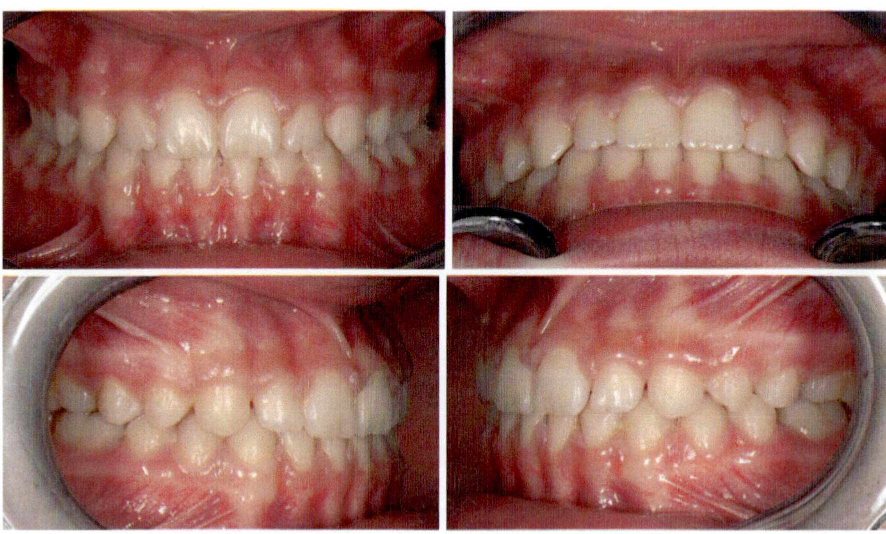

Fig. 12.83 Intraoral photos after treatment

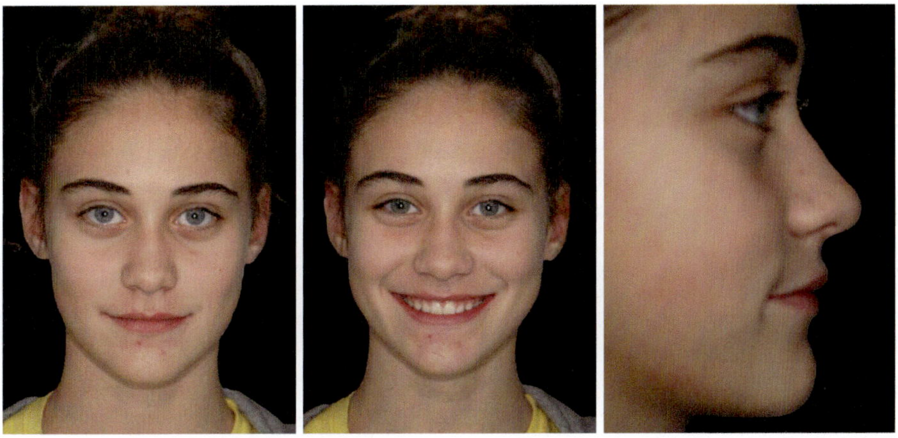

Fig. 12.84 Extraoral photos after treatment

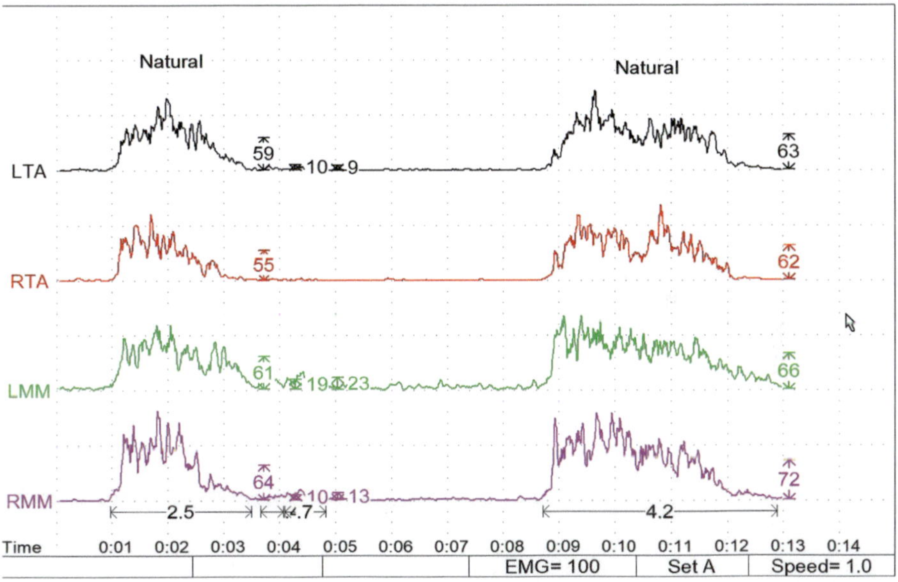

Fig. 12.85 Scan 11 (post-treatment) shows the surface EMG results in sweep mode. The patient was instructed to clench in CO (first burst and second burst). Output s-EMG is still low but indicates that muscle activity is better than at the start of treatment (LMM: left masseter muscle; LTA: left anterior temporalis; RMM: right masseter muscle; RTA: right anterior temporalis)

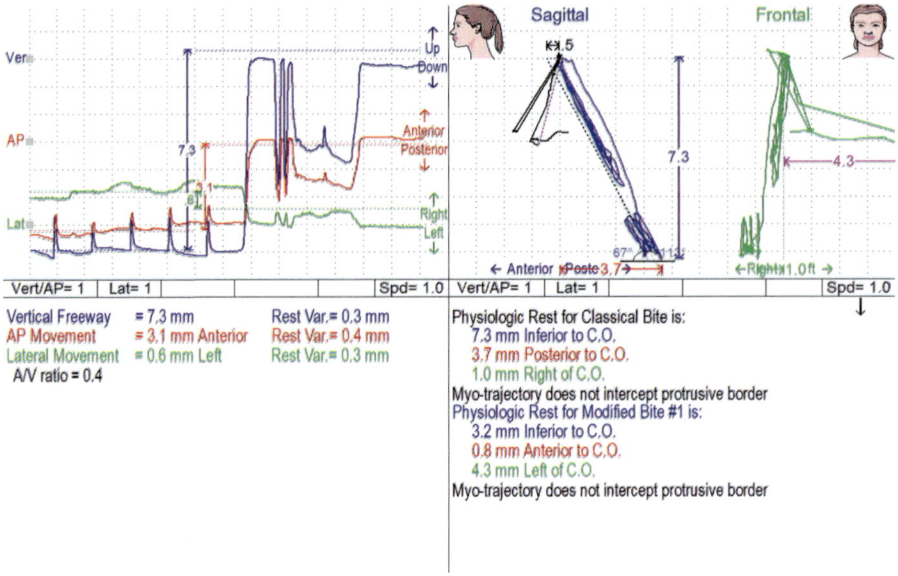

Fig. 12.86 Post-treatment. Scan 4/5 in split screen modality. On the left sweep V, AP, and Lat lines. The patient is instructed to rest mandibular posture and the instructed to close to Centric Occlusion. Note the TENS spikes on V and AP lines. On the right, the corresponding Sagittal/frontal scan 5 shows a 0.5-mm. AP discrepancy on HP (Horizontal Plane of Occlusion). The vertical freeway space is 7.3 mm. AP: anterior-posterior; CO: centric occlusion; Lat: lateral; Spd: speed; Vert: vertical

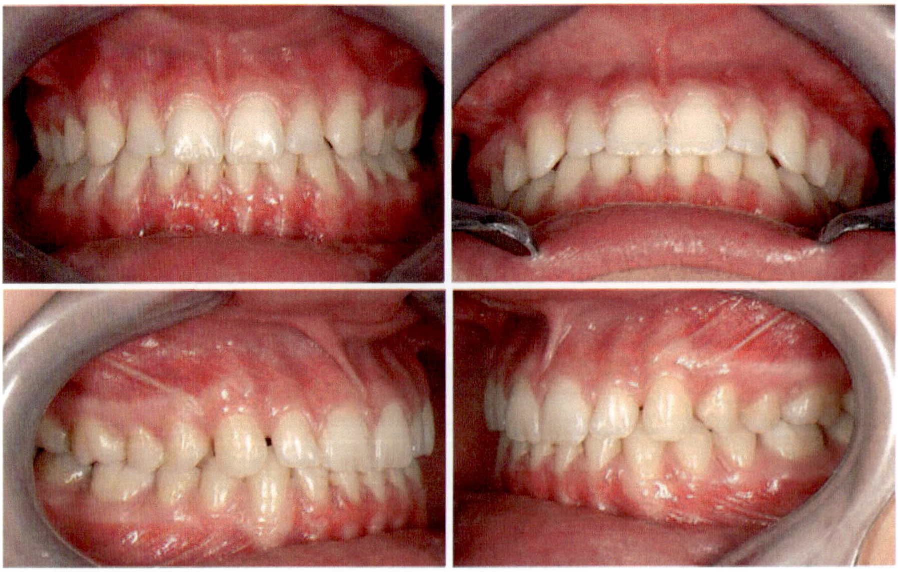

Fig. 12.87 Intraoral photos at 5.5 years after treatment

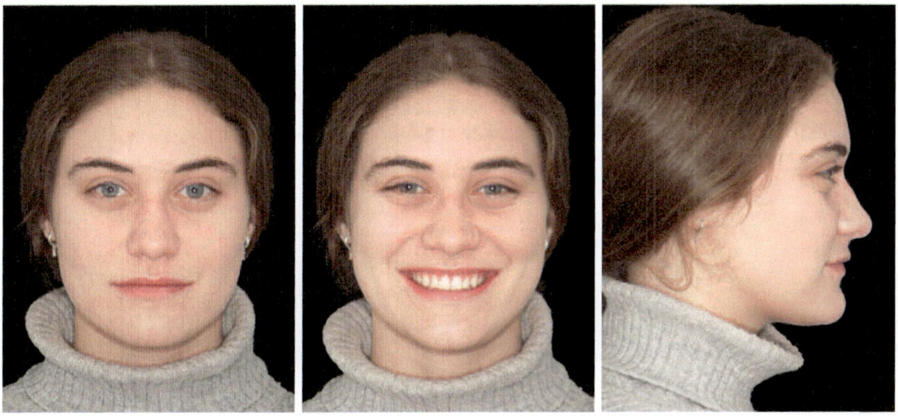

Fig. 12.88 Extraoral photos at 5.5 years after treatment

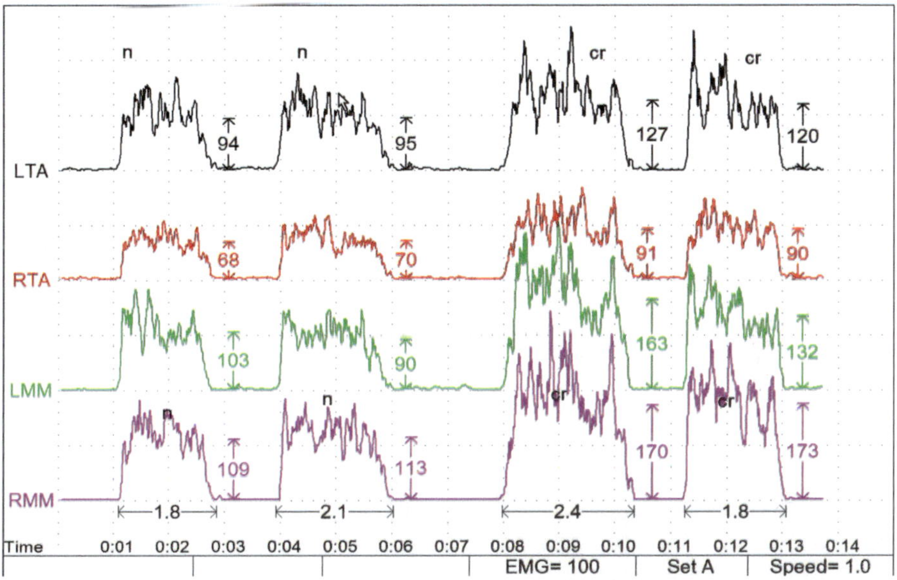

Fig. 12.89 Scan 11 (post-treatment follow-up at 5.5 years) shows the surface EMG results in sweep mode. The patient was instructed to clench in CO (first burst and second burst), and then clench with cotton rolls between the teeth, which temporarily prevented occlusion (third burst and fourth burst). Output s-EMG is now very good indicating muscle fatigue/malocclusion is resolved and muscle function restored. Note the masseter muscles are firing more than the temporalis muscles. Balance is good

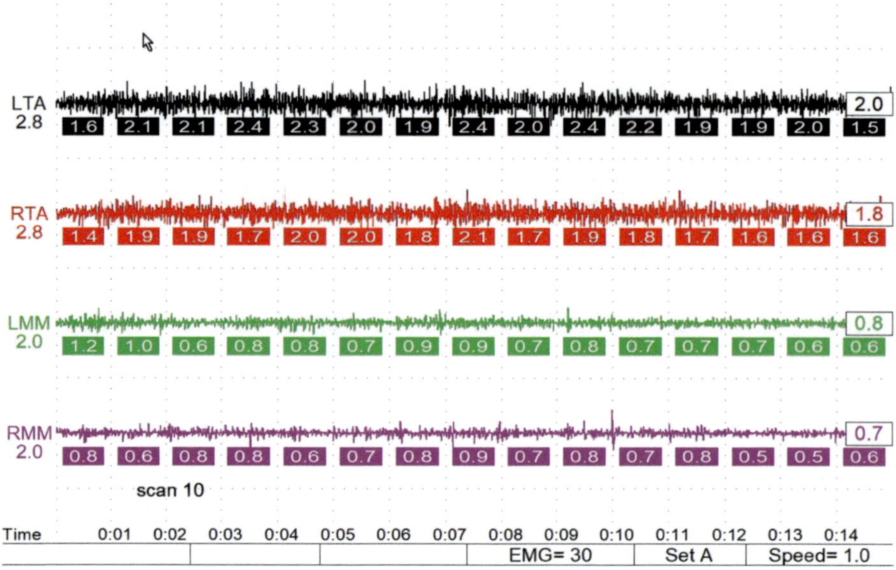

Fig. 12.90 Scan 10 shows that the muscles were relaxed (after TENS). An Aqualizer was used to avoid tooth contact for CNS deconditioning. CNS: central nervous system; LMM: left masseter muscle; LTA: left anterior temporalis; RMM: right masseter muscle; RTA: right anterior temporalis; TENS: transcutaneous electrical nerve stimulation

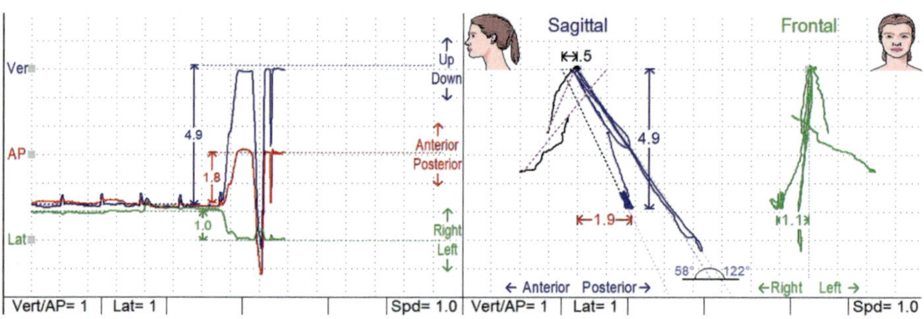

Fig. 12.91 Scan 4/5 (post-treatment follow-up at 5.5 years) in split screen modality. On the left sweep V, AP, and Lat lines. The patient is instructed to rest mandibular posture and the instructed to close to Centric Occlusion. Note the TENS spikes on V and AP lines. On the right, the corresponding Sagittal/frontal scan 5 shows a 0.5-mm. AP discrepancy on HP (Horizontal Plane of Occlusion). The vertical freeway space is 4.9 mm. AP: anterior-posterior; CO: centric occlusion; Lat: lateral; Spd: speed; Vert: vertical

stabilized. It is important to note that there is a period of time after orthodontic treatment during which the rehabilitation of muscular function takes place, and it is only after this that satisfactory results can be obtained through surface electromyography (S-EMG).

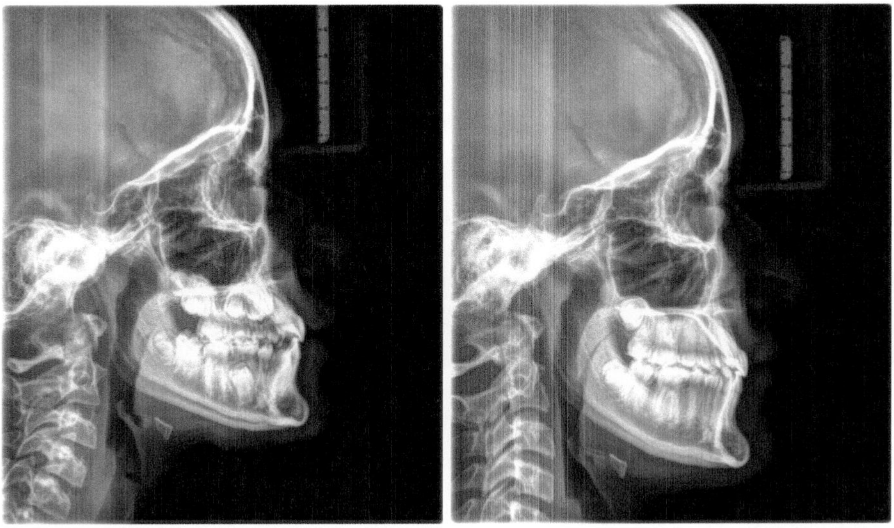

Fig. 12.92 Initial (2014) lateral cephalogram and after treatment lateral cephalogram (2017). Vertical development is crucial in Class III therapy to reduce sagittal discrepancy and to increase aesthetic outcome

Retention is a crucial aspect of post-treatment care of Class III skeletal with excess freeway space, and it should be geared toward *allowing for some posterior extrusion*. This is particularly important for skeletally mature patients who possess all the necessary anatomical features that increase deep bite. There will always be a constant and stable increase of freeway space, which is maintained throughout the completion of growth and development.

It is important to exercise caution when treating Class III individuals with small upper diastemas. Attempting to close these gaps may inadvertently result in condylar retrusion, which can be a significant setback in achieving optimal treatment outcomes. As such, careful consideration should be given to the most appropriate course of action in such cases.

Case 12.6

Class II Occlusion with Increased Freeway Space. Slight Functional Asymmetry

Summary A 8-year-old Caucasian child presented with a concern regarding misaligned teeth and sought orthodontic treatment. The orthodontic consultation was part of a regular dental check-up.

Pre-treatment	
Extraoral analysis	
Facial profile orthognathic/flat	
Facial height	
Occlusal plane Normal	
Facial symmetry right side bending	
Lips competent	
Mandibular posture	
Head posture no apparent deviation	
Intraoral analysis (Fig. 12.96)	
Teeth	
Molar	Class II right, class I left
Canine	Class II right, class I left
Overjet	Positive
Overbite	3
Oral hygiene	Fair
Rotations	
Crossbite first molars, right	
Diastemas	
Crowding	
Agenesis	
Missing teeth	
Intraoral functional analysis (Fig. 12.97)	
Swallow	Normal
Tongue tie	No
Tongue posture	
Slurred speech	
Neuromuscular diagnosis	
Freeway space increased	
Skeletal class	I
Anterior wall	Yes
TMJ	No signs or symptoms
Problem list • Mandible is blocked posteriorly from anterior wall. • Functional asymmetry by right working side.	
Neuromuscular treatment objectives • Mandibular Freedom. • Increase vertical functional discrepancy on right.	

Introduction

When dealing with functional asymmetries in clinical orthodontic management, it is important to approach the issue with caution, especially in cases where habits, such as unilateral mastication, are involved. The use of functional appliances, like the Frankel appliance, can prove beneficial in re-educating mandibular movement and encouraging more symmetric function, but a practical approach should also consider the possibility of anatomical differences between the right and left condyles. In such cases, increasing the vertical occlusion on the affected side (working side) could potentially stimulate partial recovery of the condyle's anatomical structure.

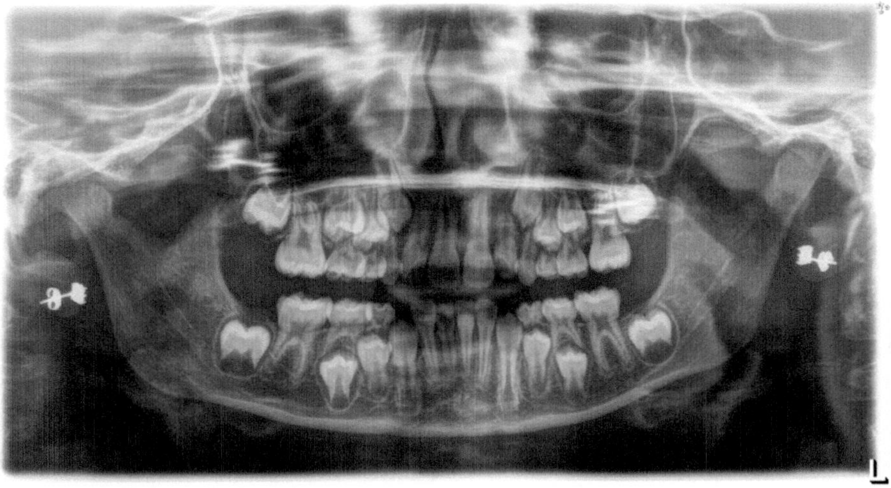

Fig. 12.93 Panoramic x-ray before treatment

It's essential to understand that the goal of treatment should not only be to improve morphology but also to modify or re-adapt function to a more symmetric mandibular anatomy. However, achieving this can be challenging and requires a high degree of patient cooperation, as compliance is especially critical in *functional rehabilitations*, which have no non-compliance treatment options available.

The case in question involves an attempt to reduce the freeway space in general, with a particular focus on the right side. Figure 12.93 depicts a panoramic X-ray, which highlights a shortened length of the right condyle. Additionally, the posterior-anterior cephalogram indicates facial asymmetry, with involvement in cervical vertebrae and their alignment. This could be suggestive of an ascending-like problem that could potentially limit ideal cervical/head posture, further emphasizing the complexity of the case (Figs. 12.94 and 12.95).

Intra- and extraoral photos are shown in Figs. 12.96 and 12.97. Intraoral photos show a Class II molar occlusion on the affected side and a Class I molar occlusion on the balancing side. The extraoral photos show a notable lateral deviation of the lower third of the face toward the right. This is even more visible when the young patient smiles.

Rapid palatal expansion (RPE) was applied by 11/2016 and expansion lasted about 21 days. By October 2017, an upper fixed appliance was applied, and the results can be seen in Fig. 12.98.

Upper alignment continued and lower fixed appliance was delayed. A tentative K7 evaluation was carried out in November 2018. Unfortunately, the young patient did not tolerate TENS, but some valuable information was taken from the scans. Figures 12.99 and 12.100 show a sagittal/frontal scan of swallow from HRP and scan 3.

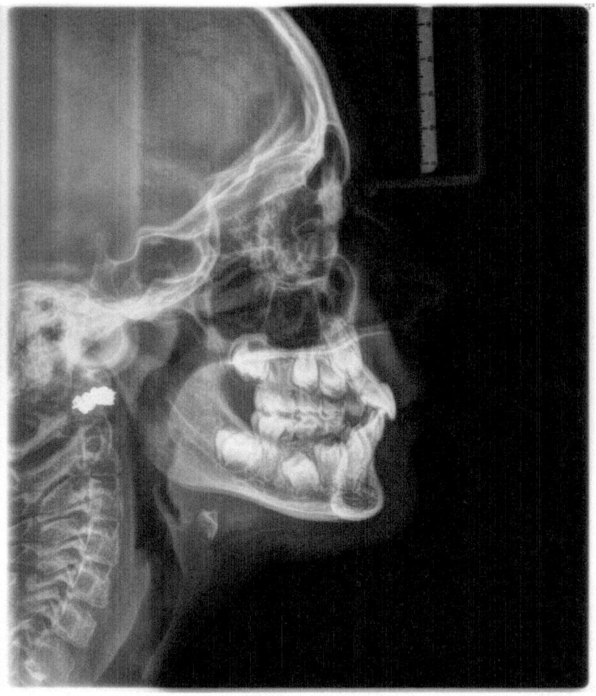

Fig. 12.94 Lateral cephalogram x-ray before treatment

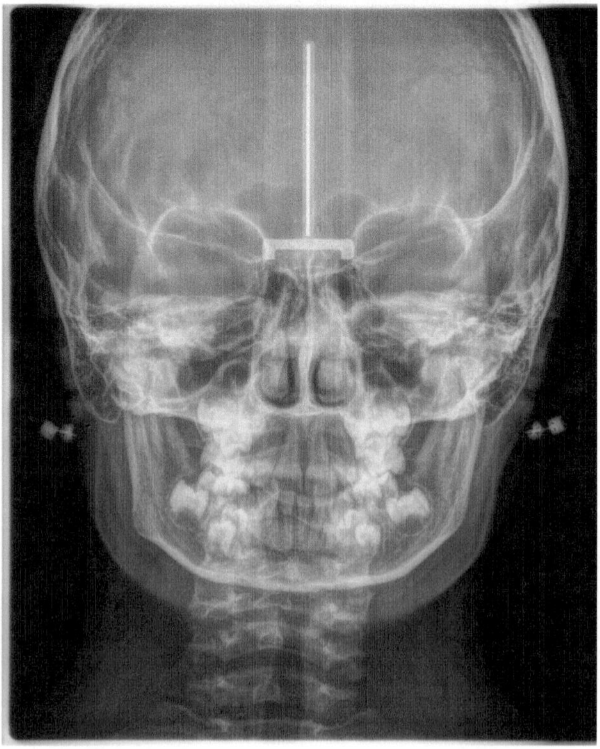

Fig. 12.95 Posterior/anterior cephalogram X-ray before treatment

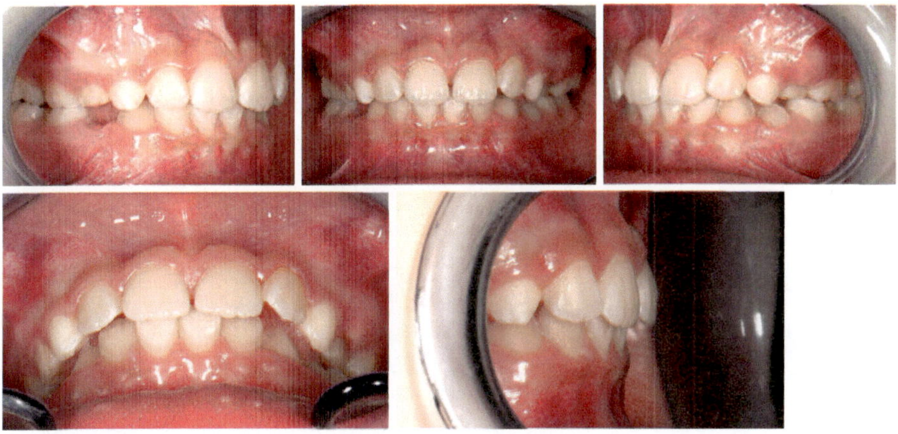

Fig. 12.96 Intraoral photos before treatment, 10/2016. Note the lower midline deviation to the patient's right

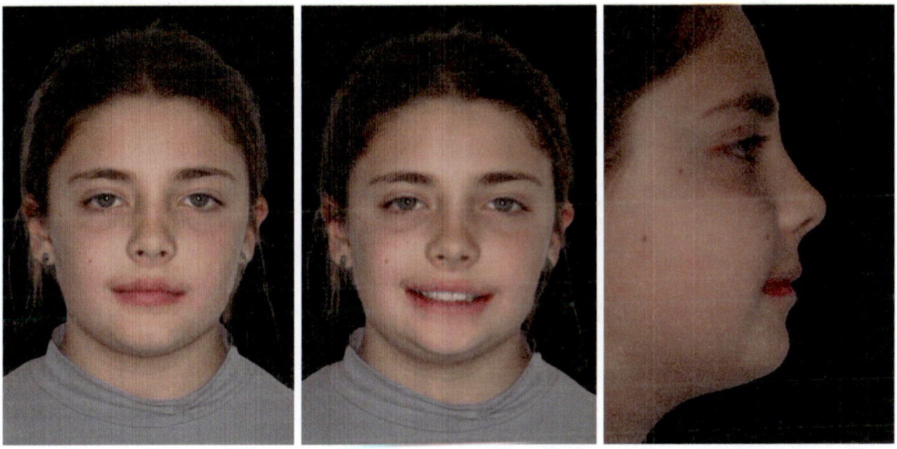

Fig. 12.97 Extraoral photos before treatment, 10/2016. Note the smile directed as maxillary canting

Figure 12.99 shows that the HRP is slightly in front of the V line. This is very important information because we assume that unless muscles ***naturally*** work for a vertical movement to CO (which is impossible), there is an anterior wall that is a clear obstacle to mandibular postural advancement. As swallow starts (red arrow) the mandible advances vertically together with an anterior movement (red AP line in sweep mode). This continues until swallow has started at that specific level and mandibular position (green box). When finally, the patient is instructed to "tap tap" in CO, the first contact is on front incisors; eventually sliding back and up to reach CO.

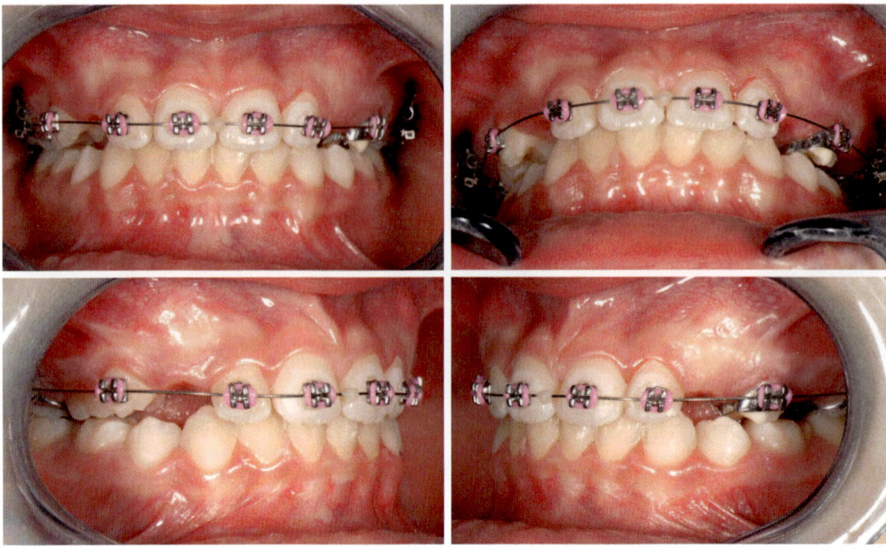

Fig. 12.98 Intraoral photo after RPE and upper fixed appliance, 10/2017

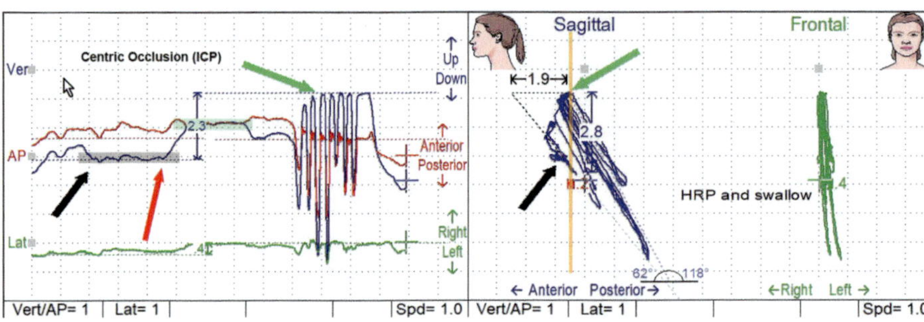

Fig. 12.99 Follow-up. Sweep and sagittal/frontal scan of **swallow from HRP,** 11/2018. Black arrows = HRP. Gray box = HRP level in sweep. Green box = vertical height level of swallow. Red arrow: start of swallow sequence (VSS), Green arrows = Centric Occlusion (CO). Orange line = Vertical V line through CO. AP: anterior-posterior; CO: centric occlusion; Lat: lateral; Spd: speed; Vert: vertical

If HRP is on or slightly in front of the V line, our neuromuscular objectives are to bring forward the CO point on our scan 5 and to consume freeway space by extrusion to reduce the Sagittal requests. Obviously, the vertical freeway space is practically unknown at this point of treatment, but since TENS application was not possible due to compliance issues, clinical judgment is crucial.

Uneven build-ups were constructed with composite on lower first molars, favoring a lower build-up on the working side. This permits the operator to extrude more on the working side than the balancing one. Once teeth come in contact, the extrusion will be greater on the affected, working side. This should reduce or erase right

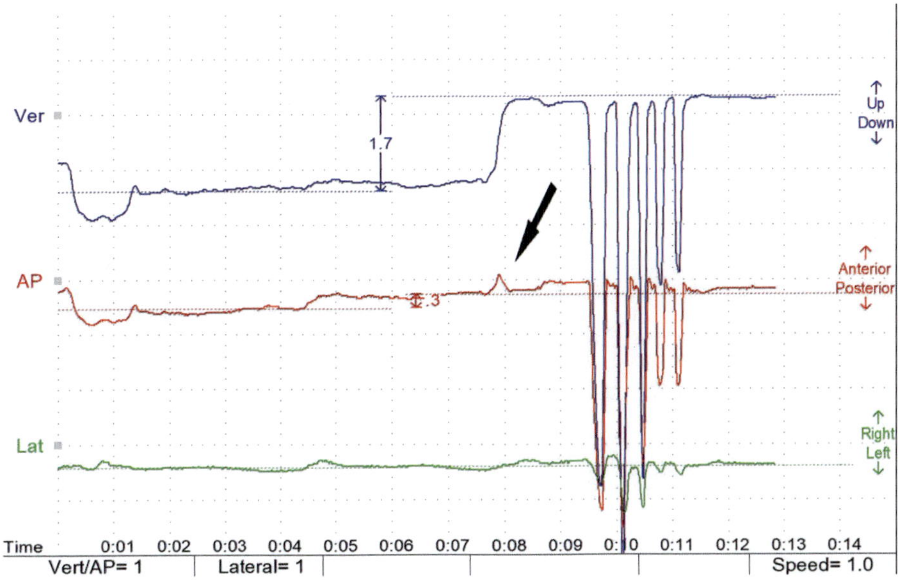

Fig. 12.100 Follow-up. Scan 3. The black arrow indicates that RP is approximately on the V line. Scan 3 (pre-treatment) shows the vertical, anterior-posterior, and lateral movements of the mandible in sweep mode. The patient was instructed to maintain the mandible in the rest position and then to close it to CO. There was a normal freeway space (1.7 mm). When closing, there was no apparent anterior-posterior movement, a slight movement forward upon closure (which was immediately converted to a backward movement [black arrow]). AP: anterior-posterior; Lat: lateral; Ver: vertical

dentoalveolar maxillary canting and distract vertically the condyle on the affected side.

Since the asymmetry is not severe, a possible rapid orthodontic solution with vertical correction of the affected side may be sufficient. The other orthodontic objective remains a reduction of the sagittal discrepancy by means of torque correction of the upper anterior teeth, by extrusion of the posterior and mid sectors. The mid sectors were aggressively extruded favoring the right working side. In September 2019, treatment was terminated after a final incisor advancement and torque correction. Final radiology, intra and extraoral photos were taken and can be seen in Figs. 12.101, 12.102 and 12.103.

Discussion

Posterior-anterior cephalogram taken at the end of treatment confirms an ascendent postural problem that has not been addressed during orthodontic therapy. The patient is asymptomatic and in good general health. She is an avid horseback rider and has gone through common traumas from horseback riding. The panoramic X-ray (Fig. 12.101), although not taken in CO, shows a somewhat improvement in right condylar length, although the author does not believe this is an ideal method for condylar length measurement.

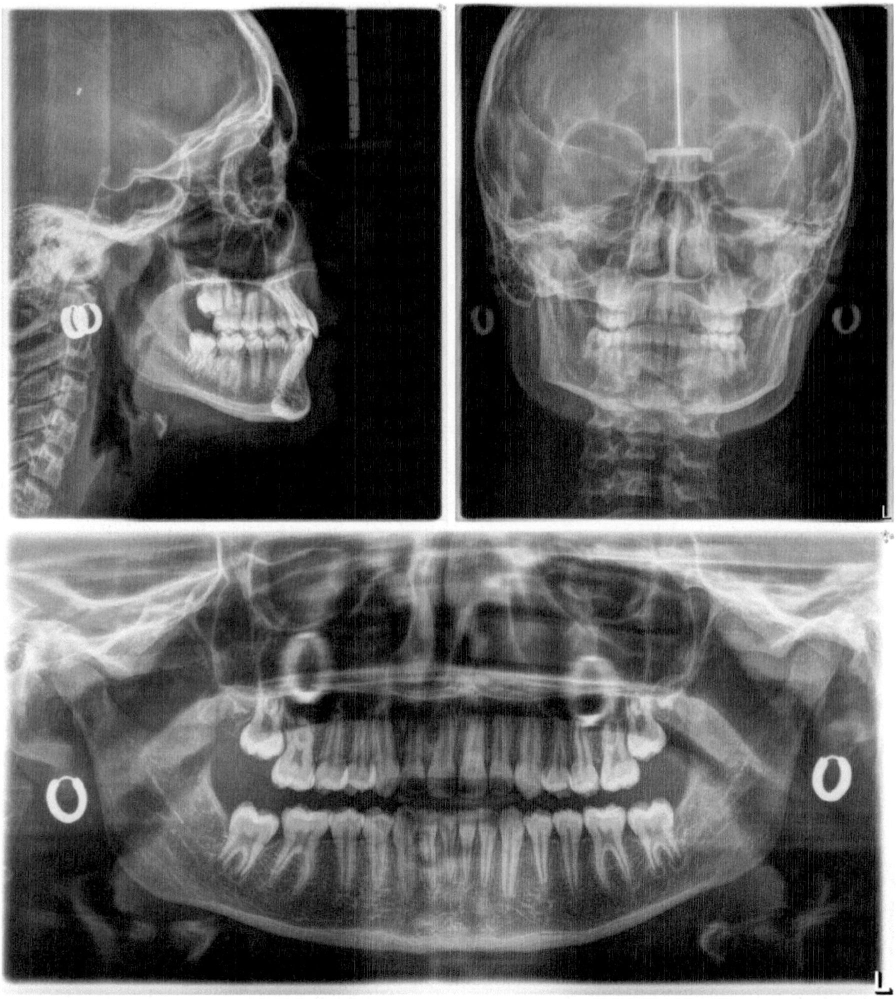

Fig. 12.101 Lateral cephalogram and posterior/anterior cephalogram and panoramic X-ray after treatment

Intraoral photos at the end of treatment (Fig. 12.102) show an overall improvement of the occlusal symmetry, and more importantly, a vertical gap between the occlusal surfaces of the right first molars. This is due to the aggressive extrusion of the pre-molar sector at the end of treatment and to the removal of the posterior build-ups. It will be necessary sometime before there is a closure of the posterior gap, and retention must not limit this unforced extrusion. A pre-built positioner/finisher was applied on a 12-h/day application (8 h during sleep and 4 h during the day with multiple MVC exercises).

By December 2019 (3 months after treatment), the first complete k7 scan was taken and the patient collaboration was good. It was so far possible to apply TENS

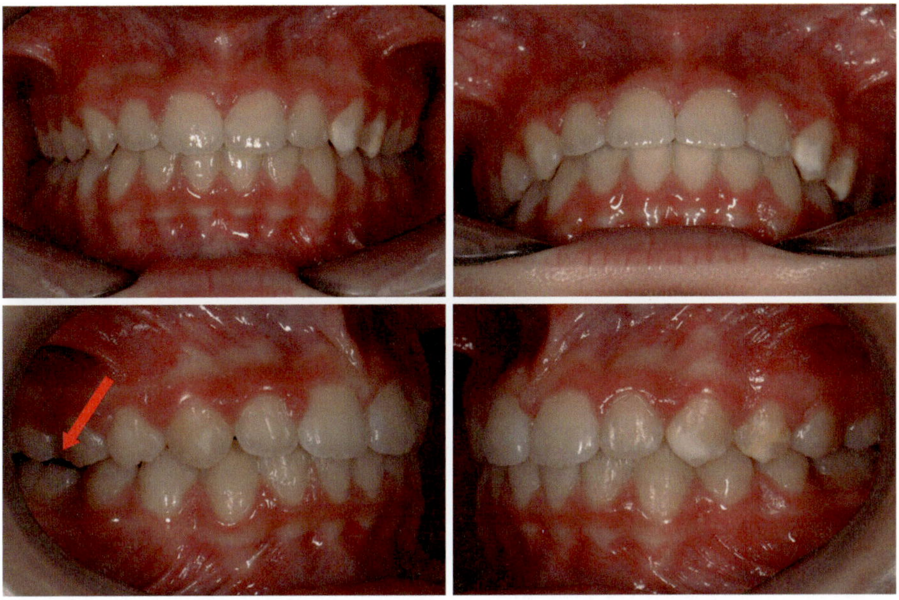

Fig. 12.102 Intraoral photo after treatment. Note vertical gap at upper right molar due to a major right upper pre-molar extrusion (red arrow)

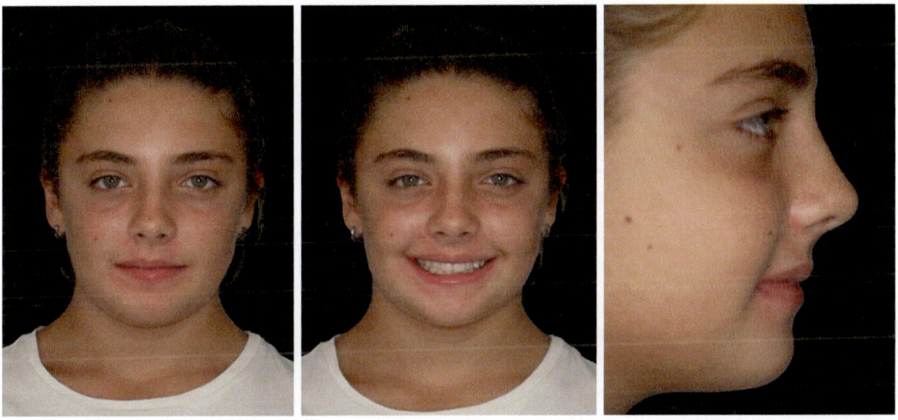

Fig. 12.103 Post-treatment extraoral photos

as indicated and finally the K7 results of post-orthodontic treatment can be seen in Figs. 12.104, 12.105, 12.106 and 12.107.

Scan 104 confirms that the patient swallows correctly in CO, although there is a slight premature activation of the masseter muscles, indicating a probable tongue posture slightly between the dental arches at HRP. What comes as a surprise, is the AP line that is still indicative of a vertical or almost vertical movement to CO. The

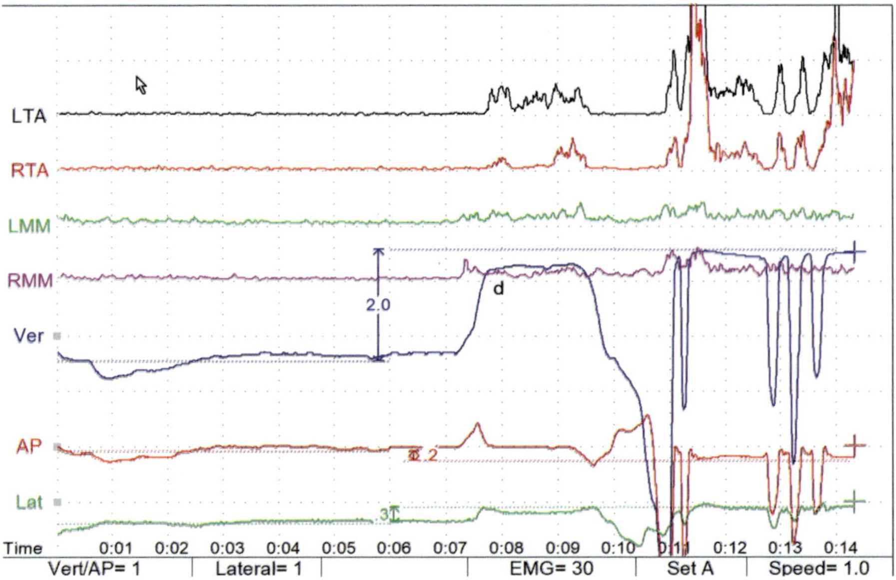

Fig. 12.104 Polygraphic scan (scan 3 + S-EMG filtered, scan 21) Post-treatment shows a VSS (Voluntary Swallow of Saliva, indicated with "d"). The vertical blue line shows mandibular closure (upward) when swallow starts. There is a premature activation of the masseter muscles at the start of deglutition sequence indicating that the patient swallows initially with tongue between the teeth but then maintains ICP during swallow). There is absence of AP movement. (LMM: left masseter muscle; LTA: left anterior temporalis; RMM: right masseter muscle; RTA: right anterior temporalis). AP: anterior-posterior; Lat: lateral; Ver: vertical

ideal (AP) anterior movement should result at a 50% ratio in respect of the Vertical movement, that is around 2 mm.

The same can be seen in Fig. 12.105, scan 3, repeated several times. Figure 12.106 is a functional confirmation that there is still something to address in this occlusion. In fact, even though well-balanced output favors the asymmetry correction, a reduced output during MVC of the masseters in respect of the temporalis muscles is indicative of a posterior occlusion. Further confirmation comes from scan 4/5 in Fig. 12.107 where the AP discrepancy is 1.3 mm on HP. Vertical freeway space is slightly augmented (4 mm).

So besides the frustration of not retrieving better news from the first K7 evaluation, the question is: what is going on? Applying a very sensitive eye (bioelectric instrumentation) shows us more than what we can clinically assess. Once again, the excessive use of a positioner has a resulted in a negative and unpredictable effect on occlusion. **Generalized intrusion** caused by gummy positioners determines the following effects:

1. Increase in freeway space. This is a direct consequence of the generalized intrusion of the upper and lower teeth.
2. Increase in anterior occlusion. As an effect of intrusion, the CO point (and HP line) elevates (vertical increase of HP) on scan 5, this is the exact opposite

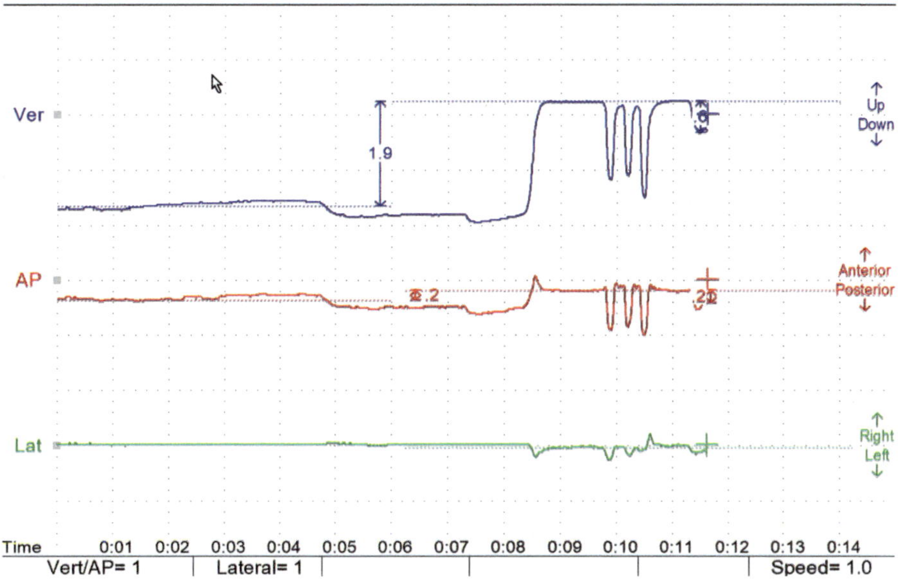

Fig. 12.105 Scan 3 (post-treatment) shows the vertical, anterior-posterior, and lateral movements of the mandible in sweep mode. The patient was instructed to maintain the mandible in the rest position and then to close it to CO. There was a normal freeway space (1.9 mm). When closing, there was no apparent anterior-posterior movement, a slight movement forward during closure, 0.2 mm), and a lateral movement that was initially to the left 0.2 mm. AP: anterior-posterior; Lat: lateral; Ver: vertical

desired in Class III treatments in which extrusion favors a lowering of HP and CO thus reducing the sagittal discrepancy. For this reason, *the 1.3 mm increase in the HP can be corrected by treating the opposite way, with extrusion.*

3. Muscle fatigue is sometimes reported by patients. The gummy-like positioner also works as a stimulation to serrate. Besides muscle fatigue, this can be a positive effect sometimes desired to increase muscle function on hypotonic face musculature.
4. Sometimes there can be TMJ pain. Meaning that the standard aperture for the prefabricated positioners does not fit all. Meaning that the individual aperture recorded for the construction of a more sophisticated positioner does not either. Probably the best aperture is the PRP taken with neuromuscular techniques.

The complete interruption of the positioner as retention must have beneficial effects. If so, subsequent scans on follow-up checks must show some kind of improvement. This improvement is not expected to be immediate but has to come somewhat naturally as occlusion sets by itself. After suspension of positioner use, an upper removable appliance from 3–3 was constructed to inhibit posterior occlusal contact, thus permitting spontaneous extrusion of the posterior teeth.

Intra- and extraoral photos were taken in February 2022 (3.5 years after treatment Fig. 12.108).

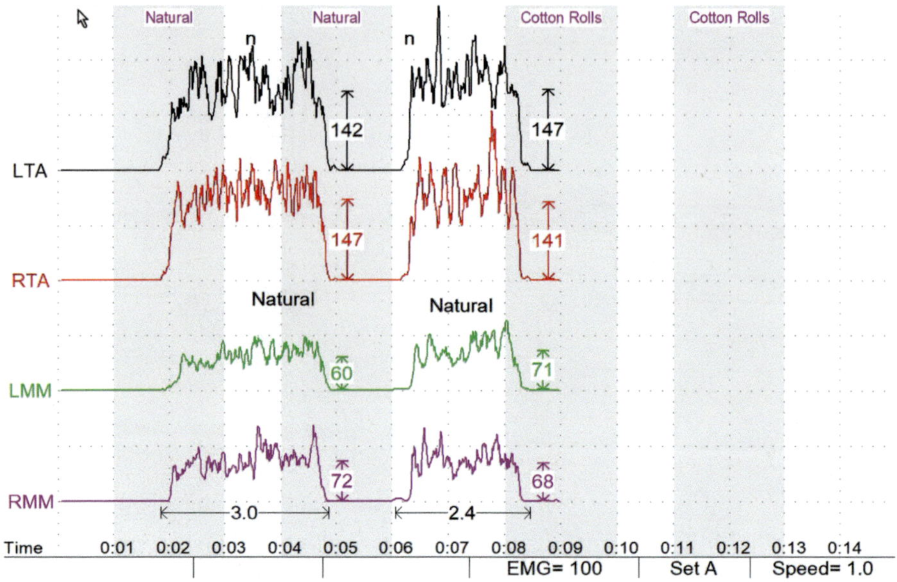

Fig. 12.106 Scan 11 (post-treatment) shows the surface EMG results in sweep mode. The patient was instructed to clench in CO (first burst and second burst). Output s-EMG is unsatisfactory for the masseter muscles and the general there is a symmetric balancing. The Temporalis have a stronger output during clench in respect of the masseters. CO: centric occlusion; EMG: electromyography; LMM: left masseter muscle; LTA: left anterior temporalis; RMM: right masseter muscle; RTA: right anterior temporalis

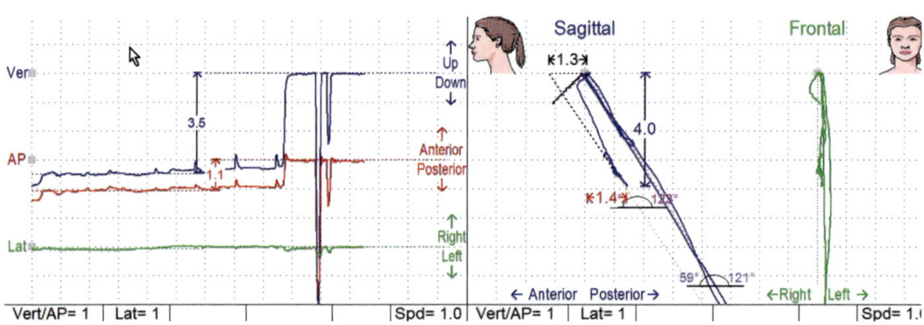

Fig. 12.107 Scan 4/5 (post-treatment) in split screen modality. On the left sweep V, AP, and Lat lines. The patient is instructed to rest mandibular posture and the instructed to close to Centric Occlusion. Note the TENS spikes on V and AP lines. On the right, the corresponding Sagittal/frontal scan 5 shows a 1.3-mm. AP discrepancy on HP (Horizontal Plane of Occlusion). The vertical freeway space is 4.0 mm. AP: anterior-posterior; CO: centric occlusion; Lat: lateral; Spd: speed; Vert: vertical

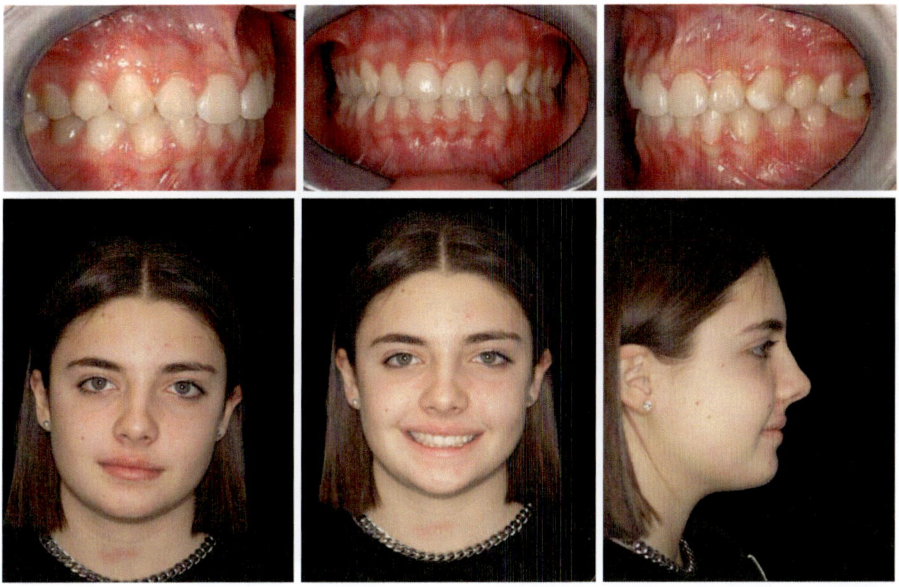

Fig. 12.108 Intra- and extraoral photos were taken at 3.5 years after treatment

Figure 12.108 confirms the visual difference caused by skeletal/functional asymmetry. The patient has been instructed to chew as much as possible on the left side and to suspend any upper retention. Lower fixed retention has been applied in the previous check-up. During the month of November 2022, a new K7 evaluation was necessary to evaluate progress. An abstract of the most significant scans can be seen in Figs. 12.109, 12.110, 12.111, 12.112 and 12.113.

Figures 12.109 and 12.110 show scan 21 and that the patient swallows in CO during VSS. There is no pre-activation of the masseter muscles as seen previously. These two scans 21 are the same scan but at different gains to verify even the slight muscular activation at initial mandibular elevation for the swallowing process. 111 represents scan 11. These results are very positive if compared with the previous results. Finally, the masseter muscles are picking up their function. It can be noted that there is an increase in the right masseter which is proportional to the asymmetry found in the patient. The working side has stronger muscles. Figure 12.113 represents scan 4/5 after 45′ of Tensing with Aqualizer®. Vertical freeway space looks increased (4.8 mm) while the AP discrepancy has been reduced. This result is considered satisfactory and should become better with time. For this reason, it was decided to follow up with scan 11 every 4 months or so to evaluate progress in muscle function. Re-educating functional balancing (chewing on balancing side) might reserve positive results. The following scan 11 represents the latest follow-up scan (Fig. 12.114), February 2023):

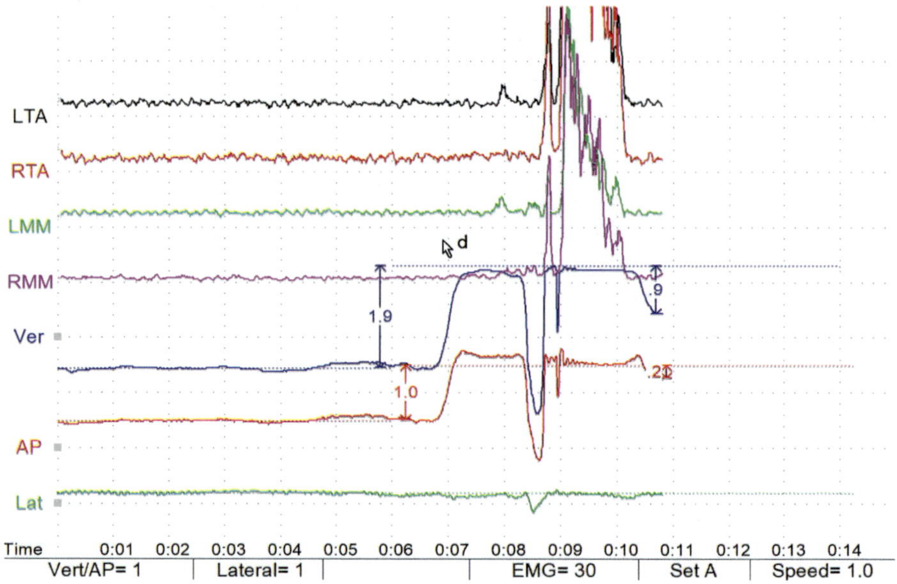

Fig. 12.109 Polygraphic scan (scan 3 + S-EMG filtered, scan 21) Post-treatment, 4 years after treatment, showing a VSS (Voluntary Swallow of Saliva, indicated starting point in "d"). The vertical blue line shows mandibular closure (upward) when swallow starts. There is no premature activation of the masseter muscles at the start of deglutition sequence indicating that the patient swallows correctly in CO. The AP red line indicates a forward mandibular movement during swallow. (LMM: left masseter muscle; LTA: left anterior temporalis; RMM: right masseter muscle; RTA: right anterior temporalis). AP: anterior-posterior; Lat: lateral; Ver: vertical

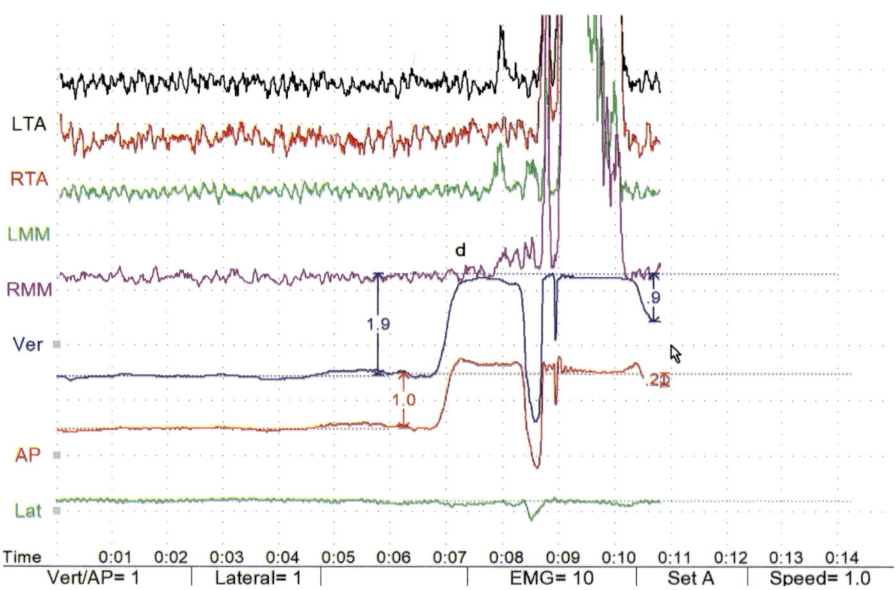

Fig. 12.110 Same scan as previous but with different gains (EMG = 10 MicroVolts), Post-treatment 4 years after treatment

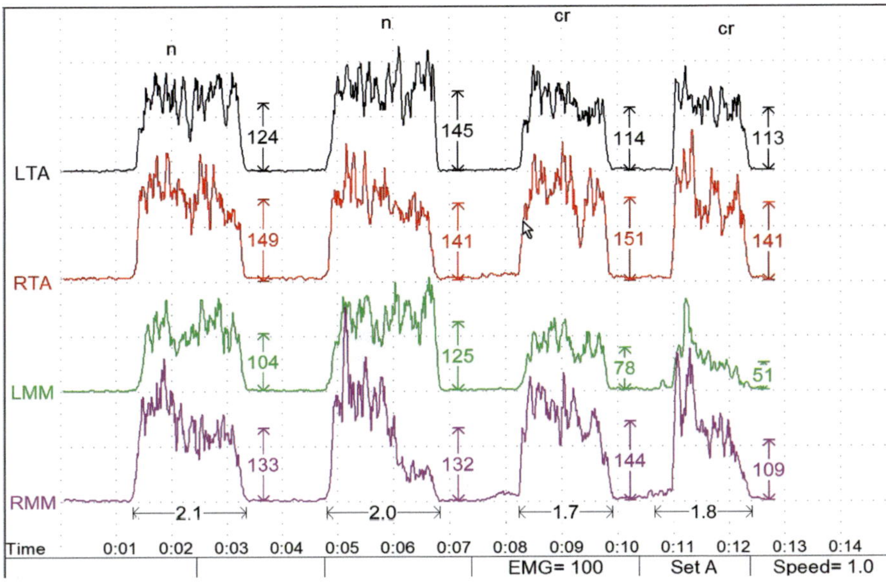

Fig. 12.111 Post-treatment 4 years after treatment. Scan 11 (post-treatment) shows the surface EMG results in sweep mode. The patient was instructed to clench in CO (first burst and second burst), and then clench with cotton rolls between the teeth, which temporarily prevented occlusion (third burst and fourth burst). Output s-EMG is satisfactory. and the general there is a symmetric balancing except for the marginal increase of right masseter over the left masseter. The Temporalis have a slightly stronger output during clench in respect of the masseters. CO: centric occlusion; EMG: electromyography; LMM: left masseter muscle; LTA: left anterior temporalis; RMM: right masseter muscle; RTA: right anterior temporalis

These last scans show a stable and constant increase, balance and correction of the muscular activation sequence as requested by neuromuscular standards. Fig. 12.114 shows clench one and two with a correct sequence of activation, with the temporalis muscles activating before the masseters. The rehabilitation process in asymmetry is difficult and slow. Further studies are needed to evaluate the long-term effectiveness of functional voluntary rehabilitation in developing asymmetries. This patient has been instructed to chew *mainly on her left to promote muscle compensation*. These scans demonstrate that it is possible to voluntarily re-equilibrate muscle function of the stomatognathic system.

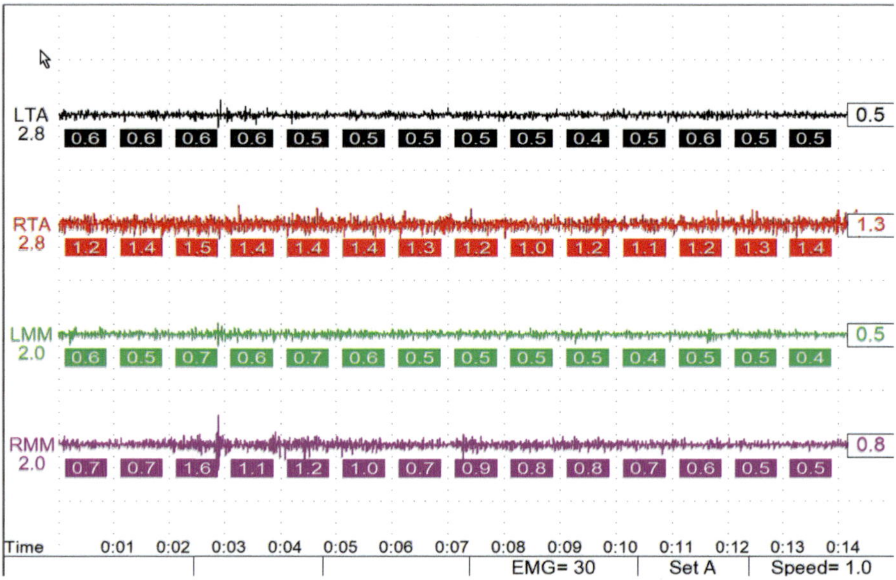

Fig. 12.112 Post-treatment 4 years after treatment. Scan 10 shows that the muscles were relaxed (after TENS). An Aqualizer was used to avoid tooth contact for CNS deconditioning. CNS: central nervous system; LMM: left masseter muscle; LTA: left anterior temporalis; RMM: right masseter muscle; RTA: right anterior temporalis

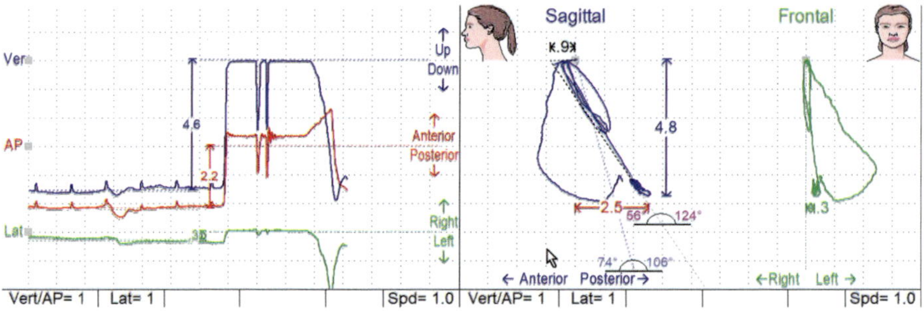

Fig. 12.113 Scan 4/5 (Post-treatment 4 years after treatment) in split screen modality. On the left sweep V, AP, and Lat lines. The patient is instructed to rest mandibular posture and the instructed to close to Centric Occlusion. Note the TENS spikes on V and AP lines. On the right, the corresponding Sagittal/frontal scan 5 shows a 0.9-mm. AP discrepancy on HP (Horizontal Plane of Occlusion). The vertical freeway space is 4.8 mm. AP: anterior-posterior; CO: centric occlusion; Lat: lateral; Spd: speed; Vert: vertical

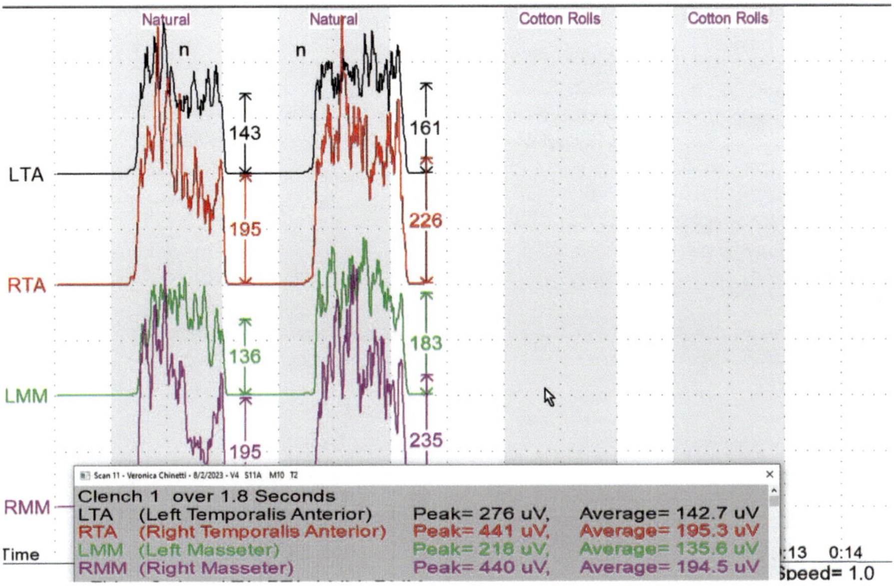

Fig. 12.114 Scan 11 (post-treatment follow-up at 4.3 years) shows the surface EMG results in sweep mode. The patient was instructed to clench in CO (first burst and second burst). Output s-EMG is satisfactory. and the general there is a better general output. The Temporalis do not have a complete stronger output during clench in respect of the masseters. CO: centric occlusion; EMG: electromyography; LMM: left masseter muscle; LTA: left anterior temporalis; RMM: right masseter muscle; RTA: right anterior temporalis

Case 12.7

Class II Long Face Syndrome with Loss of Freeway Space. Increased OJ

Summary A 8-year-old Caucasian child presented with the mother with a concern regarding misaligned teeth and facial development.

Pre-treatment	
Extraoral analysis	
Facial profile	Concave, long face
Facial height	Increased
Occlusal plane	Normal
Facial symmetry	
Lips	Incompetent
Mandibular posture	
Head posture extended	
Intraoral analysis (Fig. 12.12)	
Teeth	
Molar	Class II right, class I left
Canine	Class II right, class I left
Overjet positive	9 mm
Overbite	3 mm
Oral hygiene	Good
Rotations	
Crossbite	
Diastemas	
Crowding	Lower
Agenesis	
Missing teeth	
Intraoral analysis (Fig. 12.13)	
Swallow	Deviated
Tongue tie	No
Tongue posture	Good
Slurred speech	No
Neuromuscular diagnosis	
Freeway space decreased or absent	
Skeletal class	II
Anterior Wall	No
TMJ	No signs or symptoms

Problem list

- Absence of freeway space produces head extension.
- OJ and lower crowding.
- Open bite morphology.

Neuromuscular treatment objectives

- Mandibular Freedom by creating freeway space.
- Correction of mandibular plane to create long-term stability.

Introduction

Open bite morphology is widely recognized as a challenging condition to treat in orthodontics due to the limited room for dental compensation resulting from skeletal morphology. To achieve a stable occlusion without risking condylar resorption and arthrosis, it is crucial to apply interceptive therapy during a child's growth phase. This skeletal morphology often leads to unsuccessful orthodontic treatment, making interceptive therapy even more essential to reduce the need for surgery at a later age. The neuromuscular approach, which utilizes bioelectrical instrumentation, may provide an advantage over other diagnostic or evaluation techniques in orthodontics. The ability to measure freeway space is a critical factor in addressing vertical discrepancies. Although the anatomy of the condyle and glenoid fossa is not always conducive to successful treatment, the optimal solution is to rely on musculature to determine condylar repositioning.

Figures 12.115 and 12.116 show intra- and extraoral photos before treatment. Fig. 12.117 show lateral ncephalogram and panoramic X-rays.

Lateral cephalogram and panoramic X-rays had been taken in late 2003 and can be seen in Fig. 12.117.

This case holds significant importance as it showcases the usefulness of bioelectric instrumentation in evaluating neuromuscular treatment goals. Open bite cases, such as the one presented, often lack freeway space and can cause symptomatic issues, even in children, such as cervicalgia and TMJ noises. In such cases, measuring freeway space using TENS is unnecessary since there is no freeway space available and there is only one direction for treatment. The Teuscher appliance can prove

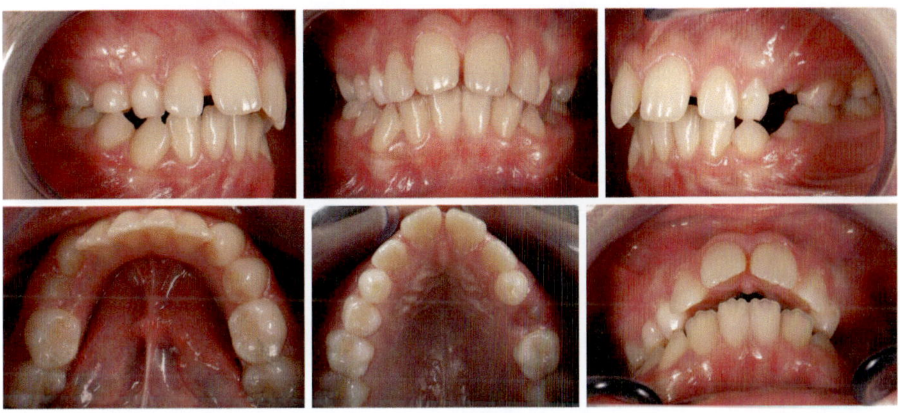

Fig. 12.115 Intraoral photos before treatment (12.2006)

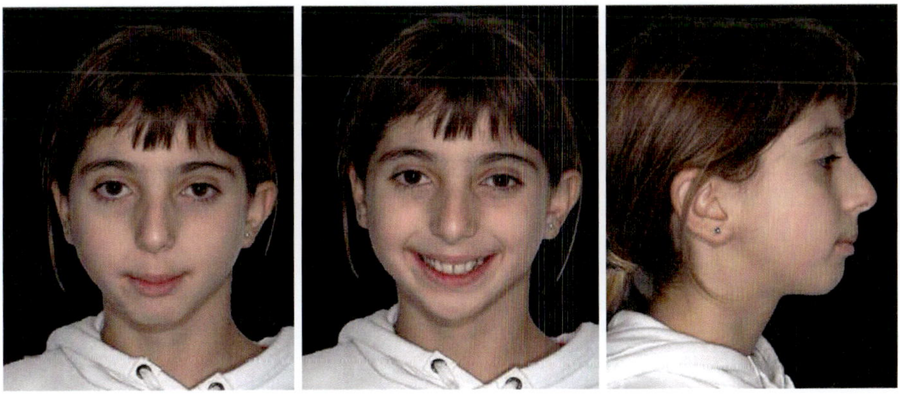

Fig. 12.116 Extraoral photos before treatment (12.2006)

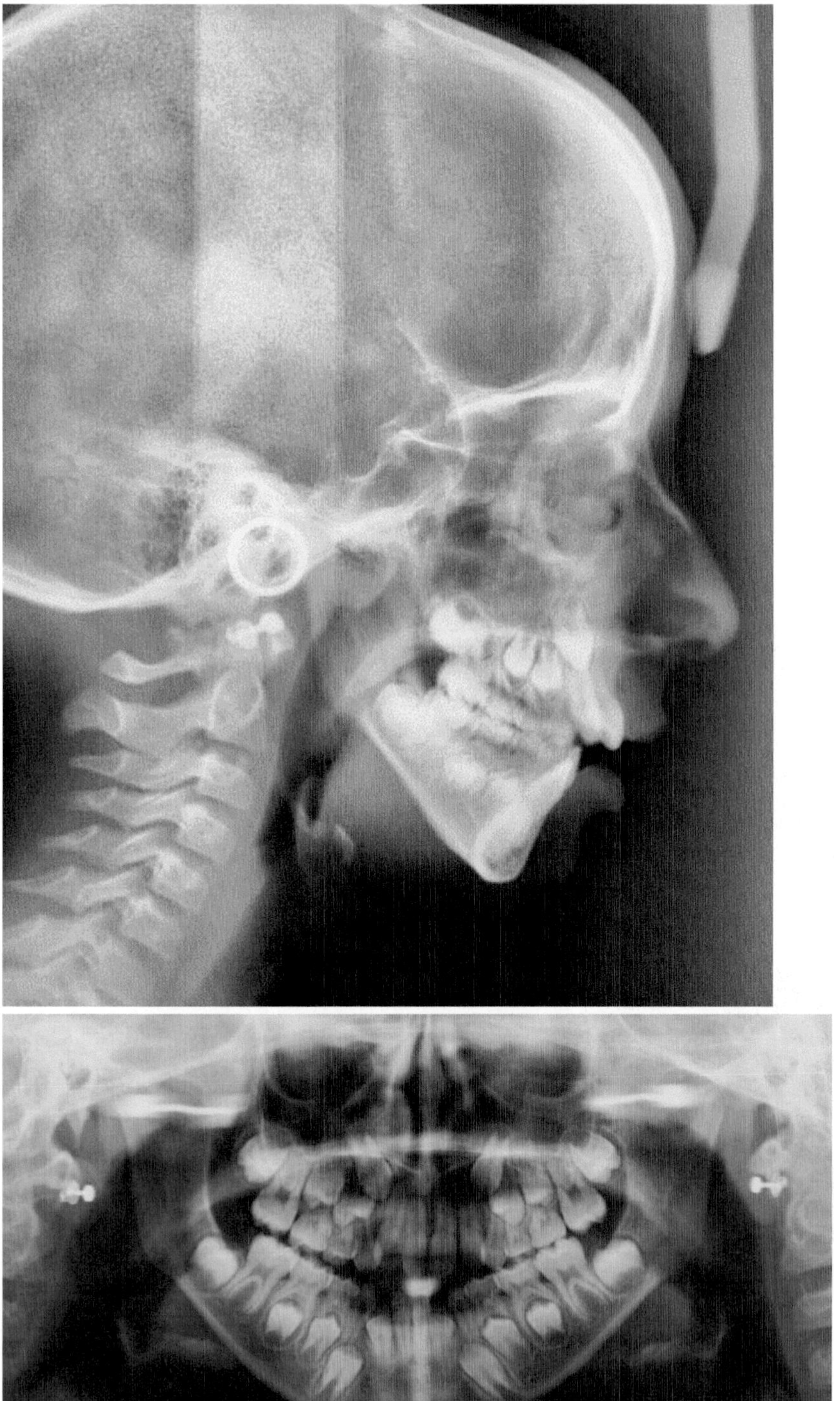

Fig. 12.117 Lateral cephalogram and panoramic X-rays taken before treatment (12.2003)

to be very effective in applying orthopedic forces to the upper maxilla, reducing vertical discrepancy. If treatment mechanics are applied efficiently, a positive functional outcome can be achieved by creating freeway space through upper intrusion and reduction of vertical growth. This can lead to a stable occlusion, forward mandibular advancement through increased mandibular closure, and absence of cervical compensation.

The following steps clarify the orthodontic procedure:

1. 1/2007 Applied Teuscher, 500 gr. pull.
2. 7/2007 RPE.
3. 3/2008 removal of RP-expander.
4. 4/2008 Intraoral photos taken (Fig. 12.118), applied upper fixed appliance.
5. 6.2008 Applied lower fixed appliance.
6. May 2009, treatment was terminated (Figs. 12.119, 12.120, 12.121 and 12.122), applied retention with premade positioner and instructed for 12-h use (8 h nighttime and 4 h daytime) for 3 months. Lower fixed 3–3 lingual retainer applied in May 2009.

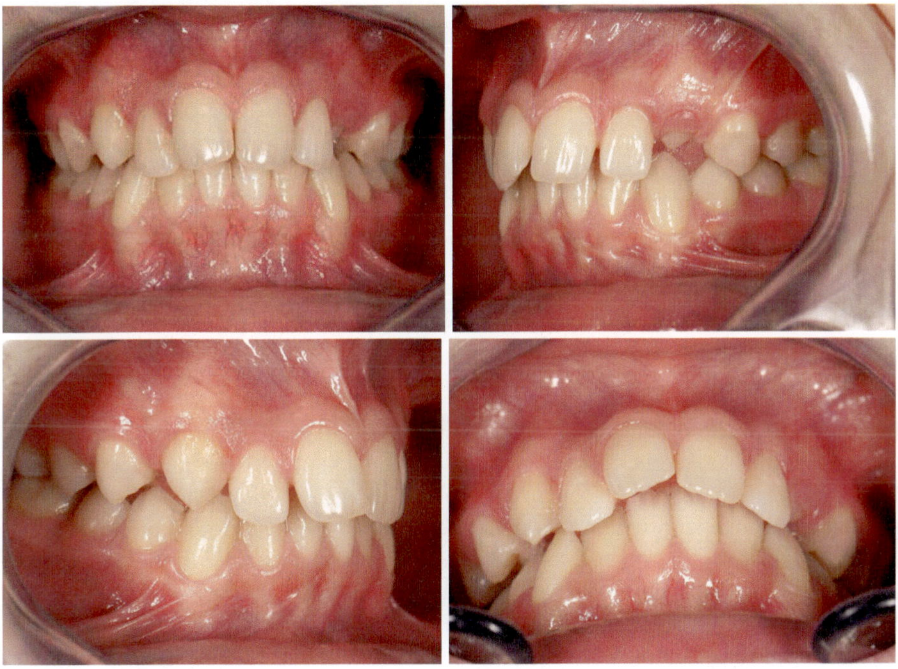

Fig. 12.118 Intraoral photos after Teuscher and RME treatment, 4.2008. Note Class I dental occlusion on the left side and a Class III dental occlusion on the right side. The overjet has been reduced by increased mandibular closure

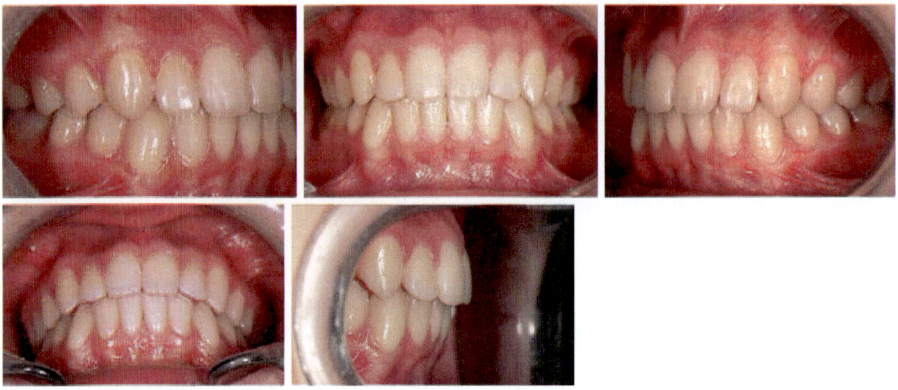

Fig. 12.119 Intraoral photos after treatment. 5.2009

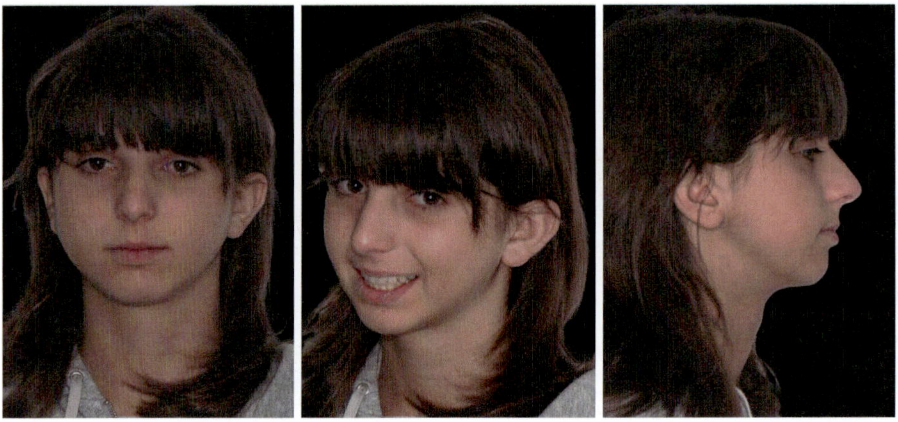

Fig. 12.120 Extraoral photos after treatment. 5.2009

Discussion

In addition to improving the aesthetic appearance of dental occlusion and facial features, addressing certain issues is crucial. From a neuromuscular perspective, the primary objective in cases of severe open bite is to utilize orthopedic forces to counteract the negative auto-feeding loop that perpetuates the posterior eruption of molar sectors, worsening the open bite both dentally and skeletally. The therapy should aim to create freeway space that is not solely a result of head extension, allowing for the retrieval of a normal postural attitude of the craniofacial complex. In theory, freeway space is essential for the growth of the mandibular ramus because reducing the compression of anatomical components (teeth and bone) decreases the strain on tensional components (muscles and fascia), which no longer apply tensile forces that may hinder the vertical growth of the ramus.

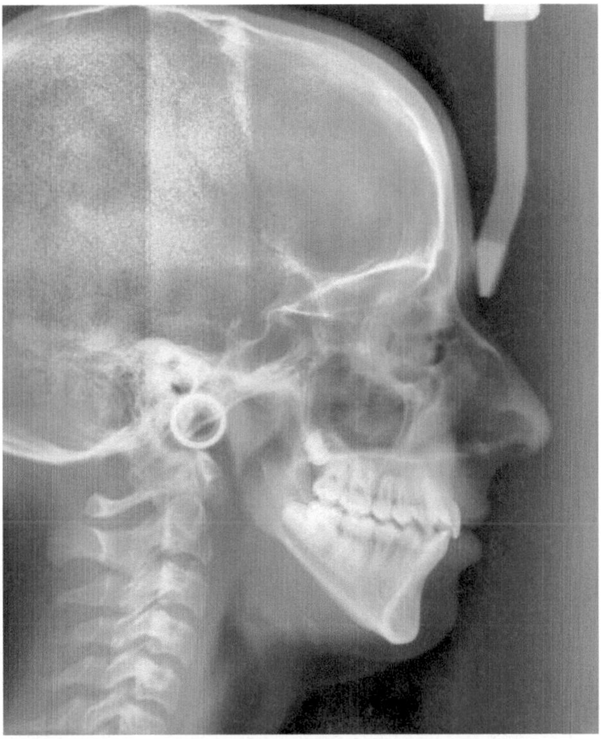

Fig. 12.121 Lateral cephalogram after treatment. 5.2009

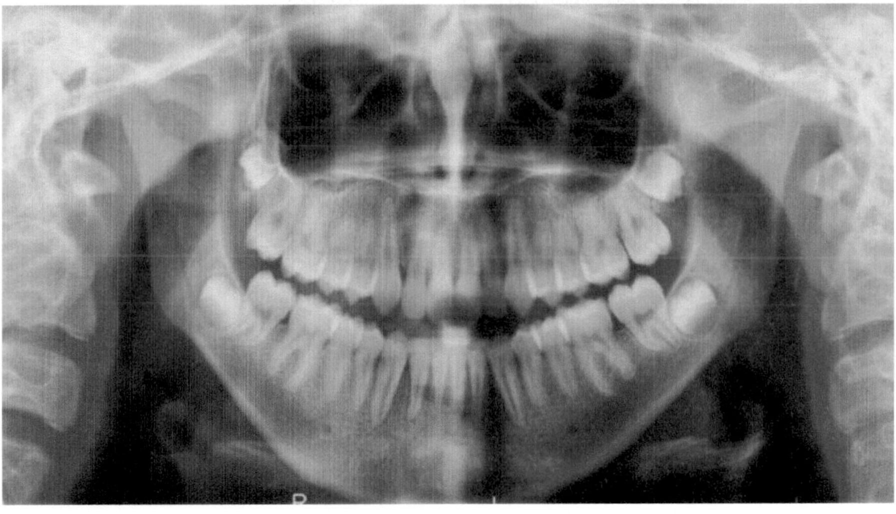

Fig. 12.122 Panoramic X-ray, after treatment, 5.2009

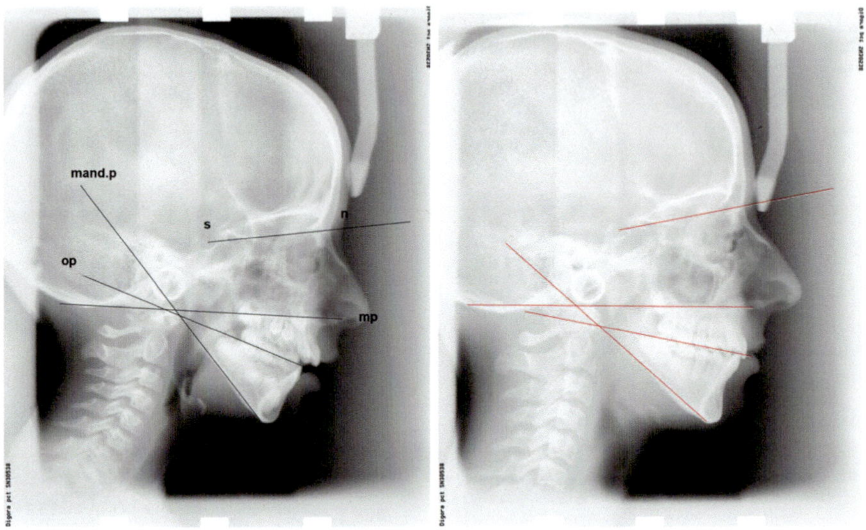

Fig. 12.123 Lateral cephalograms before (left) and after treatment (right). Tracings in black before treatment and in red after treatment. Mand.p = mandibular plane; s = sella; n = nasion; op = occlusal plane; mp = maxillary plane

The development of skeletal open bite is a complex process influenced by several factors, including epigenetic factors that arise from the environment, such as orthodontics. As chronic mouth breathing has been shown to negatively affect facial development, it is crucial to recognize the potential impact of orthodontic and orthopedic treatments on facial growth. Unfortunately, such treatments cannot be sustained throughout childhood, making it necessary to intervene at any age and interrupt any epigenetic influences that may impede facial development or sustain oral dysfunction. Therefore, this patient has undergone several consultations with an ear, nose, and throat specialist to improve breathing during treatment.

Figures 12.123, 12.124 and 12.125 show lateral cephalograms before and after treatment with several measurements that demonstrate changes due to treatment and growth. Figures 12.124 and 12.125 show two different superimpositions, on S-N line and on maxillary plane.

This superimposition (Fig. 12.124) is indicative of important changes from a cephalometric point of view. The following summarizes the results of a comparison of before and after treatment:

1. The mandibular plane rotated counterclockwise.
2. The occlusal plane rotated counterclockwise.
3. The angle between the two maxillary planes opened, meaning that a posterior clockwise rotation accompanied vertical limitation.

The following tracings are superimposed also on the maxillary plane to highlight the changes on the lower third of the facial skeleton (Fig. 12.125).

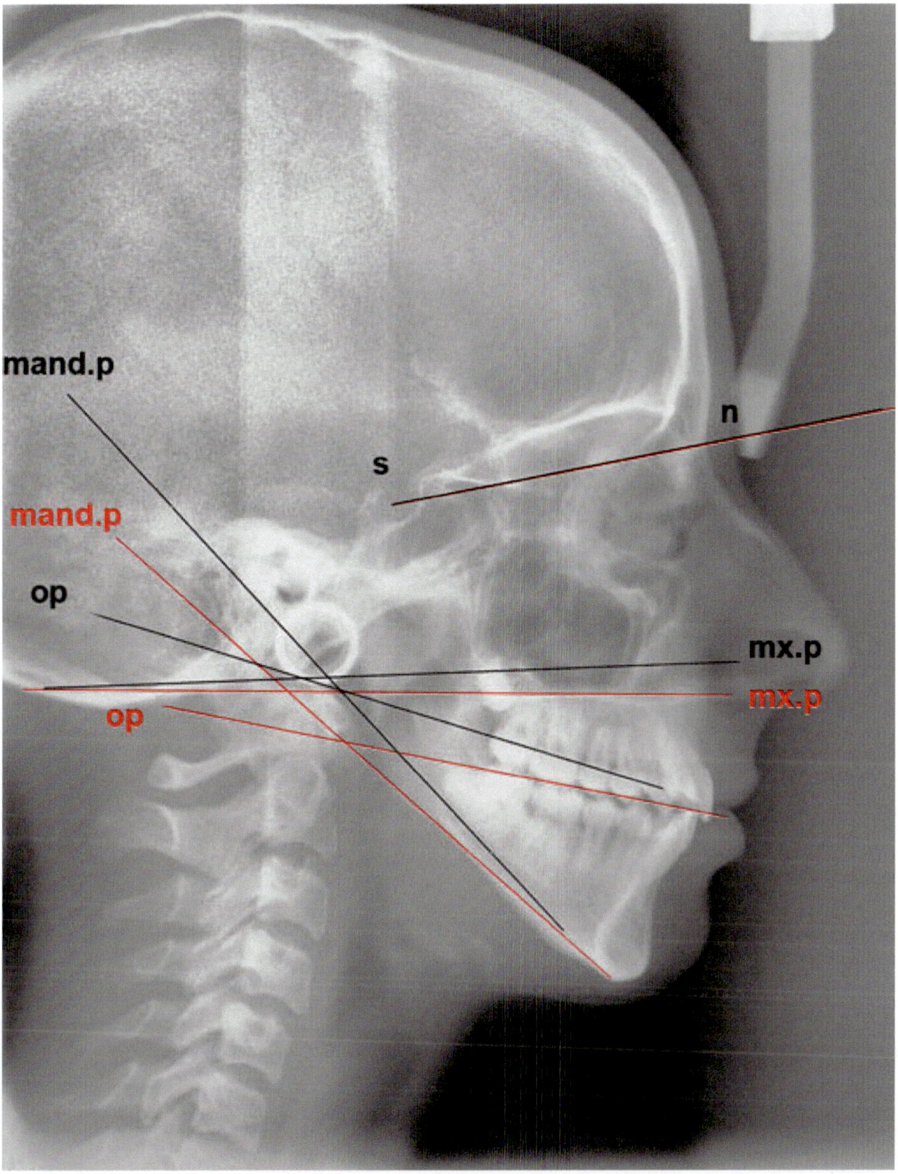

Fig. 12.124 Superimposition of initial tracings (black) from initial lateral cephalogram with tracings from final lateral cephalograms (red) on the s-n line (sella-nasion) and showing final lateral cephalogram. Mand.p = mandibular plane; s = sella; n = nasion; op = occlusal plane; mp = mandibular plane; mx.p = maxillary plane

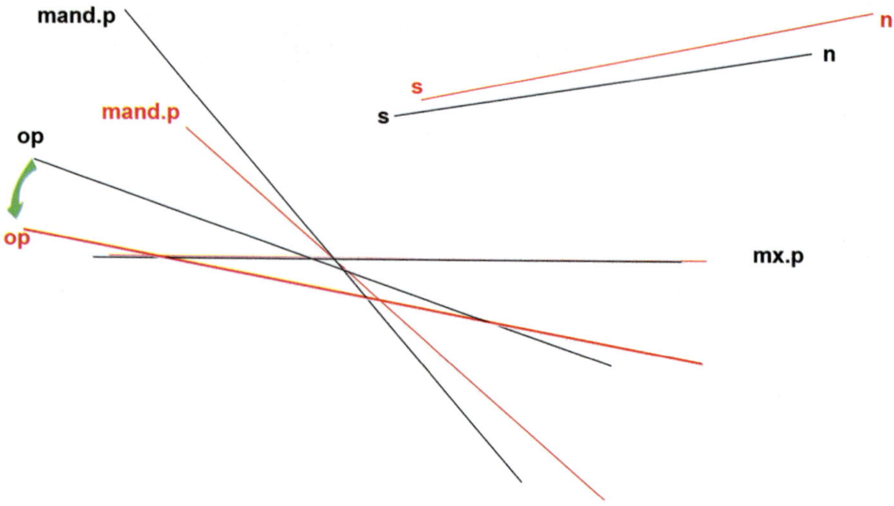

Fig. 12.125 Superimposition of tracings before and after treatment on maxillary plane. The green arrow shows the positive counterclockwise rotation of the occlusal plane. In black: before treatment; in red: after treatment; Mand.p = mandibular plane; s = sella; n = nasion; op = occlusal plane; mp = mandibular plane; mx.p = maxillary plane

The counterclockwise rotation of the occlusal plane and the mandibular plane relative to the maxillary plane is indicative of an increase in the posterior facial height relative to the anterior facial height. The positive outcome was the result of proper programming linked to patient collaboration.

Follow-up check-ups were conducted on a yearly basis. Retention was suspended by the patient 2 years after treatment. Follow-up documentation can be seen in Figs. 12.126 and 12.127 at 14 years after treatment.

During this check-up at 14 years after treatment, a complete k7 study was conducted to assess long-term stability and results. Figures 12.128, 12.129, 12.130 and 12.131 show some selected tracings from the K7-system evaluation.

After 14 years from treatment, this patient reported no cervical or TMJ or pain. The only occasional complaint was a right-sided headache. Figure 12.128 shows that muscles at rest are not completely relaxed and that the right anterior temporalis is slightly above the resting limits. Figure 12.129 shows a limited output of the right masseter during MVC. For this reason, some occlusal adjustments were performed (coronoplasty), but the reports are not yet included in this report. After coronoplasty, the neuromuscular system takes quite some time to adjust, react, and

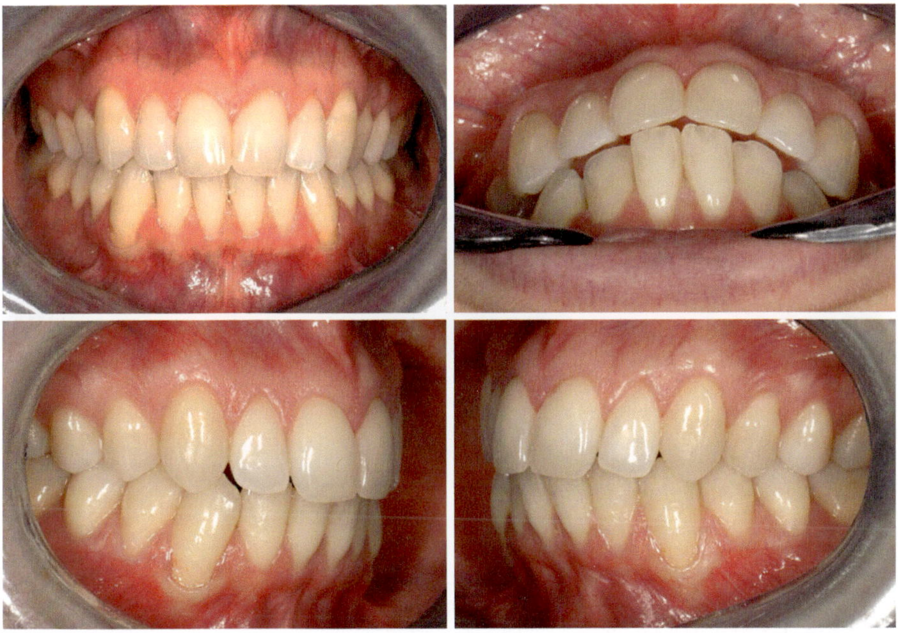

Fig. 12.126 Intraoral photos at 14 years after treatment

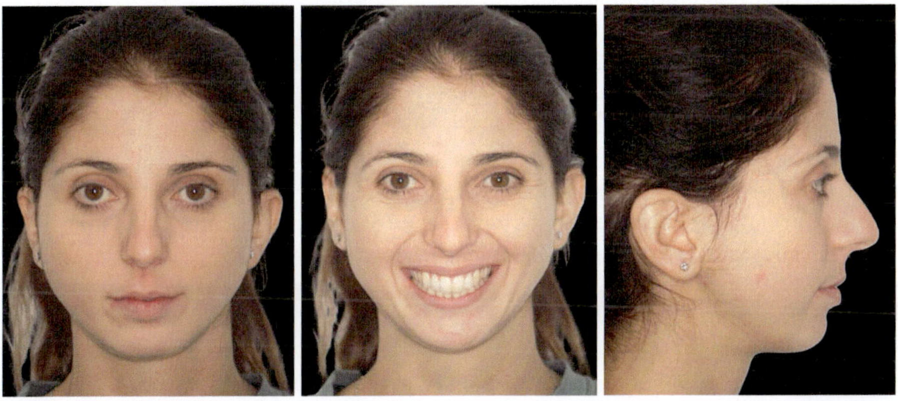

Fig. 12.127 Extraoral photos at 14 years after treatment

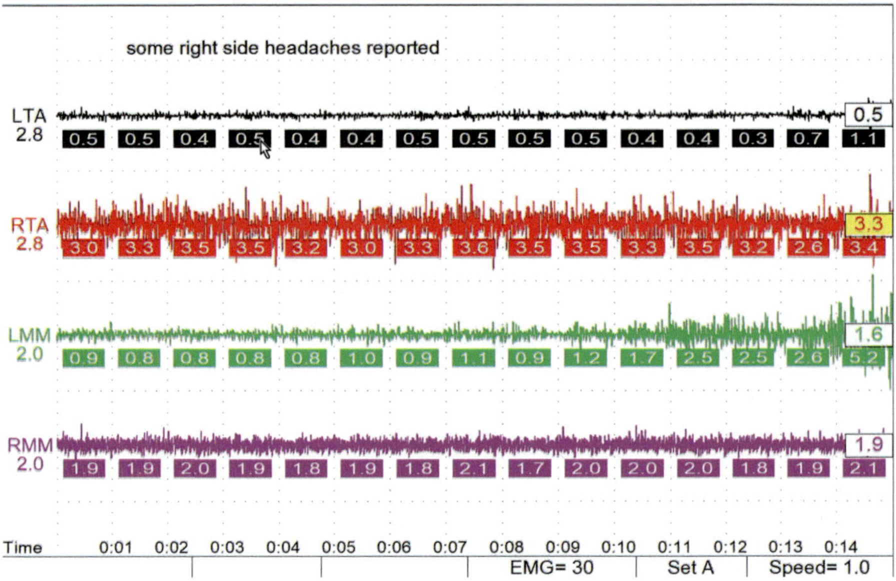

Fig. 12.128 Scan 9 (post-treatment follow-up at 14 years from treatment) shows the surface EMG results for the LTA, RTA, LMM, and RMM. The muscle outputs at rest were within the normal limits except for RTA slightly over. CO: centric occlusion; EMG: electromyography; LMM: left masseter muscle; LTA: left anterior temporalis; RMM: right masseter muscle; RTA: right anterior temporalis

stabilize occlusion to the anatomical change in dental anatomy. Just like the changes and stabilization of occlusion takes several months after orthodontic treatment. Figure 12.130 shows that there is some activation of the perioral musculature during VSS, but it is not a strong activation (this is frequent in open-bite morphology). Figure 12.131 shows the results of scan 21 for a SSS. It is notable that the submental musculature is activated before the perioral musculature, indicating that there is only a residual activation of the perioral musculature due to secondary tongue thrust (author's hypothesis).

Scan 4/5 can be seen in Fig. 12.132 and shows that there is a vertical freeway space of 0.9 mm and forward mandibular movement to CO. These scan results are to be considered acceptable even if freeway space is minimal.

Figure 12.133 shows the differences in occlusion before and at 14 years after orthodontic treatment.

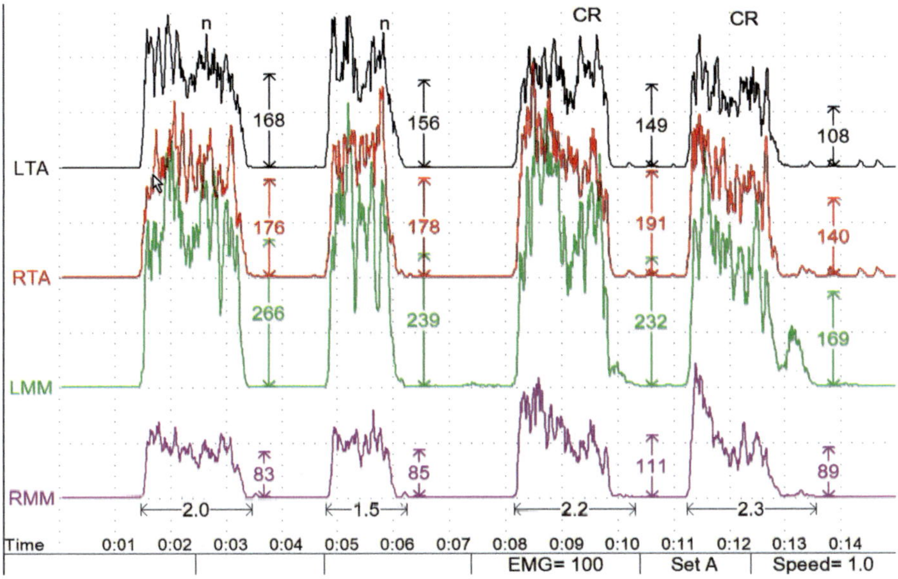

Fig. 12.129 Scan 11 (post-treatment follow-up at 14 years) shows the surface EMG results in sweep mode. The patient was instructed to clench in CO (first and second bursts), and then clench with cotton rolls between the teeth, which temporarily prevented occlusion (third burst and fourth burst). Output s-EMG is very good for open bite morphology indicating muscle fatigue is not present. RMM output is low and not balanced with LMM. LMM: left masseter muscle; LTA: left anterior temporalis; RMM: right masseter muscle; RTA: right anterior temporalis

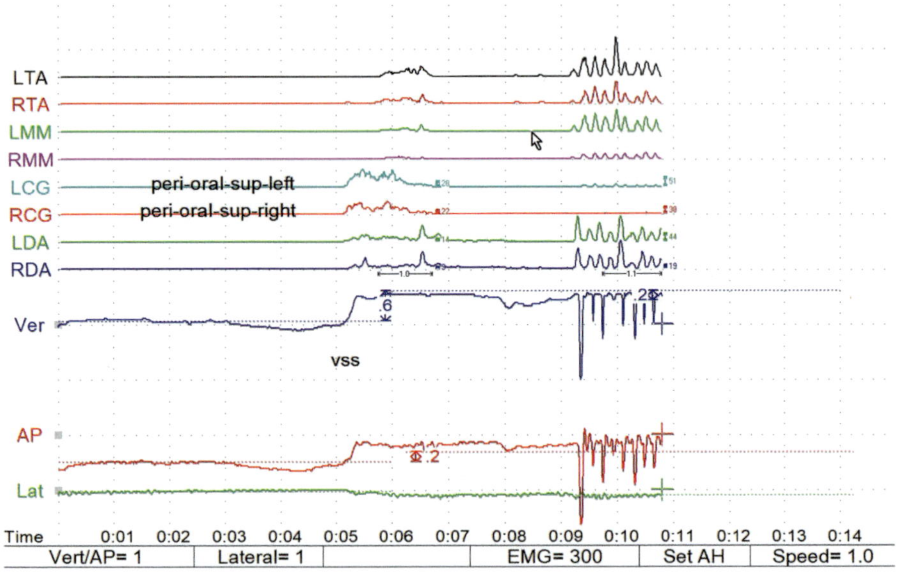

Fig. 12.130 Polygraphic scan (scan 3 + S-EMG filtered, scan 21) Post-treatment follow-up at 14 years after treatment, showing a VSS (Voluntary Swallow of Saliva, indicated with "VSS"). The vertical blue line (Ver) shows mandibular closure (upward) when swallow starts. There is no premature activation of the masseter muscles at the start of deglutition sequence indicating that the patient swallows correctly in CO and does not put the tongue between the teeth. The perioral musculature is activated together with the sub-mental musculature. (LMM: left masseter muscle; LTA: left anterior temporalis; RMM: right masseter muscle; RTA: right anterior temporalis). AP: anterior-posterior; Lat: lateral; Ver: vertical;; LDA = sub-mental musculature (red arrows for activation); LCG = perioral musculature upper left; RCG = perioral musculature upper right

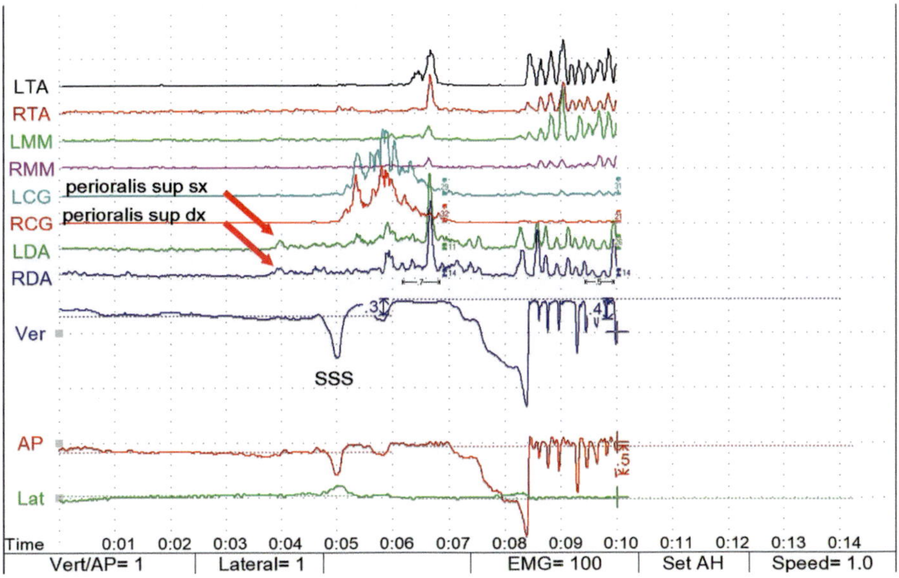

Fig. 12.131 Polygraphic scan (scan 3 + S-EMG filtered, scan 21) Post-treatment follow-up at 14 years after treatment, showing a SSS (Spontaneous Swallow of Saliva, indicated with "SSS"). The vertical blue line shows mandibular closure (upward) when swallow starts. There is no premature activation of the masseter muscles at start of deglutition sequence indicating that the patient swallows correctly in CO and does not interpose the tongue between the teeth. The perioral musculature is activated after the sub-mental musculature (red arrows). LMM: left masseter muscle; LTA: left anterior temporalis; RMM: right masseter muscle; RTA: right anterior temporalis. AP: anterior-posterior; Lat: lateral; Ver: vertical; LDA = sub-mental musculature (red arrows for activation); LCG = perioral musculature upper left; RCG = perioral musculature upper right

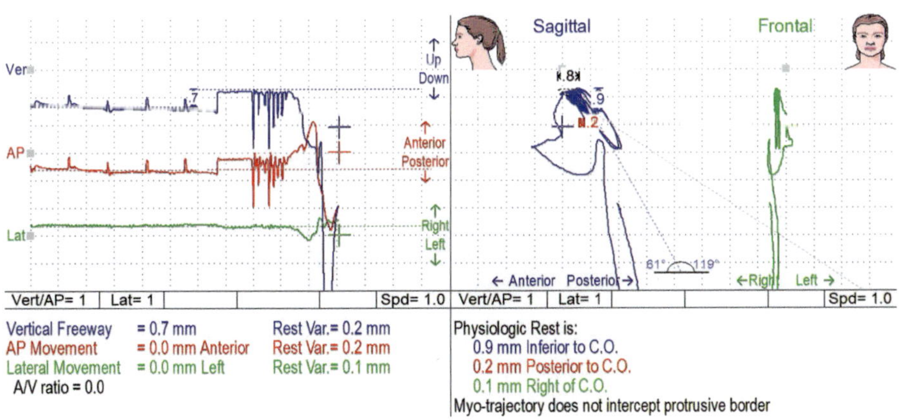

Fig. 12.132 Scan 4/5 (post-treatment follow-up at 14 years) in split screen modality. On the left sweep V, AP, and Lat lines. The patient is instructed to rest mandibular posture and instructed to close to Centric Occlusion. Note the TENS spikes on V and AP lines. On the right, the corresponding Sagittal/frontal scan 5 shows a 0.8-mm. AP discrepancy on HP (Horizontal Plane of Occlusion). The vertical freeway space is 0.9 mm. AP: anterior-posterior; CO: centric occlusion; Lat: lateral; Spd: speed; Vert: vertical

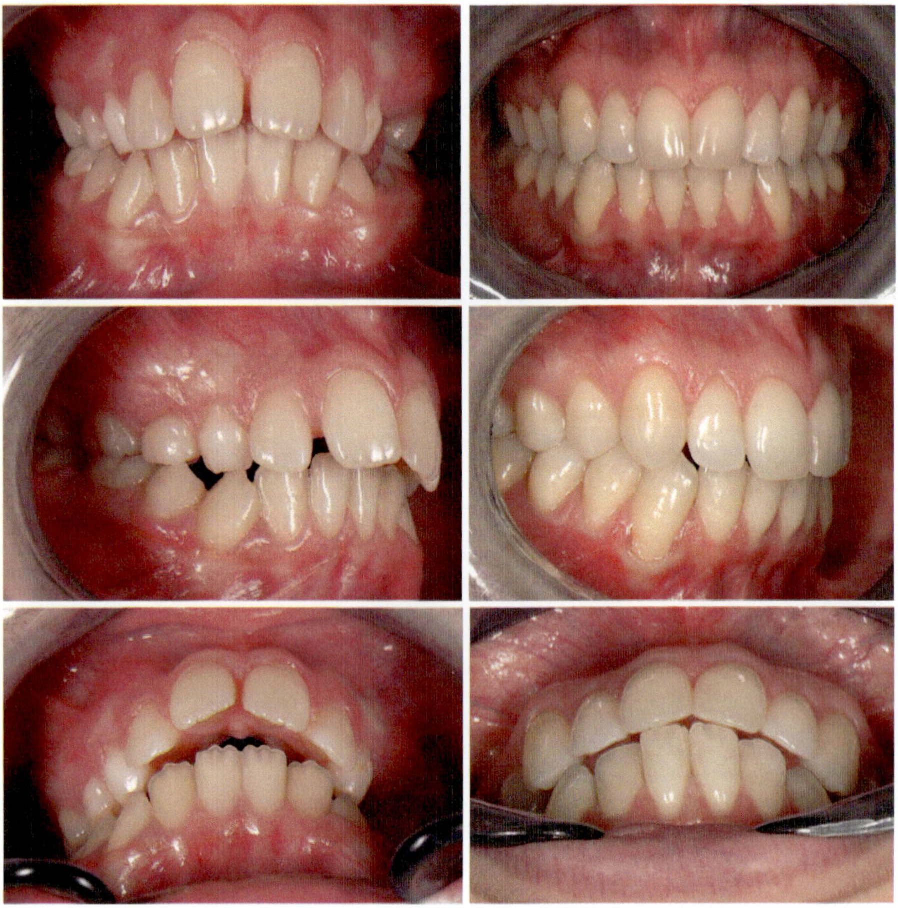

Fig. 12.133 Intraoral photos before treatment and after 17 years. Left column before treatment and right column after treatment

Case 12.8

Skeletal Class I and Dental Class I: Distal Occlusion and Anterior Wall

Summary A 12-year-old Caucasian child (and mother) were concerned regarding deep bite occlusion and suspected associated symptomatology: continuous shoulder pain and cervicalgia.

Pre-treatment	
Extraoral analysis	
Facial profile	Straight
Facial height	Normal
Occlusal plane	Normal
Facial symmetry	
Lips	Competent
Mandibular posture	
Head posture	
Intraoral analysis (Fig. 12.134)	
Teeth	
Molar	Class I
Canine	Class I
Overjet	0
Overbite	4 mm
Oral hygiene	Good
Rotations	
Crossbite	
Diastemas	
Crowding lower	
Agenesis	
Missing teeth	
Intraoral analysis (Fig. 12.134)	
Swallow	Deviated
Tongue tie	No
Tongue posture	Good
Slurred speech	No
Neuromuscular clinical diagnosis	
Freeway space	
Skeletal class	I
Anterior wall	Yes
TMJ	
Related signs of initial TMD: Cervicalgia and shoulder pain	
Problem list	
• Front wall is responsible for distal occlusion.	
• Anterior incisal contact with 0 mm OJ.	
Neuromuscular treatment objectives	
• Mandibular freedom by eliminating front wall.	
• Vertical freeway space correction and mandibular repositioning.	

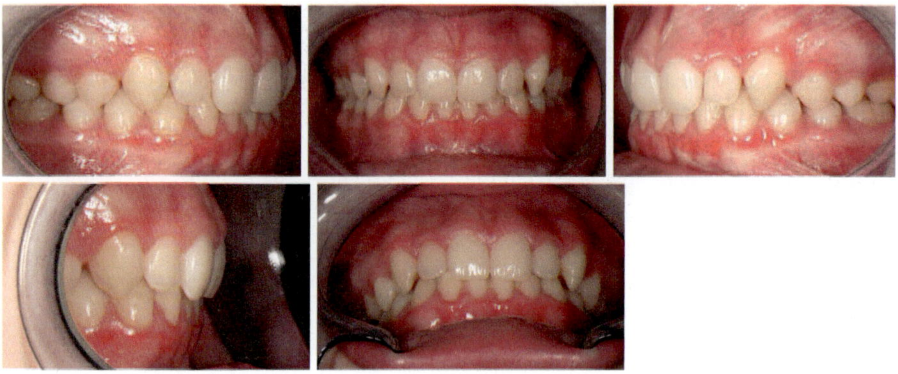

Fig. 12.134 Intraoral photos before treatment

Introduction

Academically speaking, professional athletes demonstrate a heightened sensitivity to changes in anatomy, postural instability, and alterations in their surrounding environment. In comparison to the general population, they typically possess a greater threshold for pain and exhibit a greater degree of pain tolerance [6, 7]. This particular case centers around a young volleyball athlete who has expressed concern over the recent onset of cervical and shoulder pain. While a cursory examination of the dental occlusion may not necessarily raise any alarm bells for most orthodontists, a closer inspection may reveal underlying dysfunctions that have the potential to progress into more complicated pathologies, such as TMD. It is imperative that healthcare professionals not overlook symptoms such as neck and shoulder pain in children, as they may be indicative of larger issues at play.

Figures 12.134 and 12.135 show intra- and extraoral photos before treatment (11.2018).

Since this young patient is symptomatic, it is necessary to verify quantitively the amount of anterior wall restriction. Should scan 5 show an excess of freeway space, then this case will have a positive prognostic outcome because extrusion after mandibular freedom will be sufficient to maintain a Class I dental relationship. A complete functional analysis was carried out in November 2018 and some selected scans can be seen in Figs. 12.136, 12.137 and 12.138.

Discussion

Scan 11 (Fig. 12.136) shows that the overall output of the right masseter is low in respect of the contralateral masseter while the temporalis muscles seem more balanced. Figure 12.137 shows that there is an activation of the masseter muscles at start of swallow. This muscle activation occurs before the temporalis muscles do, indicating that the patient swallows with tongue between the teeth at start of deglutition. The other sign showing that the tongue occupies space between the arches during swallow is represented by the blue vertical line that never reaches CO level (determined by tap-tap procedure). Not without surprise, scan 5 shows that there is a

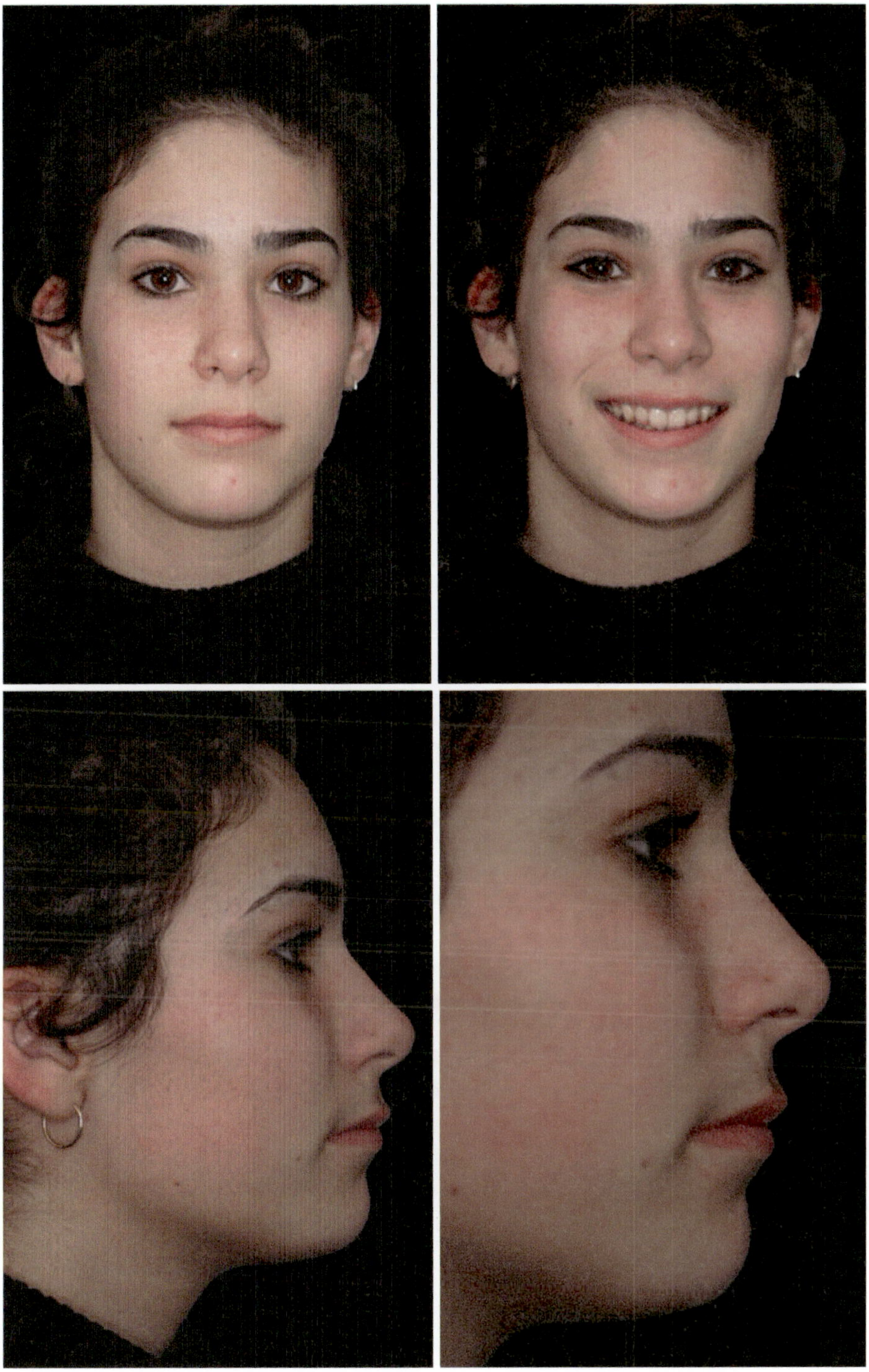

Fig. 12.135 Extraoral photos before treatment

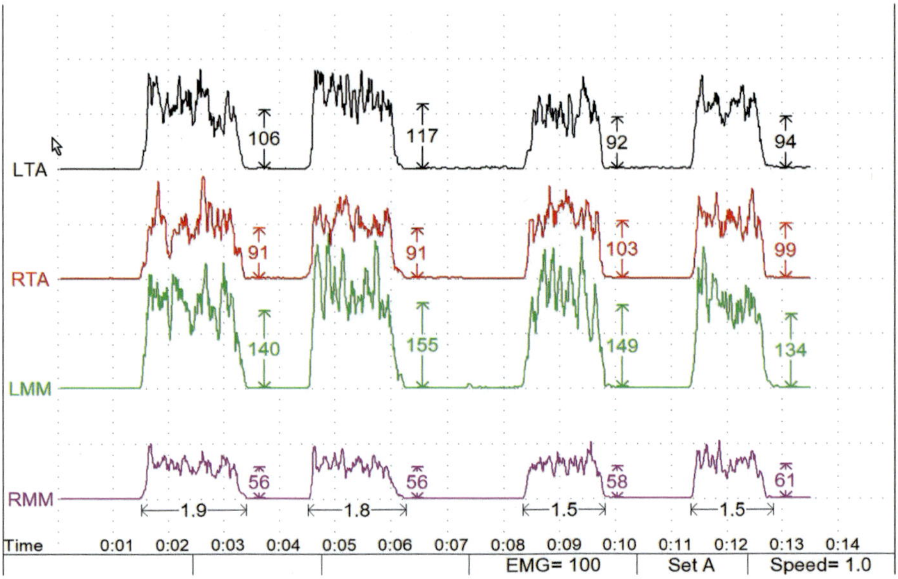

Fig. 12.136 July 2021 Scan 11 (pre-treatment) shows the surface EMG results in sweep mode. The patient was instructed to clench in CO (first burst and second burst), and then clench with cotton rolls between the teeth, which temporarily prevented occlusion (third burst and fourth burst). Output s-EMG is not satisfactory, and the general output is low. There is a discrete balance of output for the temporalis muscles only; the RMM seems to be under-activated during MVC. CO: centric occlusion; EMG: electromyography; LMM: left masseter muscle; LTA: left anterior temporalis; RMM: right masseter muscle; RTA: right anterior temporalis

notable sagittal and vertical discrepancy between the muscular request for an ideal centric (Myocentric) and actual CO (Fig. 12.138). This high degree of sagittal push-back on the mandible reflects at condylar level, thus creating disk compression in the TMJ. The results seen in scan 21 (Fig. 12.137) reflect a protective feature of the stomatognathic system: to avoid CO (ICP) during swallow, the tongue is called to act as "bite" to avoid dental occlusion. Swallowing with the tongue between the dental arches takes some effort too, but at some point, during the swallow, while the mandible attempts to come to ICP vertically, there is also a distalizing action the tongue cannot avoid doing to the mandible (and to the condyle) because of the suction and closure of the anterior opening it must comply with (green box in Fig. 12.137). ***Yet the condylar position is still protected even though slightly distalized: if occluding in CO during swallow, the condylar position would be even more posterior***.

The kinesiographic and neuromuscular objectives are to move the CO point more anteriorly and down vertically. The vertical movement is obviously obtained by dental extrusion that lowers the HP, while the sagittal correction is gained by a slight

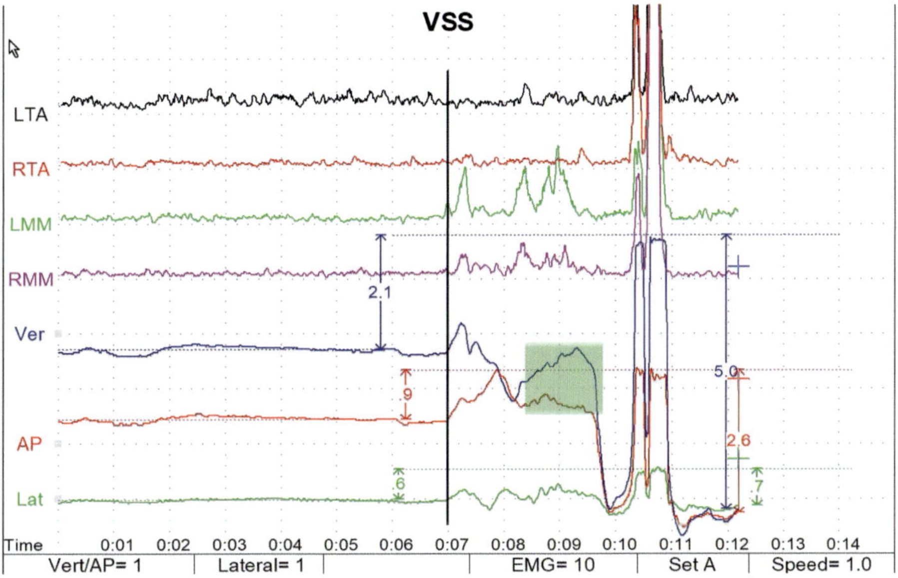

Fig. 12.137 Polygraphic scan (scan 3 + S-EMG filtered, scan 21) Pre-treatment shows a VSS (Voluntary Swallow of Saliva, indicated with "VSS"). The vertical blue line shows start of mandibular closure (upward) when swallow starts. There is an activation of the masseter muscles at start of deglutition sequence indicating that the patient swallows with tongue between the teeth. (LMM: left masseter muscle; LTA: left anterior temporalis; RMM: right masseter muscle; RTA: right anterior temporalis). AP: anterior-posterior; Lat: lateral; Ver: vertical, black vertical line indicates start of swallow sequence. Green box: see text for explanation

expansion and correction of the low torque present before treatment of the upper incisors. As seen in Fig. 12.138, the Myocentric can be calculated on the Myotrajectory and intercepting the V line (in green). This could make this case very easy to resolve by correcting anterior torque and extruding 3 mm. Care should be taken to align any low anterior teeth that might have compensated the anterior wall by lingual tipping. Class III elastics will be a good treatment mechanic for these cases. The extrusion provided accompanies lower distal tipping. Forces should be gentle, continuous, and long lasting.

By February 2019, a fixed appliance was applied to the upper arch, and leveling started with a low-force NiTi wire. By December 2019, the lower arch had been engaged with a 0.016 NiTi while the upper arches were engaged with .017x.025 NiTi wire. Upper Turbos were applied to favor extrusion of the mid-sectors (premolar region) as seen in Fig. 12.139.

Treatment was terminated in August 2020. Photos taken in January 2021 can be seen in Figs. 12.140 and 12.141.

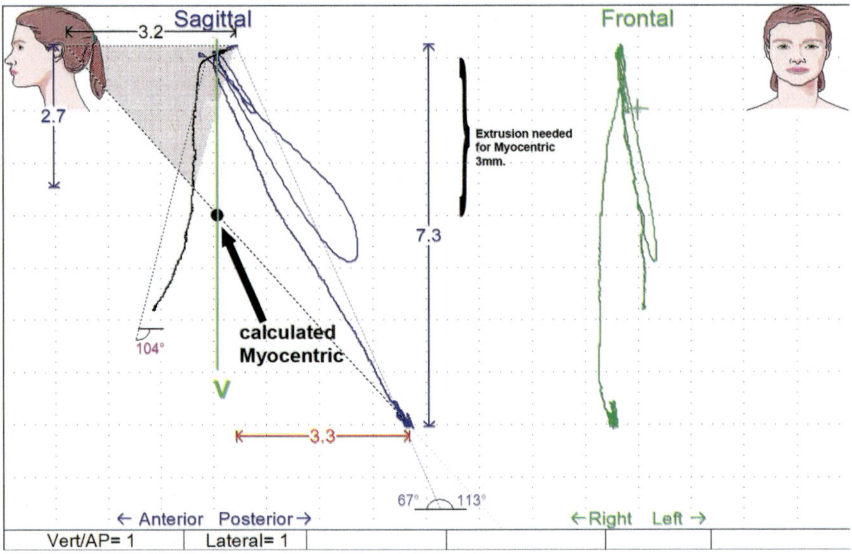

Fig. 12.138 Scan 5 in sagittal/frontal modality. The patient is instructed to rest mandibular posture and the instructed to close to Centric Occlusion. Sagittal/frontal scan 5 shows a 3.2-mm. AP discrepancy on HP (Horizontal Plane of Occlusion). Vertical freeway space is 7.3 mm. AP: anterior-posterior; CO: centric occlusion; Lat: lateral; Spd: speed; Vert: vertical; In green vertical V line passing through CO. Black dot = calculated Myocentric; in black right curly bracket explained amount of extrusion needed (see text)

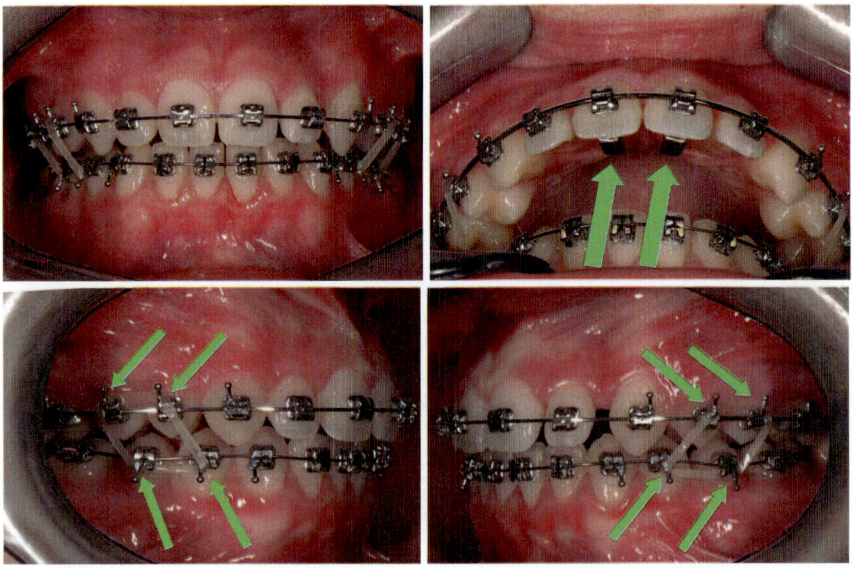

Fig. 12.139 Follow-up intraoral photos showing pre-molar box elastics (3/16, 4 oz.) for extrusion on pre-molar teeth. Green arrows show how elastics are passed across bracket hooks (lower photos) while green arrow on upper photo show bite turbos. Note how upper expansion/alignment has created upper diastemas

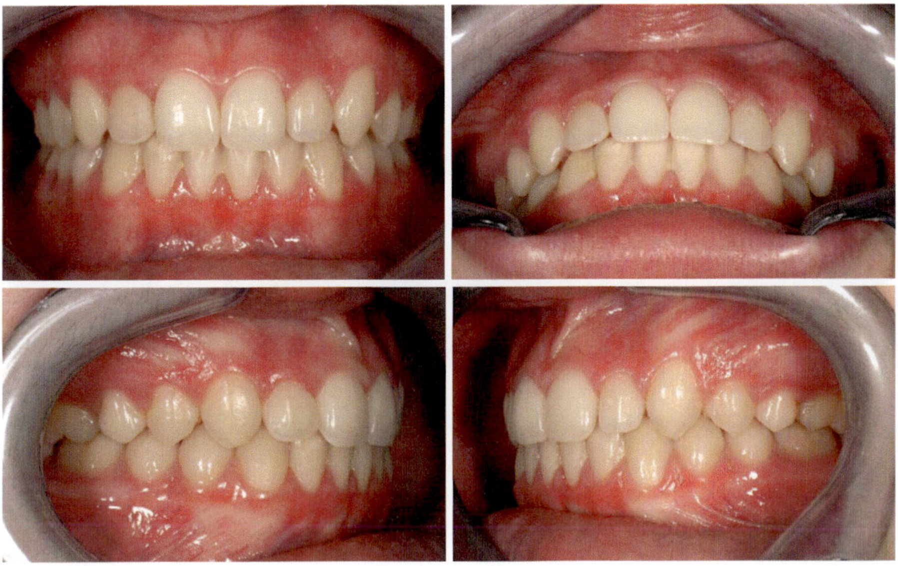

Fig. 12.140 intraoral photos after treatment. January 2021

A series of k7 functional evaluations were done over the last 24 months to monitor treatment outcomes. These evaluations can be seen in Figs. 12.142, 12.143, 12.144 and 12.145 (July 2021), Figs. 146 and 147 (August 2022) and Figs. 12.148, 12.149 and 12.150 (April 2023).

Follow-up intra- and extraoral photos can be seen in Figs. 12.151 and 12.152, April 2023.

The kinesiographic scans show that she is functionally a deep-bite with excess freeway space. All malocclusions are accompanied by tongue dysfunction, in other words, only a well-balanced occlusion and a good mandibular posture can guarantee the ideal environment for a correct tongue function. The correction of the habitual path of closure on the Myotrajectory (acceptable 0.7 mm discrepancy on HP) is sometimes not sufficient to regain a correct swallow sequence immediately (Fig. 12.143), the improvement seen for VSS (Fig. 12.142) is though a good indication of a progressive rehabilitation of tongue function towards an ideal function. This small but notable problem is visualized during SSS which is noticeably linked to sub-cortical mechanisms; the delay in swallow correction durin SSS could be explained because the tongue posture is still adapting to a new occlusion.

The sagittal relationship benefitted the most from this therapy. The extrusion of the pre-molar sectors did use up some freeway space, but probably not sufficiently to be ideal. If analyzed, scan 4/5 in Fig. 12.150, the ideal freeway space and thus the Myocentric, would be behind the vertical V line. This means that in order to be in an ideal Myocentric, treatment should distalize the upper arch and extrude about 5 mm. In other words, there is no neuromuscular orthodontic correction on the ideal MyoCentric as of scan 4/5 of Fig. 12.150. The best possible result would be an extrusion of about 1.8 mm to retain a Myocentric on the Myotrajectory (Fig. 12.153).

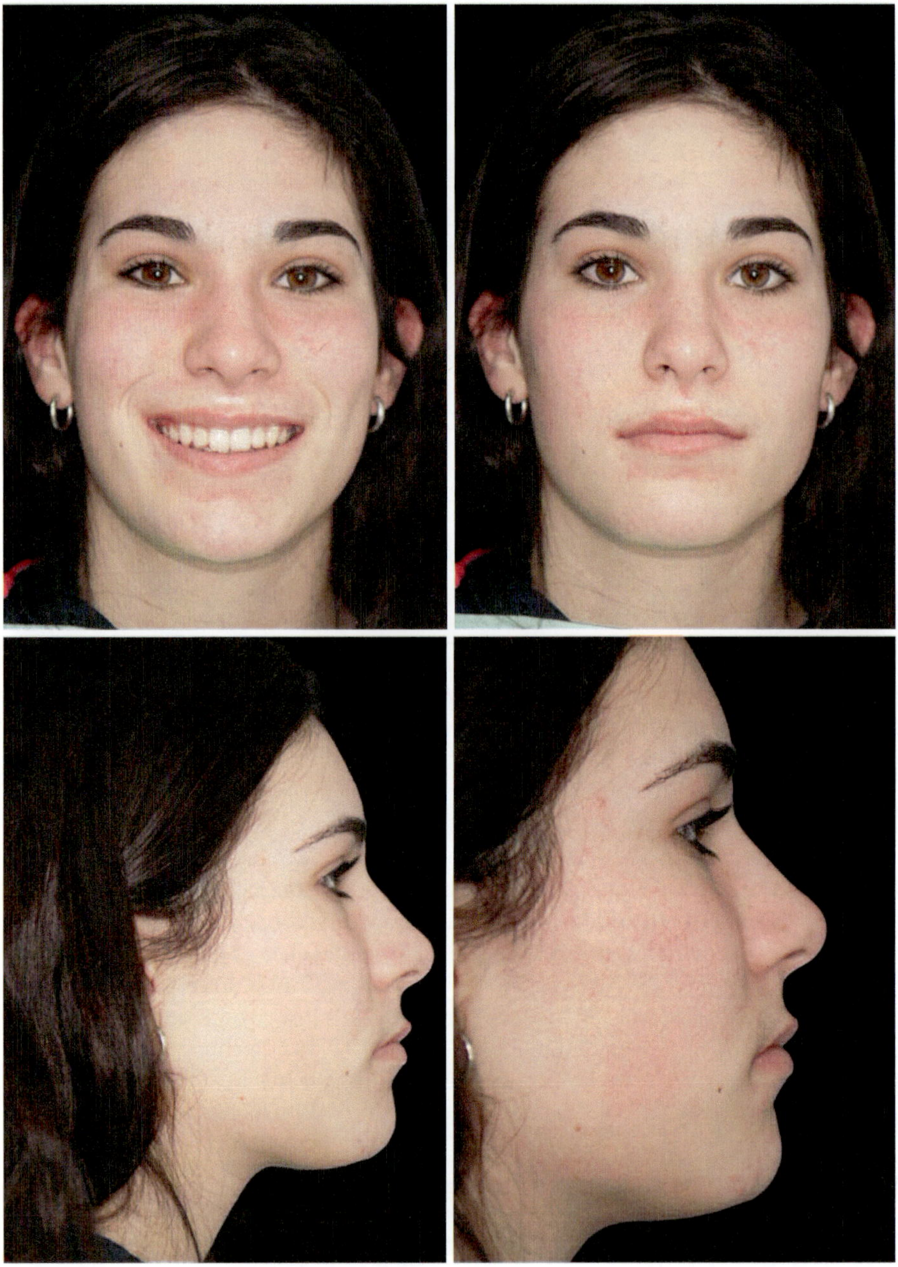

Fig. 12.141 Extraoral photos after treatment. January 2021

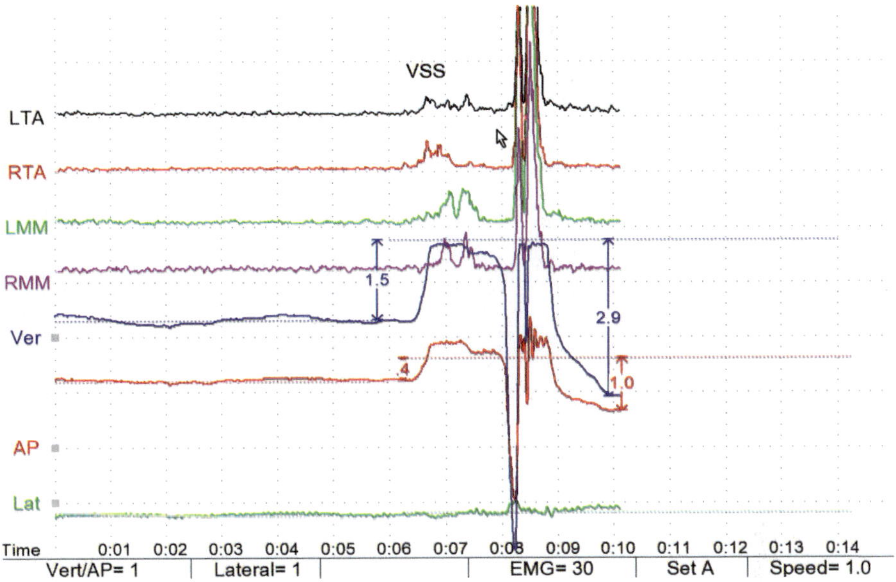

Fig. 12.142 July 2021 Polygraphic scan (scan 3 + S-EMG filtered, scan 21) Post-treatment follow-up at, showing a VSS (Voluntary Swallow of Saliva, indicated with "VSS"). The 1 blue line (vertical) shows mandibular closure (upward) when swallow starts. There is no premature activation of the masseter muscles at start of deglutition sequence indicating that the patient swallows correctly in CO. (LMM: left masseter muscle; LTA: left anterior temporalis; RMM: right masseter muscle; RTA: right anterior temporalis.). AP: anterior-posterior; Lat: lateral; Ver: vertical

Figures 12.154, 12.155 and 12.156 show the final lateral cephalograms and a cephalometric superimposition on the s-n line. It is notable that there has been an increase in the vertical relationship of the third lower of the face. Mandibular advancement could have improved airway, even if lateral cephalograms are not considered the optimal diagnostic method for this kind of evaluation.

The patient has been pain free since January 2019. No other signs of oral dysfunction are notable. Currently on an upper removable appliance as retention.

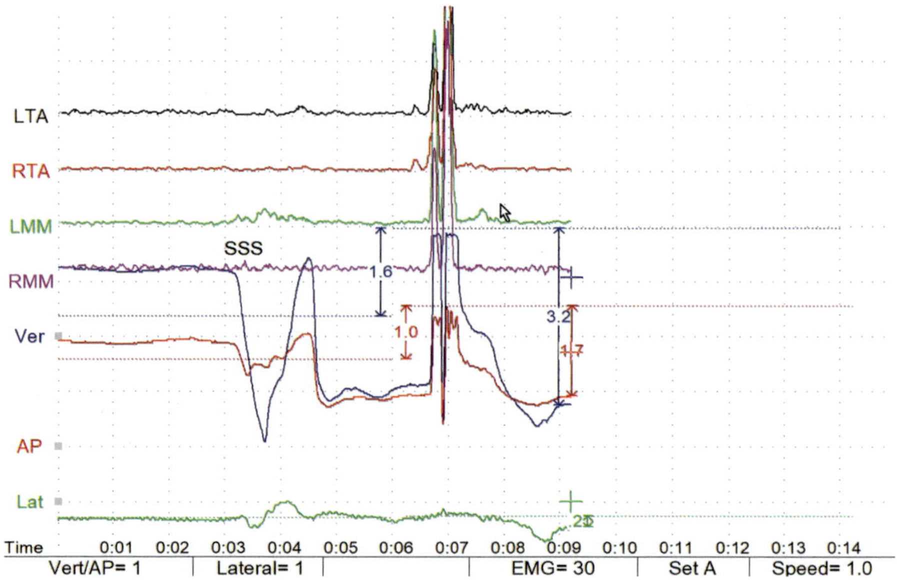

Fig. 12.143 July 2021 Polygraphic scan (scan 3 + S-EMG filtered, scan 21) Post-treatment follow-up shows a SSS (Spontaneous Swallow of Saliva, indicated with "SSS"). The vertical blue line shows mandibular opening (downward) when swallow starts. There is a slight premature activation of the masseter muscles at start of deglutition sequence indicating that the patient does not swallow correctly in C.O. Vertical and AP lines do not reach CO. (LMM: left masseter muscle; LTA: left anterior temporalis; RMM: right masseter muscle; RTA: right anterior temporalis.). AP: anterior-posterior; Lat: lateral; Ver: vertical

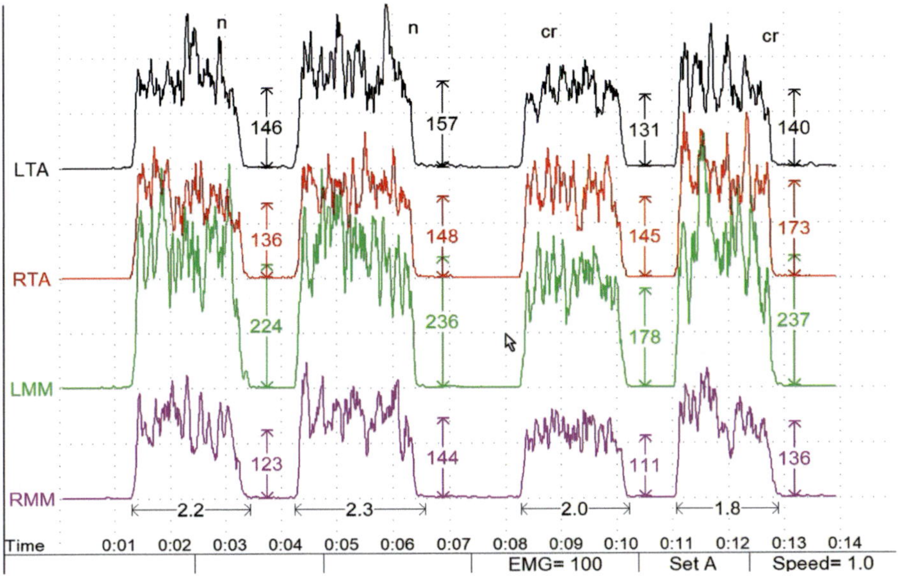

Fig. 12.144 July 2021 Scan 11 (post-treatment follow-up) shows the surface EMG results in sweep mode. The patient was instructed to clench in CO (first burst and second burst), and then clench with cotton rolls between the teeth, which temporarily prevented occlusion (third burst and fourth burst). Output s-EMG is satisfactory and the general output is high. There is balance of output for the temporalis muscles only; the RMM seems to be underactivated during MVC. CO: centric occlusion; EMG: electromyography; LMM: left masseter muscle; LTA: left anterior temporalis; RMM: right masseter muscle; RTA: right anterior temporalis

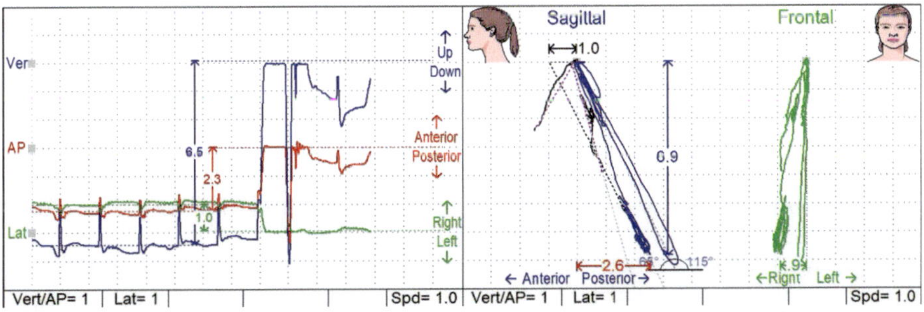

Fig. 12.145 July 2021 Scan 4/5 in split screen modality. On the left sweep of V, AP, and Lat lines. The patient is instructed to rest mandibular posture and the instructed to close to Centric Occlusion. Note the TENS spikes on V and AP lines. On the right, the corresponding Sagittal/frontal scan 5 shows a 1.0-mm. AP discrepancy on HP (Horizontal Plane of Occlusion). Vertical freeway space is 6.9 mm. AP: anterior-posterior; CO: centric occlusion; Lat: lateral; Spd: speed; Vert: vertical

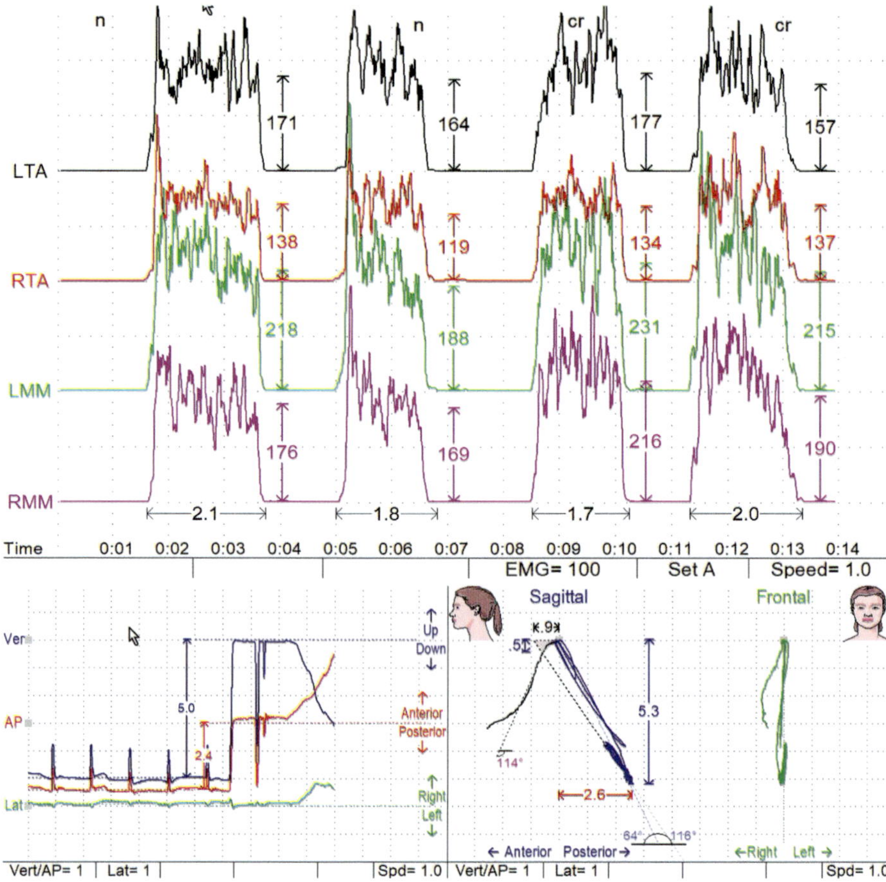

Figs. 146 and 147 August 2022 *Upper:* Scan 11 (Post-treatment) shows the surface EMG results in sweep mode. The patient was instructed to clench in CO (first burst and second burst), and then clench with cotton rolls between the teeth, which temporarily prevented occlusion (third burst and fourth burst). Output s-EMG is satisfactory, and the general output is high. The RMM that previously was low in output has slowly regained a normal output. CO: centric occlusion; EMG: electromyography; LMM: left masseter muscle; LTA: left anterior temporalis; RMM: right masseter muscle; RTA: right anterior temporalis. *Lower:* Showing scan 4/5 in split screen modality. On the left sweep of V, AP, and Lat lines. The patient is instructed to rest mandibular posture and the instructed to close to Centric Occlusion. Note the TENS spikes on V and AP lines. On the right, the corresponding Sagittal/frontal scan 5 shows a 0.9-mm. AP discrepancy on HP (Horizontal Plane of Occlusion). Vertical freeway space is 5.3 mm. AP: anterior-posterior; CO: centric occlusion; Lat: lateral; Spd: speed; Vert: vertical

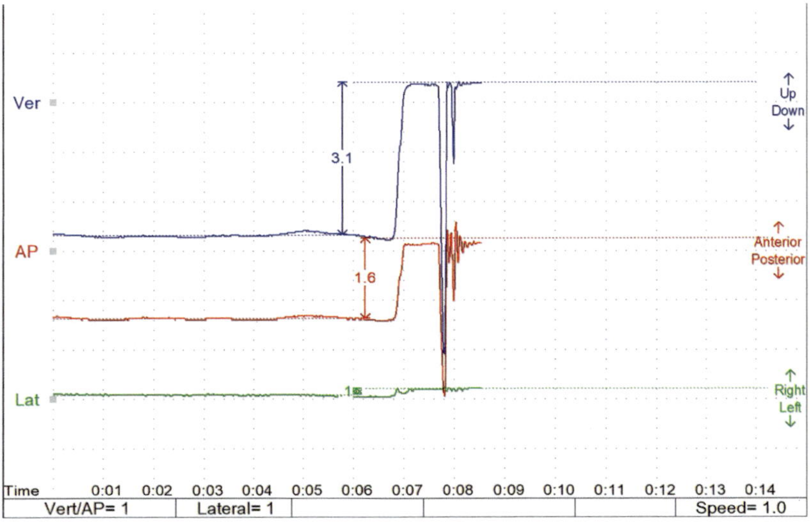

Fig. 12.148 (April 2023). Scan 3 (post-treatment) shows that the freeway space was 3.1 mm, the mandible moved forward during closure (A/V ratio: 0.5), and the lateral movement was 0.1 mm to the right. AP: anterior-posterior; A/V: anterior/vertical ratio; Lat: lateral; Vert: vertical

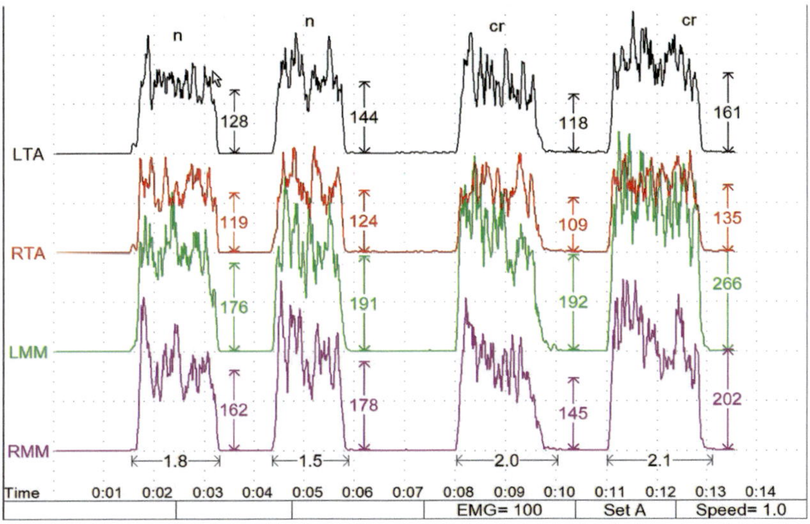

Fig. 12.149 (April 2023). Scan 11 (post-treatment follow-up) shows the surface EMG results in sweep mode. The patient was instructed to clench in CO (first burst and second burst), and then clench with cotton rolls between the teeth, which temporarily prevented occlusion (third burst and fourth burst). Output s-EMG is satisfactory, and the general output is high. **The RMM that previously was low in output has slowly regained a normal output**. All muscles are balanced and masseter output is greater than temporalis. **Note muscle output and balancing increase at regular check-ups in** Figs. 12.136, 12.144, and 146. CO: centric occlusion; EMG: electromyography; LMM: left masseter muscle; LTA: left anterior temporalis; RMM: right masseter muscle; RTA: right anterior temporalis

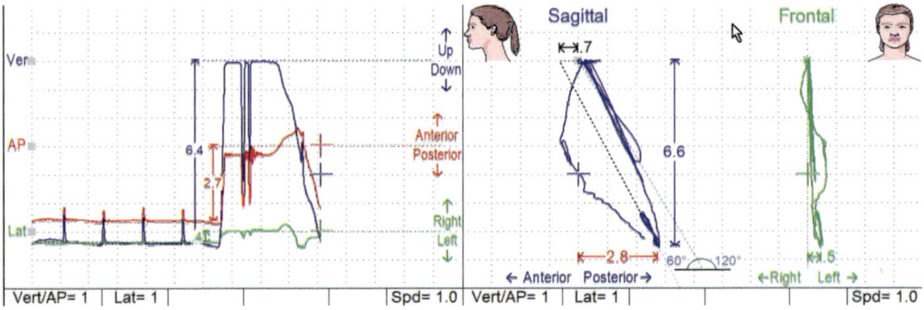

Fig. 12.150 (April 2023). Scan 4/5 in split screen modality. On the left sweep of V, AP, and Lat lines. The patient is instructed to rest mandibular posture and the instructed to close to Centric Occlusion. Note the TENS spikes on V and AP lines. On the right, the corresponding Sagittal/ frontal scan 5 shows a 0.7-mm. AP discrepancy on HP (Horizontal Plane of Occlusion). Vertical freeway space is 6.6 mm. AP: anterior-posterior; CO: centric occlusion; Lat: lateral; Spd: speed; Vert: vertical

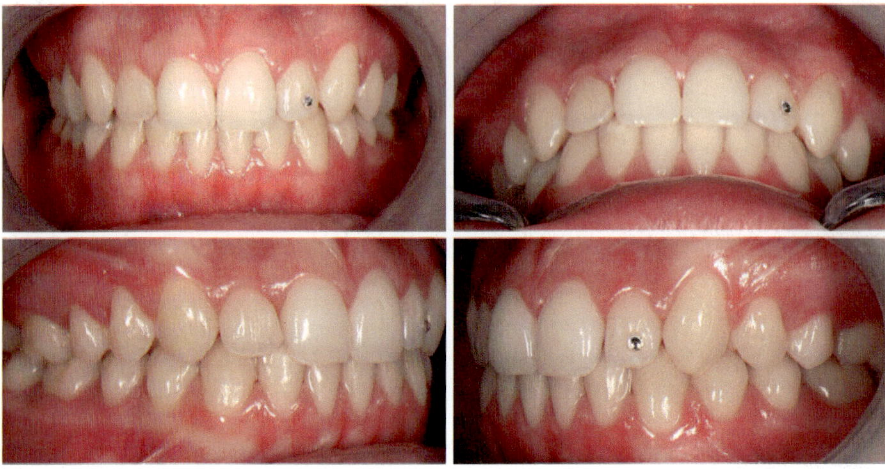

Fig. 12.151 April 2023. Intraoral photos at 28 months after therapy

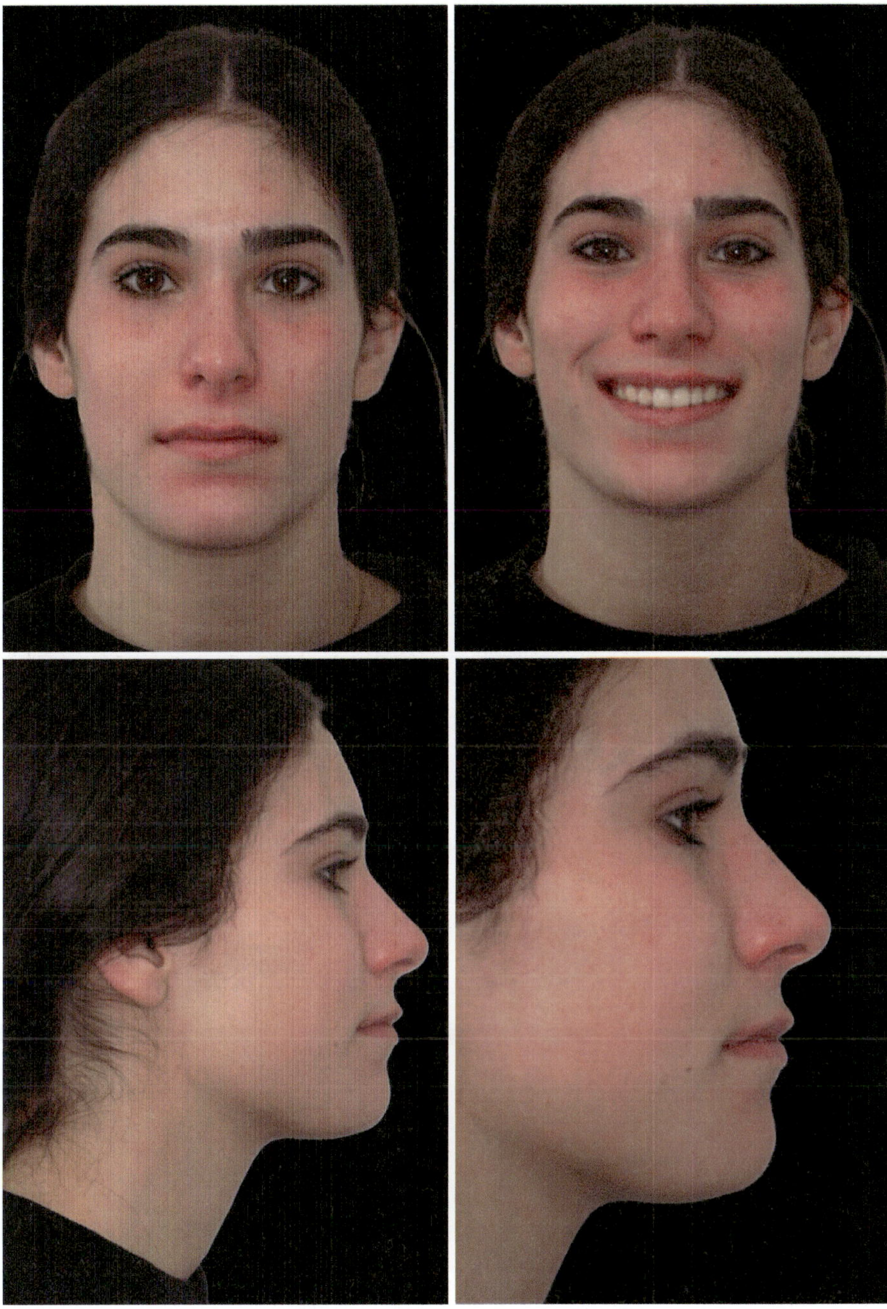

Fig. 12.152 April 2023 Extraoral photos at 28 months after therapy

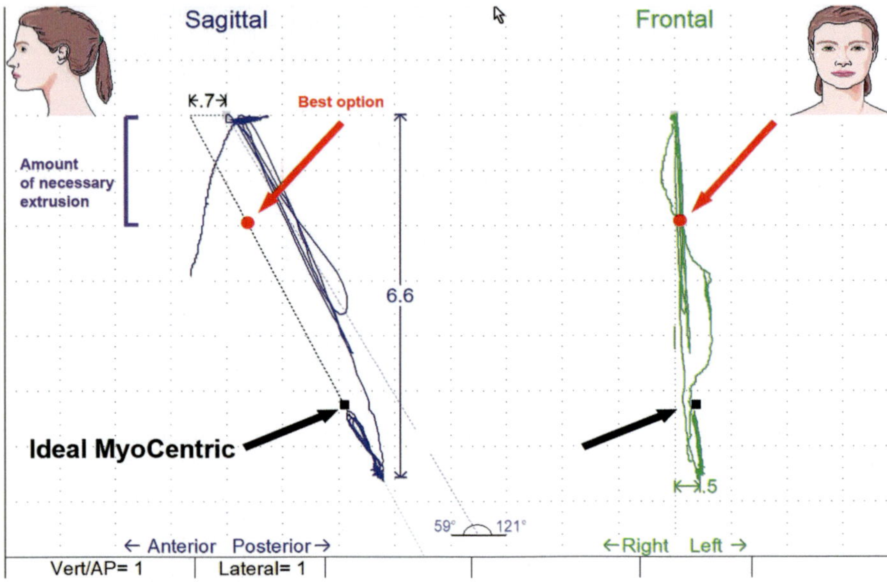

Fig. 12.153 Scan 5 in sagittal/frontal mode. Black arrows and black dots indicate the ideal Myocentric. Red arrows and red dots indicate the best possible option on the Myotrajectory. In purple the amount of necessary dental extrusion necessary to lower the HP (horizontal plane of occlusion), 2 mm, to adjust the Myotrajectory to the best centric (red dot). The ideal MyoCentric is an improbable task with orthodontics alone and would require almost 5 mm of further extrusion and about 1.8 mm of retractive orthodontics

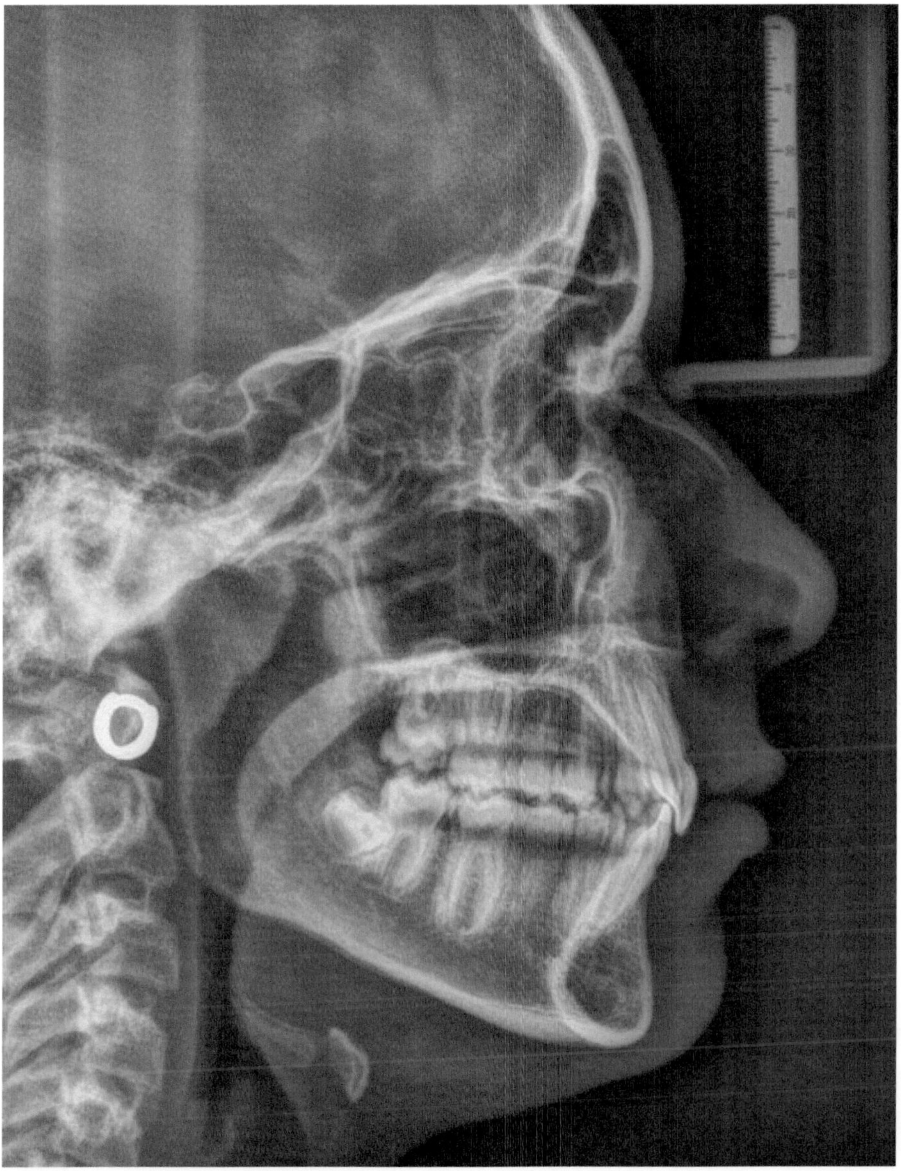

Fig. 12.154 Lateral cephalogram before treatment

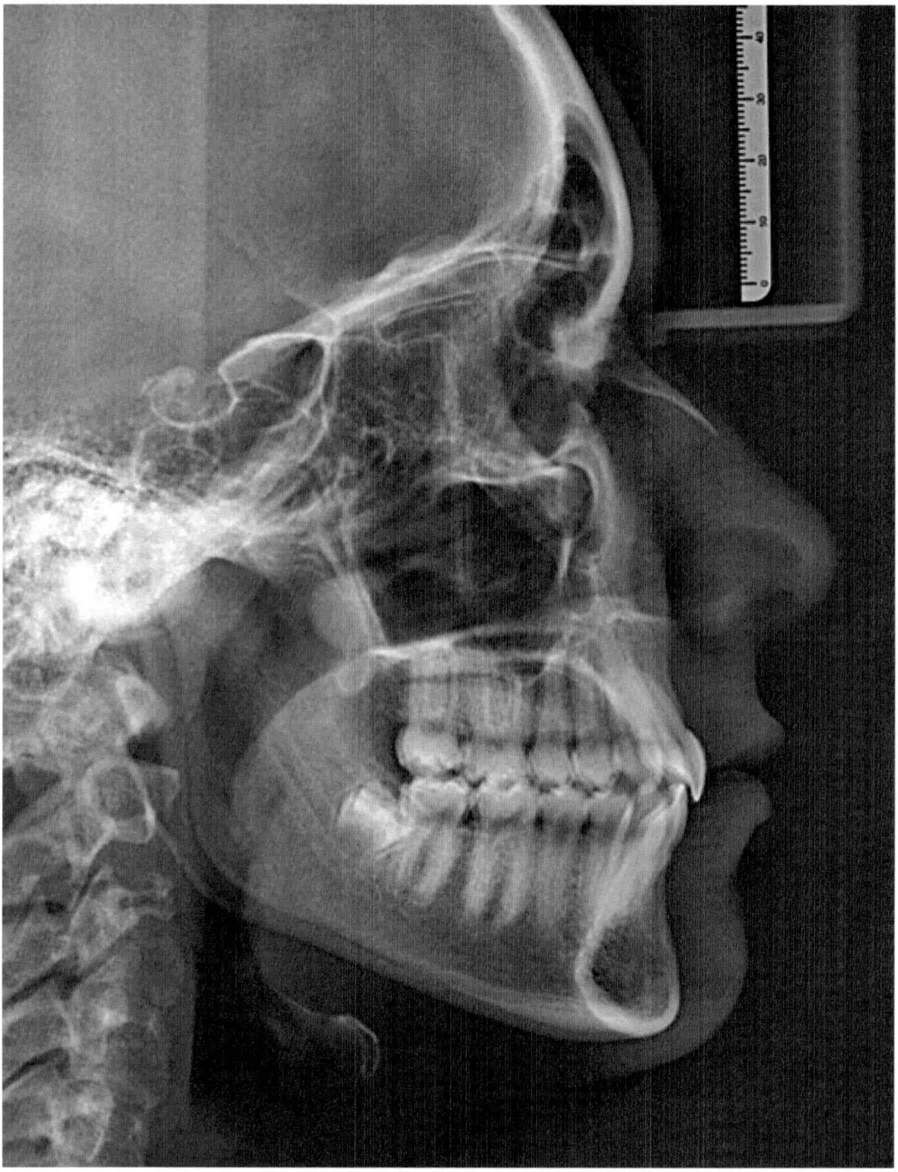

Fig. 12.155 Lateral cephalogram after treatment

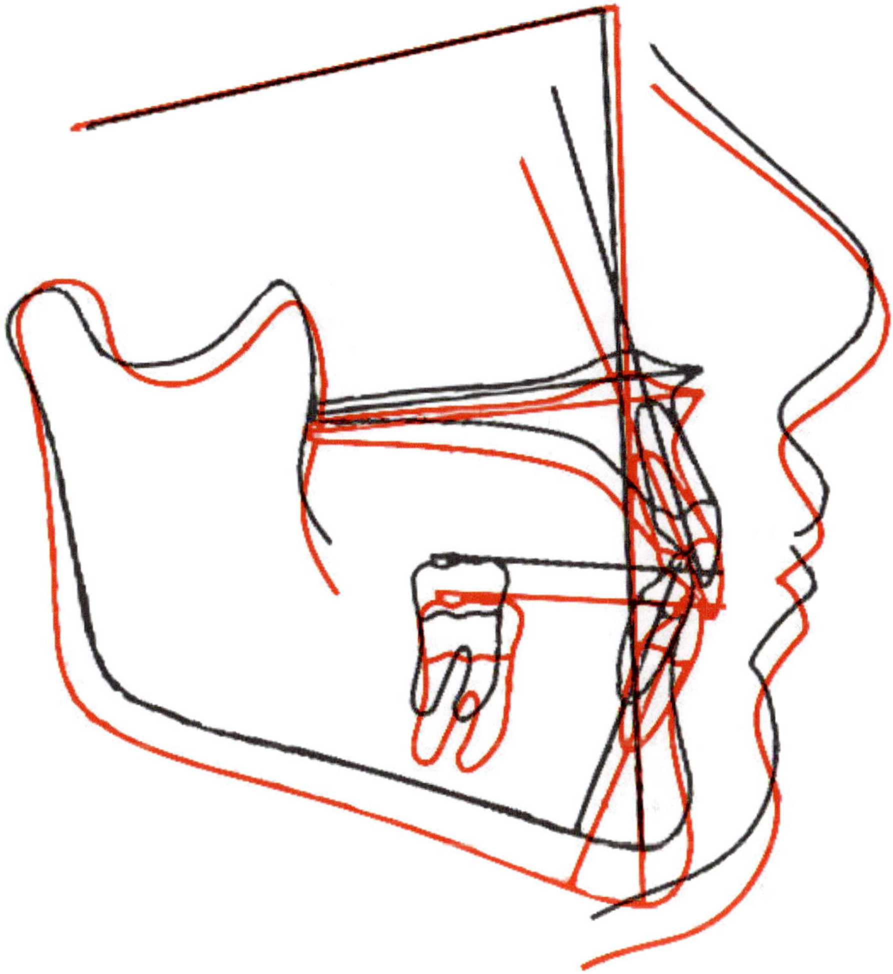

Fig. 12.156 Superimposition on s-n line before (black) and after (red) treatment

References

1. Fabio S. Applying neuromuscular techniques in the orthodontic setting. South Eur J Orthod Dentofac Res. 2017;4:31–42.
2. Melgaco CA, et al. Immediate changes in condylar position after rapid maxillary expansion. Am J Orthod Dentofac Orthop. 2014;145(6):771–9.
3. Lapatki BG, et al. The importance of the level of the lip line and resting lip pressure in Class II, division 2 malocclusion. J Dent Res. 2002;81(5):323–8.
4. Westwood PV, et al. Long-term effects of class III treatment with rapid maxillary expansion and facemask therapy followed by fixed appliances. Am J Orthod Dentofac Orthop. 2003;123(3):306–20.
5. Zimmer B, Nischwitz D. Therapeutic changes in the occlusal plane inclination using intermaxillary elastics. J Orofac Orthop. 2012;73(5):377–86.
6. Pettersen SD, Aslaksen PM, Pettersen SA. Pain Processing in Elite and High-Level Athletes Compared to Non-athletes. Front Psychol. 2020;11:1908. https://doi.org/10.3389/fpsyg.2020.01908. PMID: 32849117; PMCID: PMC7399202.
7. Tesarz J, Schuster AK, Hartmann M, Gerhardt A, Eich W. Pain perception in athletes compared to normally active controls: a systematic review with meta-analysis. Pain. 2012;153(6):1253–62. https://doi.org/10.1016/j.pain.2012.03.005. PMID: 22607985.

Printed by Printforce, the Netherlands